Pass Finals

THIRD EDITION

GEOFF SMITH
MD FRCP

Consultant Physician and Gastroenterologist,
Imperial College Healthcare NHS Trust, London

ELIZABETH CARTY
MD FRCP

Consultant Physician and Gastroenterologist,
Whipps Cross Hospital, Barts Health NHS Trust, London

LOUISE LANGMEAD
MD FRCP

Consultant Physician and Gastroenterologist,
The Royal London Hospital, Barts Health NHS Trust, London

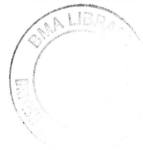

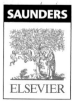

SAUNDERS

ELSEVIER

Edinburgh   London   New York   Oxford
Philadelphia   St Louis   Sydney   Toronto 2013

SAUNDERS

ELSEVIER

© 2013 Elsevier Limited. All rights reserved.

First edition 2004
Second edition 2008
Reprinted 2009
Third edition 2013
   Reprinted 2014

ISBN 9780702046209

British Library Cataloguing in Publication Data
A catalogue record for this book is available from the British Library

Library of Congress Cataloging in Publication Data
A catalog record for this book is available from the Library of Congress

Notices

Knowledge and best practice in this field are constantly changing. As new research and experience broaden our understanding, changes in research methods, professional practices, or medical treatment may become necessary.

Practitioners and researchers must always rely on their own experience and knowledge in evaluating and using any information, methods, compounds, or experiments described herein. In using such information or methods they should be mindful of their own safety and the safety of others, including parties for whom they have a professional responsibility.

With respect to any drug or pharmaceutical products identified, readers are advised to check the most current information provided (i) on procedures featured or (ii) by the manufacturer of each product to be administered, to verify the recommended dose or formula, the method and duration of administration, and contraindications. It is the responsibility of practitioners, relying on their own experience and knowledge of their patients, to make diagnoses, to determine dosages and the best treatment for each individual patient, and to take all appropriate safety precautions.

To the fullest extent of the law, neither the Publisher nor the authors, contributors, or editors, assume any liability for any injury and/or damage to persons or property as a matter of products liability, negligence or otherwise, or from any use or operation of any methods, products, instructions, or ideas contained in the material herein.

ELSEVIER your source for books, journals and multimedia in the health sciences

www.elsevierhealth.com

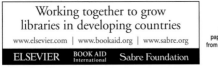

Working together to grow libraries in developing countries

www.elsevier.com | www.bookaid.org | www.sabre.org

ELSEVIER   BOOK AID International   Sabre Foundation

The publisher's policy is to use paper manufactured from sustainable forests

Printed in China

Series Preface

Medical students and doctors in training are expected to travel to different hospitals and community health centres as part of their education. Many books are too large to carry around, but the information they contain is often vital for the basic understanding of disease processes.

The *Pocket Essentials* series is designed to provide portable, pocket-sized companions for ntials series is designed to provide portable, pocket-sized companions for larger texts like our own *Kumar and Clark's Clinical Medicine*. They are most useful for clinical practice, whether in hospital or the community, and for exam revision.

All the books in the series have the same helpful features:

- succinct text
- simple line drawings
- emergency and other boxes
- tables that summarise causes and clinical features of disease
- examination questions and answers

They contain core material for quick revision, easy reference and practical management. The modern format makes them easy to read, providing an indispensable 'pocket essential'.

Parveen Kumar and Michael Clark
Series Editors

Preface to the Third Edition

In this new edition of *Pass Finals* we have brought the text up-to-date, aligning it with the 8th edition of Kumar and Clark's *Clinical Medicine*. The example questions have been expanded and we have focused on clinical medicine and its assessment. The layout of the book has changed to make it more 'pocketable'.

Our thanks go to Lynn Watt at Elsevier for her patience in the face of adversity and slipping deadlines, and our families for their tolerance as we spent our 'free time' in front of a computer screen.

As ever, good luck – and remember: they want to pass you, whatever it feels like on the day!

G.S.
E.C.
L.L.
June 2012

Acknowledgements

Our thanks go to Dr Nick Reading (Consultant Radiologist, Whipps Cross University Hospital) for supplying images for the radiology chapter.

Preface to the First Edition

The range and depth of knowledge that medical students seem to be expected to retain grows continuously. This is despite the stated policy of many medical schools that the 'information load' should be reduced in undergraduate teaching. Over the last decade many traditional styles of examination have become less common, replaced by multiple-choice style examinations based on clinical scenarios and OSCE examinations, in place of long and short cases.

The advance of molecular medicine and the increasing links between basic sciences and clinical medicine have led us to include these topics in the text. Common radiological investigations are also included as they are becoming a key part of many examinations. The use of evidence-based medicine demands an understanding of statistics and trial design and these topics are, as a result, also included.

In this book we have tried to distil a core dataset in general and speciality medicine. The information is provided as bulleted lists and is supported by diagrams and self-assessment questions. By its nature, therefore, this is not a definitive textbook of clinical medicine and the page references to the 6th edition of Kumar and Clark's *Clinical Medicine* are designed to point the reader towards a more in-depth explanation of the subject. We hope, however, that it will act as a source of rapid access information for the important disease processes and thereby act as a useful revision aid.

Finally we would like to thank those individuals that have supported our efforts – notably Ellen Green and Siân Jarman at Elsevier for their efforts and Sarah Russell for the design work. Also to Parveen Kumar and Michael Clark for their critique of the text and for writing *Clinical Medicine* in the first place, and to our families for support and coffee during the writing. Finally, we should thank the Good Samaritan for ongoing inspiration.
Good Luck!

G.S.
E.C.
L.L.

Contents

How to pass medical finals

There are, and always have been, several truisms about sitting final exams in medicine. At the end of the day, the vast majority of students pass their final exams and earn the right to call themselves 'Doctor'. There are, however, tactics and techniques that you can use to make the process less painful.

WRITTEN EXAMS

Much of this sounds obvious, but 'schoolchild errors' are commonly made in the stress of final exams.

Be prepared

- Exam technique is a learned skill
- Know the distribution of marks for the paper
- Make sure you know the format of the exam
- Practise questions from past papers
- Practise keeping to time

Directed learning

- The vast majority of questions are about common and important areas of medicine
- Rare syndromes are very unlikely to come up
- Medical emergencies are often asked about
- Remember the classic pitfalls in medicine (Table 1.1)

Read the instructions

- Make sure you are quite clear on how many questions you have to answer and how much time you have for each one
- If need be, write the start and finish times for each section on the top of the paper and stick to them

Answer the question asked

- Read the question carefully – preferably twice
- Answer the question asked, not the one you want to answer – don't just write down everything that you remember about the topic

Answer all the questions

- Attempt the correct number of questions
- If you are running out of time, try to put something down on paper, even if it is only an essay plan – you may get some credit

Presentation

- Clear, neat handwriting is easier to mark
- Structure your answer: headings and subheadings speed up marking
- Spell accurately

> **Table 1.1** The structured answer
>
> For any disease, outline:
> Incidence – common/rare
> Distribution
>   Age
>   Sex
>   Geographical
>   Racial
> Pathology
> Aetiology
> Clinical features
> Associated conditions
> Investigations
> Therapeutic options
> Outcome or prognosis
> Complications

Anonymous papers

● Many exams require you to put a name or candidate number on each page – make sure you do

MULTIPLE CHOICE PAPERS

● Several different formats exist (see Ch. 2)
● Make sure that you know what question type is used
● Keep to time and answer all of the questions
● Do not spend long on a question you have no idea about – you can always go back to it
● Most questions have some obvious wrong answers – shortening the odds
● Practise as many questions as you can
● Questions are often re-used – do as many past papers as you can

Negative marking

● Rarely used
● Mark deducted for a wrong answer
● Aims to deter 'wild guesses'
● Informed guesses are risky but on balance worth it

CLINICAL EXAMS

Clinical exams can be more nerve-racking than written papers. The 'performance' in front of examiners is stressful. Again, basic tactics will help you out.

Dress code

Go for smart, conservative and comfortable dress. Loud waistcoats and cartoon ties will not help.

Equipment

● The vast majority of the equipment you will need for a clinical examination will be provided

- You will need:
  - A stethoscope – make sure it is clean and working
  - A pen – most important for long cases
- Ophthalmoscopes should be provided, but if you have your own and are comfortable using it, take it with you. Make sure the batteries are fresh
- Everything else is a luxury. Pockets bulging with equipment are uncomfortable and heavy

Three key aims

- Do not hurt or embarrass the patient
- Ensure the examiner sees you carry out all parts of the examination competently
- Synthesize a diagnosis, differential and management plan

The order of importance of the above depends upon the examiner and the case. If the diagnosis is straightforward, the examiner will want you to reach it without too much of a performance. If the diagnosis is difficult, he or she will want you to demonstrate your ability to elicit clinical signs, even if the underlying cause escapes you.

Examination technique

- Make sure that your examination technique is swift and professional
- Do what you are asked
  - 'Examine the cardiovascular system' means a full examination starting with the hands
  - 'Listen to the heart' means just auscultation
  - Examiners should make it clear what they want

Dignity

- *NEVER* hurt or embarrass the patient
- *ALWAYS* introduce yourself
- *ALWAYS* ask permission to examine
- *ALWAYS* ask whether the area you are going to examine is painful or tender
- *THANK* the patient at the end of the examination

Scoring points

- A professional introduction, followed by an examination technique that is fluent and clearly well practised, is as important as reaching a diagnosis
- Even if the diagnosis eludes you, describe your findings
- Outline the positive findings at examination and the important negatives
- If you can, come up with a diagnosis and differential
- The longer you can talk, the fewer questions can be asked (although talking rubbish does not help)

VIVA VOCE EXAMS

Vivas or oral examinations still make up a part of final examinations in some medical schools. They may be routine for all candidates or used specifically to re-examine a borderline candidate. If you are called for a viva in the latter situation, remember that honours students may be examined as well and that a selection of candidates across the whole range of marks will be examined to provide a standard range of scores.

In general, it is difficult to fail the whole exam because of a poor performance in a viva.

Dress

- Be smart and conservative

Format

- There are usually two examiners – one may be external

You may be:

Asked questions

- e.g. What classes of drug are useful in the management of hypertension?

Given a case scenario

- e.g. Outline the management options for a 74-year-old woman who comes to see you with rheumatoid arthritis

Asked about medical emergencies

- e.g. A 55-year-old man is admitted with haematemesis and a blood pressure of 90/50. What would you do?

Asked to report the results of an investigation

- e.g. A chest X-ray, ECG or blood test results

Identify an object

- Pathological specimen
- Piece of equipment (e.g. nasogastric tube, urinary catheter)

Tactics

- 'Engage your brain before your mouth'
- Structure your answer (Tables 1.1 and 1.2)
- Do not dig holes; if you realize that you are completely wrong, apologize and start again – the examiners expect you to be nervous
- When giving lists of causes, start with the commonest first
- When giving lists of investigations, start with the least invasive and explain how they help with the diagnosis
- Make sure the tests are appropriate; if you are going to mention a blood count, chest X-ray and so on, make sure you state why you are discussing them

LAST-MINUTE REVISION

What to revise

- Revising facts you already know is easier than learning new information in the weeks prior to the exam. Consistent learning throughout the course is the best preparation
- Target the revision to the exam. Base revision around past papers and the type of exam you are sitting
- In the last week, go over notes and take timed practice exams rather than trying to learn new data

---

Table 1.2 Disease aetiology

For any clinical symptom or sign (e.g. diarrhoea[a]), classify the causes into:

Infective
  Viruses
    Rotavirus
    Adenovirus
  Bacteria
    Staphylococcus aureus
    Salmonella
    Cholera
  Parasites
    Giardiasis
    Ascaris
Inflammatory
  Inflammatory bowel disease
Neoplastic
  Colorectal cancer
Autoimmune
  Coeliac disease
Metabolic
  Hypercalcaemia
Endocrine
  Thyrotoxicosis
Neurological
  Autonomic neuropathy
Trauma/surgery
  Post-gastrectomy
Iatrogenic
  Drugs, e.g. laxatives
Idiopathic

[a]List is not complete.

How to revise

- Practise MCQs in a group. It is more fun and you will remember more
- Outline essay plans and fill in the essential facts. You do not need to write out complete essays except to check timings
- If your university offers mock or prize exams, sit them. They are good practice and will highlight weak areas
- Use tools such as mind maps and revision aids. The more senses you use, the better the chance of the information sinking in. Jotting down lists and notes will help you absorb what you read
- Remember to give yourself time to relax. Play sport, go out or meet your friends rather than burning the midnight oil. Learning when you are half-comatose is ineffective
- Sleep and eat properly and avoid stimulants such as caffeine tablets
- The night before the exam, do as little as possible. Find a way of relaxing and get a good (and sober) night's sleep
- And finally, do you really learn anything by frantically flicking through a book as you walk into the exam?

Question types in medical finals 2

The ideal exam question, from the examiners' point of view, is one that discriminates between different levels of knowledge or ability. A question that everybody gets right or wrong says little about an individual and is therefore a poor discriminator. Objective structured clinical examinations (OSCEs) are discussed in detail in Chapter 3.

QUESTION TYPES IN WRITTEN EXAMS

Multiple choice questions (MCQs)

- Questions usually comprise a stem that introduces the question, and five branches or options (Table 2.1)

Single best answer questions (SBAs) AKA 'Best of fives'

- Choose the branch that provides the correct or best answer

Table 2.1 MCQ styles

1. Which of the following are true of aspirin?
   A. It may cause gastric ulceration
   B. It is associated with an increased risk of transient ischaemic attacks
   C. It is associated with renal dysfunction
   D. Its use is never indicated in acute myocardial infarction
   E. It may exacerbate inflammatory bowel disease
2. Which of the following are not true of paracetamol?
   A. It is an anti-inflammatory drug
   B. It results in hepatic necrosis in severe overdose
   C. It is metabolized in the liver
   D. It is usually given intravenously
   E. It is a non-steroidal anti-inflammatory drug
3. The following drugs are associated with the stated complication
   A. Flucloxacillin: jaundice
   B. Loperamide: diarrhoea
   C. Enalapril: cough
   D. Prednisolone: weight loss
   E. Metronidazole: nausea

Answers: 1. A, C, E
2. A, D, E
3. T, F, T, F, T

Example

Which *one* of the following is a cause of liver cirrhosis?

A. Cigarette smoking
B. Alcohol
C. Heroin
D. Cannabis
E. Methadone

Answer: **B**

True (T) or false (F) questions

● For each branch, decide whether the statement is true or false:

Example

The following are recognized causes of cirrhosis:

A. Alcohol
B. Autoimmune hepatitis
C. Hepatitis C
D. Haemochromatosis
E. Cystic fibrosis

Answer: All are true

Tips and tactics

- Always ensure that you know how to complete the question paper – read the instructions carefully
- For computer-scored papers, make sure that the marks you make on the paper are clear and confined to the correct part of the paper. Always use the pencil provided. Pens may not be detected properly by the computerized reader
- Keep an eye on the time. You may only have 2–3 minutes per question
- Going through the whole paper once, answering the questions you are sure of, then going back to those that need more time may ensure that you don't miss any easy points
- Look for obvious incorrect answers. *Always* and *never* are rarely correct. Read the stem very carefully
- Check for negatives in the stem, e.g. Which of the following are *not* causes of abdominal pain? Getting this wrong could cost you 5 marks
- Even if you have no idea about the subject of a question, read the possible answers – there may be sections for which no specialist knowledge is required

Extended matching questions (EMQs)

● For a small set of questions, a common list of 15–30 options provides the list of possible answers:

Example Question 1 – Theme: Jaundice

A. Alcohol-related cirrhosis
B. Carcinoma of the pancreas
C. Hepatitis A
D. Hepatitis B

E. Hepatitis C
F. Haemochromatosis
G. Wilson's disease
H. Acute haemolysis
 I. Gilbert syndrome
J. Primary sclerosing cholangitis
K. Primary biliary cirrhosis
L. Autoimmune hepatitis
M. Budd–Chiari syndrome
N. Cystic fibrosis
O. Gallstone in the common bile duct

For each of the following questions, select the best answer from the list above:

   I. A 28-year-old man notices that his eyes have a yellow tinge following a bad cough and cold. His liver function tests are normal apart from a bilirubin of 78 μmol/L

  II. A 76-year-old woman presents with jaundice and weight loss. She denies any abdominal pain. Her bilirubin is 280 μmol/L and the alkaline phosphatase 590 U/L. The alanine aminotransferase is 87 U/L. She has a family history of ischaemic heart disease. An ultrasound of her abdomen reveals a dilated common bile duct (Table 2.2)

 III. A 45-year-old man with known diabetes presents with jaundice. He is noted to have a deep tan and hepatomegaly. His ferritin is 1201 μg/L

Answers: **I**. I, **II**. B, **III**. F

Example Question 2

A. Haemoglobin
B. Myoglobin
C. Albumin
D. Ferritin
E. Transferrin
F. Alanine aminotransferase
G. Collagen
H. Fibrinogen
 I. Factor VIII
J. Immunoglobulin
K. Serotonin (5-hydroxytryptamine, 5 HT)
L. Niacin
M. Intrinsic factor
N. Glucose-6-phosphatase
O. Lactate dehydrogenase

> **Table 2.2** Picking out key facts
>
> 'A 76-year-old woman presents with *jaundice* and *weight loss*. She denies any abdominal pain. Her bilirubin is 280 μmol/L and the alkaline phosphatase 590 U/L. The alanine aminotransferase is 87 U/L. She has a family history of ischaemic heart disease. An ultrasound of her abdomen reveals a *dilated common bile duct*'.
> Here, the classical combination of painless jaundice and weight loss gives you the diagnosis of carcinoma of the pancreas.

For each of the following questions, select the best answer from the list above:

     I. A peptide important in the absorption of vitamin B_{12} (M)
    II. An iron-containing protein derived from muscle (B)
   III. A neurotransmitter released by carcinoid tumours (K)
   IV. A helical structural connective tissue protein (G)
    V. A protein to which bilirubin is bound in the blood (C)
   VI. A protein capable of carrying oxygen in the circulation (A)
  VII. A substance the deficiency of which results in pellagra (L)
VIII. A protein precursor of bilirubin (A)
   IX. A protein released by injured hepatocytes (F)
    X. A protein that exists in five subclasses (J)

- Note that any answer from the list may be appropriate for more than one question

A second type of EMQ

● This asks for more than one answer for each question:

Example

   XI. State two molecules capable of carrying oxygen (A, B)
  XII. State two proteins secreted into the intestine (J, M)
 XIII. State three proteins found in erythrocytes or leucocytes (A, N, O)

Tips and tactics

- The examiner is usually looking for the best answer to the question; however, there may be other possible answers that will gain some marks
- Make an attempt at each part if you can, for the reasons given above. For each part of the question, underline the key facts and investigation results that may help you reach the correct answer
- Don't be put off by diseases on the list of options that you know little about. They may well not be the answer to any of the questions posed

Short answers

● These questions ask you to write notes or a short summary on three or four related topics:

Example

1. Write short notes on each of the following:
   A. Thrombolysis in myocardial infarction
   B. Risk factors for ischaemic heart disease
   C. Aspirin in ischaemic heart disease

Patient management problems

● A description of a patient history and examination is given, followed by two or three questions. For each question there is a list of options and you are asked to grade the correctness of each option:

Example

A 55-year-old man, who works for a building company, is referred complaining of a cough. The cough has been present for 3 months and

- These require short, structured answers
- If time is short, consider bulleted points or headings and lists
- Do not attempt to put down everything you know about the subject – stick to answering the question being asked and note common and important answers first before unusual or unlikely answers
- Keep a close eye on the time – it is easy to get carried away and spend far too much time on a single part of a question
- There are only a limited number of marks. Writing excessive amounts will not get you extra points

on four occasions he has coughed up some blood. He now feels breathless after mild exertion. His wife has rheumatoid arthritis and he is her main carer. He has had a previous admission for angina and attends a diabetes clinic at his local GP's. He is a smoker who drinks about 40 units of alcohol a week as beer.

He is 180 cm tall and weighs 70 kg. He has some crackles at left midzone of his lungs but no other findings on examination.

Which four of the following would be most useful in making an immediate diagnosis?

1. ECG
2. Exercise ECG
3. CT of the chest
4. MRI of the lungs
5. Peak flow measurements
6. Lung function tests
7. Full blood count
8. Blood cultures
9. Arterial blood gases
10. Chest X-ray

  Answer: **1, 5, 8, 10**

A chest X-ray reveals calcified pleural lesions and increased lung markings, most notably in the bases. Based on this, what is the most likely diagnosis?

A. Carcinoma of the bronchus
B. Chronic congestive cardiac failure
C. Streptococcal pneumonia
D. Asbestosis
E. Rheumatoid lung disease

  Answer: **D**

- The second variation of this question type asks for one-line answers to a series of questions about a case

Example

A 66-year-old man presents with chest pain. This started suddenly 2 hours previously. The pain is central and radiates to both shoulders. He is sweaty and feels very unwell. On examination, he is apyrexial and tachycardic with a blood pressure of 110/60.

1. What is the most likely diagnosis?

  Answer: Acute myocardial infarction

2. What two investigations would be of immediate use?
   Answer: ECG and troponin
3. State four immediate therapeutic steps you would institute.
   Answer: High-flow oxygen, i.v. diamorphine, morphine, aspirin and consider thrombolysis or angioplasty
4. Suggest three possible complications of the therapies you suggest.
   Answer: Haemorrhage, gastrointestinal ulceration, respiratory depression

When answering these questions, remember that although your answers may be correct, there may be a better way of answering in order to show off your knowledge.

- Give a full answer – *Acute myocardial infarction* rather than *Heart attack*
- Give investigations of different modalities – *ECG and troponin* rather than *Troponin and creatine kinase*
- Give specific rather than general treatments with differing aims – *High flow oxygen* rather than *Oxygen or i.v. access, diamorphine and aspirin* rather than *aspirin and clopidogrel*

Essay questions

- These provide a title and sometimes some specific requirements for an essay:

Example

Outline the important considerations in palliation of a patient with an inoperable lung carcinoma. In your answer, outline the important therapies you would consider using.

Tips and tactics

- Read the question carefully and underline any 'riders' or specific instructions
- Spend a minute sketching an essay plan with section headings. This allows you to order your thoughts before committing them to paper
- Headings help the examiner as they speed up marking
- Answer the specific questions being asked; do not write a general essay on the subject in the hope of getting credit
- Always include the basics. The examiner may not assume that you know something even if it seems obvious
- Time the paper carefully. Writing two 30-minute essays instead of three 20-minute essays makes passing much harder
- Read through your answer:
  - Does it all make sense?
  - Does it answer the question?
  - Is the spelling correct?
  - Is it structured and easy to read?
- If you are running out of time, write out a structured essay plan with key facts about the subject. Most marking schemes will give you some credit for this
- If the examiners cannot read your writing, they cannot mark the essay!

CLINICAL EXAMS

Short cases

- A series of patients are seen with the examiners who give you specific instructions
  - 'Look at this patient – what is the diagnosis?'
  - 'Examine this man's chest'
  - 'Listen to this woman's heart'
- You will then be expected to:
  - Introduce yourself
  - Carry out the appropriate examination
  - Present your findings and give a diagnosis, differential and management plan

Common topics for short cases

Cardiac
- Heart sounds and murmurs
- Cardiomegaly
- Dextrocardia (rare)
- Hypertensive retinopathy

Respiratory
- Chronic obstructive pulmonary disease
- Pulmonary fibrosis
- Pleural effusions
- Chest infections
- Cystic fibrosis

Gastrointestinal
- Chronic liver disease
- Ileostomy/colostomy

General tips and tactics

- Be conscientious and see as many patients as possible – examiners can easily spot students who have limited experience with patients
- Practise your verbal communication skills to improve your bedside manner
- Look enthusiastic
- Speak clearly and confidently – the examiners cannot give marks for answers they cannot hear
- Always introduce yourself and do not embarrass or hurt the patient
- Look into the examiner's eyes when you are answering
- Structure your answers sensibly, e.g. when asked for likely differential diagnosis, start with common things
- Avoid abbreviations and slang
- If you don't understand the question ask for it to be repeated
- If you don't know the answer, say so
- Don't joke with the examiner (or patient) and never argue – even if you think you are correct there is little to gain and lots to lose.

- Fistulating Crohn's disease
- Hepatosplenomegaly

Renal
- Transplanted kidney (right iliac fossa)
- Arteriovenous shunt for dialysis (left arm)
- Ileal urinary conduit (urine in the bag)
- Palpable kidneys (often polycystic kidney)

Neurological
- Multiple sclerosis
- Ophthalmoplegia
- Facial palsy
- Brachial plexus injury
- Ulnar or radial nerve damage
- Carpal tunnel syndrome
- Hemiparesis or paraparesis
- Charcot–Marie–Tooth
- Friedreich's ataxia (check speech)
- Parkinson's disease
- Cerebellar ataxia

Endocrine
- Thyroid status (Table 2.3)
- Acromegaly
- Diabetic retinopathy
- Diabetic sensory loss
- Hypopituitarism
- Cushing syndrome

Rheumatological
- Systemic sclerosis
- Rheumatoid arthritis
- Osteoarthritis
- Ankylosing spondylitis
- Paget's disease of bone

Long cases

A prolonged period with a patient prior to presenting the case to an examiner. You may be taken back to the patient in order to assess a specific part of the examination technique.

Table 2.3 'Examine this patient and assess her thyroid gland'

Hypothyroidism	Hyperthyroidism
Thick, rough, dry skin	Thin patient
Obesity	Sweaty
Bradycardia	Tachycardia ± atrial fibrillation
Slow relaxing reflexes	Exophthalmos with lid lag
Loss of outer third of the eyebrow	Tremor

- Follow the instructions you are given
- Answer the questions you are asked
- Remember, very unwell patients are unlikely to be in a clinical exam. Chronic conditions are more common. You may be given tips or a brief introduction, e.g.
  - 'This gentleman gets breathless on exertion – examine the heart'
    - → Think about heart valve murmurs and cardiac failure

- Take a detailed history
- With chronic disabling conditions, the social history is very important
- Perform a thorough clinical examination
- Keep an eye on the time and make legible notes. Divide the time into:
  - History-taking
  - Examination
  - Reviewing your findings
  - Going back to ask further questions
- When presenting, adhere to the preferred format for your medical school
- Give the positive and important negative findings
- Outline a diagnosis and a differential
- Outline the investigations that are appropriate
- Outline treatment options, including long-term care needs if appropriate.

Objective Structured Clinical Examinations (OSCEs)

3

OSCEs are now the most common form of clinical examination. They allow for standardization of the examination for all candidates and a formalized and objective marking system. They are relatively expensive in terms of the number of examiners needed, but allow a large number of candidates to be assessed in a relatively short period of time. They are also fairer, as every candidate does the same stations.

STRUCTURE

- There is a 'round robin' of test stations
- The examiner stays at the station
- Each station lasts 5–10 minutes
- Stations may be paired, e.g. a clinical examination at one station and questions about the examination and diagnosis at the next
- Each station has a strict marking sheet (Fig. 3.1)
- A wide variety of stations can be included, allowing broad testing of skills and knowledge

TYPES OF STATION

General

- Taking a targeted history for a clinical scenario
- Examining a 'patient' (may be a simulated patient) – see speciality chapters
- Patient photographs
- X-rays – see Radiology, Chapter 5
- ECGs – see Cardiology, Chapter 9
- Laboratory test interpretation – see Clinical chemistry, Chapter 6

Practical skills

- Inserting a cannula
- Inserting a urinary catheter
- Taking blood
- Taking blood gases
- Administrating i.v./i.m./s.c. injections
- Setting up an i.v. infusion
- Checking a blood transfusion
- Cardiopulmonary resuscitation
- Defibrillation
- Suturing
- Basic respiratory function tests
- Administration of a nebuliser
- Prescription and administration of oxygen therapy
- Breast/testes or rectal exam on a model
- Ophthalmoscopy

Candidate Name: Examination number:

Candidate instructions: Mrs Lewis has been referred having noticed blood in her stools. You have been asked by the consultant to take a focussedhistory of the presenting complaint. You do not need to ask about the past medical or social history, the drug history or to carry out a systems review. You do not need to present your findings to the examiner.

Examiner instructions: Please assess the candidate using the criteria listed.

		adequate	inadequate
1	Introduces self to patient, using own name, patient's name, role and a greeting		
2	States reason for the interview		
3	Obtains consent to proceed		
4	Asks patient's age		
5	Asks about occupation		
6	Obtains history of PR bleeding		
Specific information points elicited			
7	Nature of bleeding (bright red, mixed with stool) both to score		
8	Duration of symptoms		
9	Frequency of bleeding		
10	Previous episodes		
11	Recent change in bowel habit		
12	Normal bowel habit		
13	Weight loss or anorexia (both to score)		
14	Dietary changes		
15	Shortness of breath		
16	Medication history		
17	Family history		
18	Associated symptoms		
Approach to patient			
19	Active listening (verbal and non-verbal)		
20	Clarifies and reviews		
21	Avoids leading question		
22	Avoids multiple questions		
23	Does not use jargon or gives explanations		
24	Patient's rating of the candidate		

Examiner's rating

4 good	3 pass	2 borderline	1 fail

Fig. 3.1 Each station has a strict marking sheet.

Management questions

- Medical emergencies
- Writing a fluid chart
- Writing a prescription
- Reviewing a drug chart
- Writing a discharge summary

Communication

- Explaining a prescription to a patient
- Discussing a diagnosis with a patient
- Obtaining consent
- Describing a practical procedure
- Breaking bad news

Tips and tactics

- See General tips and tactics for clinical exams (Ch. 2)
- Make sure you are comfortable with the common procedures that crop up in OSCEs
- Practise the commonly needed practical skills in a clinical skills lab. These are easy marks to get
- Follow the (usually written) instructions
- At 'patient-based' stations, the examiner will have no verbal role. If you are expected to present findings, the instruction sheet will specifically tell you
- Even if a station has gone badly, you may have picked up some marks for professionalism, communication or rapport with the patient
- At the end of the station, forget it and clear your mind ready for the next one. Remember each station is a fresh start

---

EXAMPLE STATIONS

For each of the following stations, the key 'point-scoring' things that you should do are highlighted. There are general points for each type of station that are outlined at the beginning of each category. Don't forget to confirm your examination number and name with the examiner before you start.

Clinical history

Remember to:

- Read the instructions and follow them exactly
- Introduce yourself (to the patient) using your and their name
- Explain who you are and ask permission to proceed
  - This doesn't have to be too formal: 'Would you mind if I asked you a few questions?' will do
- Ask a couple of general questions, then rapidly target in on the key facts pertinent to the case
- Try not to lead the patient – 'So where do you get the pain', rather than 'So you have chest pain?'

- Give the patient a chance to expand on the answer
- Ask if there is anything else they want to tell you
- Avoid going into a long discussion about your diagnosis – these stations are about you getting the appropriate history, not explaining the diagnosis to the patient
- During the patient interaction, try to ignore the examiner unless specific instructions are given or you are asked to present your findings
- Once the bell goes, thank the patient and leave

Chest pain

Mr Davis is a 57-year-old man who attended accident and emergency with chest pain. Take an appropriate history from him. The 'patient' will have some specific pain features indicating the cause of the pain. This is most commonly acute myocardial infarction or angina. Less commonly gastro-oesophageal reflux disease (p.218). Your history needs to elicit these. The key facts that you should ask about are:

- Duration of the pain
- Previous episodes
- Character of the pain
  - Heavy/crushing in acute MI
  - Dull/tight in angina
  - Continuous or varying
- Intensity (on a range from 1–10)
- Site
- Radiation – to neck or left arm in cardiac ischaemia

Associated features

- Nausea
- Sweating
- Dizziness/faintness
- Shortness of breath
- Inducing activities
  - Exercise
  - Cold, windy days
- Relieving activities
  - Rest
  - Taking glyceryl trinitrate
- Risk factors for ischaemic heart disease
  - Family history of heart disease, stroke, hypertension or diabetes
  - Smoking history
  - Diabetes mellitus
  - Hypertension
  - Previous history of ischaemic heart disease
  - Elevated cholesterol
- Medication history
- Allergies to medication
- Risk factors for treatment
  - Recent GI bleeding
  - Recent major surgery
  - Recent cerebrovascular accident
  - Blood coagulopathy
  - Diabetic eye disease

Shortness of breath without chest pain

Mrs Jones is a 78-year-old woman with increasing shortness of breath. Take an appropriate history from her.

The initial differential
- Congestive cardiac failure/acute pulmonary oedema
- 'Silent' ischaemic heart disease
- Pneumonia/lower respiratory tract infection
- Exacerbation of chronic obstructive pulmonary disease/asthma
- Bronchogenic carcinoma

Initial questions to determine the most likely cause
- New symptom or recurrence of previous symptom
- Duration and whether getting worse
- Associated symptoms
  - Cough
  - Sputum production and type – purulent/non-purulent/frothy
  - Presence of orthopnoea and paroxysmal nocturnal dyspnoea
- History of ischaemic heart disease
- Risk factors for ischaemic heart disease or COPD
  Once the underlying cause is clear, you should target your history to the appropriate disease.

Silent ischaemic heart disease

- As for chest pain above

Congestive cardiac failure/pulmonary oedema

- Onset and severity
- Initiating, exacerbating and relieving factors
- Orthopnoea and paroxysmal nocturnal dyspnoea
- Cough/frothy sputum
- Ankle swelling
- Palpitations
- Chest pain
- Past history
  - Ischaemic heart disease
- Risk factors as for cardiac chest pain
- Medication history

Pneumonia/lower respiratory tract infection

- Cough
- Purulent sputum/colour of sputum
- Pleuritic chest pain
- Sweats/fevers
- Associated diarrhoea (atypical pneumonia)
- Risk factors
  - Smoking
  - Occupational exposure (dust/asbestos)
  - Animal exposure (birds)
  - Travel and contact history (TB)
  - HIV

Chronic obstructive pulmonary disease/asthma

- Cough
- Sputum production
- Wheeze
- Acute or insidious onset
- Exposure to precipitant
- Usual peak flow
- Usual exercise tolerance
- Exercise tolerance at present
- Previous admissions
- Previous admissions to ITU
- Smoking history
- Use of steroids
- Domiciliary oxygen cylinders/concentrator
- Home nebulizer
- Indicators of infection
  - Fevers
  - Purulent sputum

Shortness of breath with chest pain

Peter Smith is a 25-year-old man who presents with severe left-sided chest pain and shortness of breath.

Differential diagnosis
- Pneumonia (see above)
- Pleurisy
- Ischaemic heart disease (see above)
- Pulmonary embolus
- Pneumothorax

Pleurisy
- Preceding cough/sputum
- Fever
- Flu-like illness
- Pleuritic chest pain (worse on deep breathing)

Pulmonary embolus
- Sudden onset
- Pleuritic chest pain
- Shortness of breath
- Haemoptysis
- Swollen calf
- Risk factors
  - Immobility (travel/surgery/other illness)
  - Smoking
  - Oral contraceptive pill
  - Pro-coagulopathy (family history)
  - Previous miscarriages
  - Inflammatory disease
  - Malignant disease
  - Previous DVT/PE

Pneumothorax
- Classically tall thin young man
- Sudden onset
- Chest wall injury

- Short of breath with or without pain
- No fever
- No prodrome
- Risk factors
  - Asthma
  - COPD
  - Pulmonary fibrosis

Abdominal pain

Mr Flintoff is a 65-year-old man with abdominal pain. Take a history to ascertain the cause.

Basic questions
Site
- Epigastric – gastro-oesophageal reflux or dyspepsia
- Right subcostal – liver/biliary tree (e.g. gallstones)
- Left sided – diverticulosis/IBS/constipation
- Supra-pubic – bladder/pelvis
- Renal angles – renal stones/pyelonephritis

Character
- Constant
- Spasms/colicky

Associated symptoms
- Nausea
- Vomiting
- Diarrhoea
- Constipation
- Abdominal distension

Exacerbating features
- Eating
- Posture changes
- Deep breaths
- Specific foods, e.g. fatty foods (may suggest gallstones)

Relieving features
- Eating
- Vomiting
- Defaecation
- Antacids, other medications

Gastro-oesophageal reflux

- Central epigastric and retrosternal pain
- Burning/acidic in nature
- Worse with alcohol/caffeine/spicy foods
- Relieved by antacids
- Wakes from sleep at night
- Better when lying on left side
- Worse when bending over

Biliary colic

- Colicky pain (comes in waves)
- Right subcostal region
- Associated nausea/vomiting
- Associated jaundice

- Dark urine
- Pale stools

Renal colic

- Loin pain radiating to iliac fossa/testes/labia
- Vomiting
- Very severe colicky pain
- Associated symptoms
  - Haematuria
  - Anuria
- Risk factors
  - Hot weather
  - Previous stones
  - Gout
  - Crohn's disease
  - Urinary tract infections
  - Diuretics

Interpretation of results stations

Radiology

Radiology images in OSCEs tend to be simple investigations (chest X-rays, abdominal films, rarely CT scans of the head) with gross abnormalities and a short clinical history giving clues as to the diagnosis. They may also ask about the management of the abnormality. Chapter 5 covers all of the important films.

Chest X-rays

- Pneumothorax
- Tension pneumothorax
- Air under the diaphragm
- Pneumonia
- Pulmonary oedema
- Lung cancer

Abdominal films

- Renal stones
- Small bowel obstruction
- Sigmoid volvulus
- Toxic megacolon
- Pancreatic calcification

CT head

- Subdural/extradural/sub-arachnoid haemorrhage
- Mass lesions with oedema and midline shift
- Acoustic neuroma

  Example A 67-year-old man is admitted with anorexia and a productive cough. He has been feeling unwell for about 2 weeks with a cough productive of bloodstained sputum. His chest X-ray is shown in Figure 3.2.

  His temperature on admission is 36.7°C, oxygen saturation 93% on air

1. Describe the abnormality seen
   Answer: Cavitating lesion in right lung
2. Suggest three diagnoses in order of likelihood
   Answer: Lung abscess, bronchogenic carcinoma, pulmonary metastasis
3. Name two further appropriate investigations

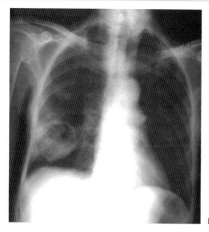

Fig. 3.2 Chest X-ray.

Answer: High resolution CT scan of the chest; sputum microscopy and culture

Example A 58-year-old woman is admitted for a CT-guided biopsy of a mass in the liver. List the important complications about which she should be advised and explain the procedure to her in order to gain informed consent

Answer: Complications about which she should be advised:

- Pain
- Bleeding
- Perforation of bowel
- Injury to right kidney
- Perforated gallbladder
- Pneumothorax

Example A 76-year-old man presents with right loin pain and haematuria. His abdominal X-ray is shown in Figure 3.3.

1. Describe the abnormality seen.
   Answer: Calcified mass in the right lateral abdomen
2. Suggest two possible diagnoses
   Answer: Calcified (porcelain) gallbladder; renal calcification (nephrocalcinosis)
3. Suggest two useful radiological investigations
   Answer: Renal ultrasound CT abdomen

Laboratory investigations

Again, these tend to be simple investigations and ask for your interpretation and management (see Ch. 6)

Example With reference to the following blood test results, answer the questions beneath:

- Hb 98 g/L WCC 7.2×10⁹/L platelets 198 MCV 101 fl
- Blood film: hypersegmented neutrophils

A. What is the haematological diagnosis?

Answer: Macrocytic (megaloblastic) anaemia

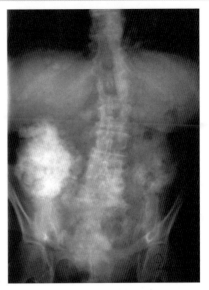

Fig. 3.3 Abdominal X-ray.

B. List 3 possible causes of your diagnosis
Answer: Vitamin B₁₂ deficiency; folic acid deficiency; chronic liver disease
C. Name two tests that would help you in determining the diagnosis
Answer: Liver biochemistry; serum haematinics

Practical procedure stations

As with clinical stations, there will be a short clinical scenario followed by an instruction. As always, introduce yourself, explain the procedure, get verbal consent and give clear instructions to the patient. You may also be asked to list possible complications or comment on the result.

Measuring peak flow
Mrs Robinson has asthma and is breathless. Please measure the peak flow.
Instructions for patient
● Please follow the student's instructions as they are given. Do not try to help or hinder the student but do try to do as they say.
Instructions to examiner
● The student introduces him/herself using his/her name and gains verbal consent
● Ensures a new disposable mouthpiece is attached
● Explains to the patient what to do, including
  ● Asking the patient to take a deep breath in
  ● Then blow out as hard and as fast as possible into the mouthpiece

- Ensures that the patient understands the lips should be tight around the mouthpiece
- Ensures that the patient can hold the meter without obstructing the linear scale
- Measures the peak flow reading using the linear scale
- Remembers to assess the best of three measurements
- Encourages and thanks the patient

Recording a 12-lead ECG

- Ensure the patient is comfortable at rest, ideally lying flat
- Turn the machine off

Limb leads

- Right leg – Black
- Right arm – Red
- Left leg – Green
- Left arm – Yellow

Chest leads

- V1–4th intercostal space, right of sternum
- V2–4th intercostal space left of sternum
- V3 – Half way between V2 and V3
- V4 – Apex of the heart
- V5 – Same horizontal plane as V4, anterior axillary line
- V6 – Same horizontal plane as V4, mid axillary line
- Turn on the ECG machine, choose: Gain 10 mm/mV, speed 25 mm/second
- Select 12-lead ECG and press start

Taking the blood pressure

- Ensure the patient is at rest and comfortable
- Explain procedure
- Choose appropriate sized cuff
- Palpate brachial artery
- Place cuff around upper right arm with the inflation bag over the brachial artery (precise location usually marked with an arrow on the cuff)
- Inflate until the radial pulse is not palpable then increase by 20 mmHg
- Place diaphragm of stethoscope over brachial artery just below the cuff
- Gradually reduce pressure until first sound is heard (Korotkoff I = systolic blood pressure)
- Continue to reduce until silence (Korotkoff V = diastolic pressure)
- *Note*: the sounds may disappear (Korotkoff II) then reappear (Korotkoff III) before becoming muffled (Korotkoff IV)

Urinary retention/catheterization

Instructions to student

- This patient is complaining of difficulty passing urine and excruciating lower abdominal pain. He is unable to keep still easily because of pain. Please take a brief history and proceed as appropriate.

Instructions to examiner

- The student is presented with a male in acute urinary retention. No complicating features. Needs urgent catheterization
- The student introduces him/herself
- Obtains hx of urinary retention

- Explains procedure of urethral catheter and gains consent
- Administers prophylactic antibiotics after checking for allergies
- Uses sterile technique
- Uses local anaesthetic gel
- Chooses appropriate size catheter
- Inserts catheter
- Obtains specimen of urine for analysis
- Attaches bag
- Documents procedure and leaves appropriate instructions for care of catheter

Taking blood cultures

- An aseptic technique is vital to avoid skin contaminants
- Repeat cultures from different sites at different times
- Wear gloves for the procedure
- Select an appropriate vein
- Thoroughly clean the overlying skin
- Do not touch the skin
- Take 15–20 mL of blood
- Open the tops of the culture bottles
- Clean the top of the bottle with a sterile wipe
- Place a fresh needle on the syringe and insert through the seal of each bottle, placing 8–10 mL of blood in each bottle
- Clearly label the samples
- Send to laboratory or place in incubator

Completion of microbiology request forms

In order to make an accurate diagnosis, the following information is vital:
- Patient details
- Clinical details: duration and type of illness, other related features
- Antibiotic therapy: duration and type of treatment
- History of foreign travel
- Type of specimen
- Requested investigation
- Clinical risks – viral hepatitis/HIV

Specific clinical examination stations

Sometimes you will be asked to demonstrate a specific piece of history-taking or examination such as those below.

Examination of a patient with Parkinson's disease
Instructions to student

- Please examine this patient, paying particular attention to the power and tone of the upper limbs. Do not examine sensation. You may undertake any further examination of the neurological system you consider appropriate. You have 5 minutes, after which you will be asked to summarize the findings and come up with a diagnosis.

Instructions to examiner

- The student introduces themselves and makes sure the patient is comfortable
- Observation (tremor, muscle bulk, fasciculation, bradykinesia, mask-like facies, lack of blinking)
- Asks about pain
- Moves arms demonstrating cogwheel rigidity
- Examines arms for power

- Tests reflexes
- Extra mark for: asking the patient to walk, glabellar tap, asking for example of handwriting, assessing function, e.g. buttons, knife and fork
- Presentation of main features
- Diagnosis

Examination of the thyroid gland and thyroid status

Mrs White has had palpitations and weight loss. Examine her thyroid gland.

- General inspection – look for signs of thyroid disease
- Examine the neck to look for a goitre
- Ask patient to take a sip of water and hold it in the mouth, then ask the patient to swallow while you watch the neck – look for movement of goitre with swallowing
- Stand behind the patient and gently feel the thyroid with both hands starting in the centre below the thyroid cartilage over the trachea, moving laterally to the two lobes which extend behind the sternomastoid muscle. Ask the patient to swallow again while you palpate. Assess the goitre for size, nodularity or diffuse enlargement, discrete nodules and firmness
- Palpate for lymph nodes
- Auscultate – listen over the thyroid for a bruit
- Assess thyroid status
- Pulse – count the rate and note presence or absence of atrial fibrillation
- Palms – warm and sweaty
- Tremor of fingers on outstretched arms
- Reflexes – slow relaxing in hypothyroidism, brisk in hyperthyroidism
- Examine the eyes for exophthalmus, lid retraction, lid lag
- Examine the reflexes for slow relaxation of in hypothyroidism

Deliberate self-harm assessment
Instructions for student

- This patient is recovering from a paracetamol overdose. Please assess her risk factors for suicide.

Instructions for patient

- Please answer the student's instructions as they are asked. You have a previous history of depression and your brother killed himself by hanging. Your husband has recently left home and your daughter has an incurable cancer. Please act withdrawn and give answers slowly. Please ensure it is clear that you did not expect your suicide plan to be discovered.

Instructions to examiner

- The student introduces him/herself and gains verbal consent
- Performs suicide assessment
- Questions to be asked:
  - Was there a clear precipitant/cause for the attempt?
  - Was the act premeditated?
  - Did the patient leave a suicide note?
  - Had the patient taken pains not to be discovered?
  - Did the patient make the attempt in strange surroundings (i.e. away from home)?
  - Would the patient do it again?
  - Concern if any answer to the above is positive

- Also establish:
  - Has the precipitant/cause for the attempt resolved?
  - Is there continuing suicidal intent?
  - Does the patient have psychiatric symptoms?
  - What is the patient's social support system?
  - Has the patient inflected self-harm before?
  - Has anyone in the family ever taken their life?
  - Does the patient have a physical illness?

Communication with patients

- This may involve explaining a diagnosis, prescription or procedure, taking consent or breaking bad news
- Always use lay language rather than medical jargon
- Allow the patient time to speak and specifically ask if there are any questions

Explanation of the diagnosis of epilepsy
Instructions to student

- A 30-year-old mother of two has been referred by her GP with new tonic clonic seizures due to grand mal epilepsy. Please explain the diagnosis to the patient and give her appropriate advice on living with epilepsy and include suggestions to start therapy with any one of the first-line single agent therapies available. You have 10 minutes.

Instructions to the patient

- You have been referred to the hospital after having had two seizures which your GP thinks are epilepsy. Tests have confirmed the diagnosis. This doctor is going to explain the diagnosis and how to live with the condition and suggest treatment with tablets to reduce the number of fits.

Instructions to examiner

- The student introduces him/herself and makes sure the patient is comfortable
- Explains the diagnosis using lay terms and medical terms
- Checks understanding
- Explains options for treatment
- Explains likely benefits of drug therapy
- Gives information on side-effects of drugs
- Discusses driving regulations
- Makes time to listen to patient's questions
- Gives extra back-up information to take home (e.g. leaflet, website address of epilepsy foundation, nurse specialist number, secretary's number).

Corticosteroid prescription and dispensing
Instructions to student

- You are giving this patient a 6-week course of prednisolone, starting at 40 mg, to treat polymyalgia rheumatica. You are aiming to reduce the dose to half or less over 6 weeks. Please write a prescription and give it to the patient with appropriate advice.

Instructions to examiner

- The student introduces him/herself
- Checks patient's details
- Asks about drug allergies

- Issues accurate prescription: date, address, name, contact number, patient's name and address and GP, legible accurate prescription and signature
- Gives patient a steroid card
- Explains to the patient that they must show this to any medical professional they see
- Advice about side-effects (psychiatric symptoms, skin changes, weight changes and fat distribution, diabetes, bone loss, immunosuppression) is given
- Warns patient not to stop the drug suddenly
- Issues a prescription for bone protection (calcium and vitamin D or a bisphosphonate)

Diabetes: starting insulin

Mr Coleman is a 21-year-old man recently diagnosed as having insulin-requiring diabetes mellitus. Explain to him how to use insulin and self-administration.

Marking sheet

- Explanation of insulin regime
- Explains and demonstrates 'stix' testing of blood glucose using a pinprick
- Instruction and demonstration of sub-cut injection, watch patient attempt to give injection; give feedback on technique
- Explain importance of varying site of injection
- Warn about hypoglycaemic episodes
- Warn about other side-effects
- Warn about failure to take insulin increasing risk of ketoacidosis
- Explain importance of taking insulin when ill
- Check understanding, listen to questions
- Arrange follow-up appointment
- Give contact detail of responsible health professional (e.g. diabetes clinical nurse specialist)

Controlled drug prescriptions

Miss Maddon is a 65-year-old woman with metastatic breast carcinoma who is taking morphine. Write a prescription for 10 mg of oral liquid morphine (Oramorph) 4 times a day for 1 month.

- Name/address/date of birth of patient
- Write out name of drug, dose regimen and total amount to be dispensed in words and numbers in indelible ink:
  - Morphine sulphate suspension ten (10) milligrams four (4) times a day for twenty-eight (28) days, total prescribed one thousand, one hundred and twenty (1120) milligrams
- Sign, print your name and date the prescription

Completion of death certificates

Personal details of the deceased

- Name
- Age – in completed years or if less than 1 year, in completed months
- Place of death – for hospital patients, this is the name of the hospital
- For patients at home, it is the private address
- For deaths elsewhere, the locality is recorded

Circumstances of certification

- Last seen alive by me – record the date that you last saw the patient alive

Information from post-mortem
- You should indicate here if the information you give takes account of a post-mortem
  - Ring option 1 if a post-mortem has been done
  - Ring option 2 if information from a post-mortem may be available later
  - Ring option 3 if a post-mortem is not being held

Seen after death
- Ring one option (a, b or c) only to indicate whether you or another medical practitioner saw the deceased after death

Cases reported to the coroner Some cases are discussed with the coroner/procurator fiscal and a certificate is completed by the attending doctor after agreement with the coroner/procurator fiscal, e.g. patients dying within 24 hours of arrival at hospital but for whom the cause of death is known. If this is the case, then ring option 4 and tick box A on the back of the certificate. Remember for cases referred to the coroner for investigation, a certificate is not completed by the attending doctor (Table 3.1).

Cause of death statement
- Remember always avoid abbreviations
- This section of the certificate is divided into 2 parts:
  Part I
- Here the immediate cause of death and any underlying cause(s) are recorded
- It is vital that this section is completed accurately and fully with as specific details as possible, e.g. histological cell types for malignancies if known

  Example A patient died from an intracerebral haemorrhage caused by cerebral metastases from a primary malignant neoplasm of the left main bronchus. This should be entered as follows:
- Disease or condition that led directly to death

  I (a) Intracerebral haemorrhage

Table 3.1 Referral decisions

A death should be referred to the coroner/procurator fiscal for investigation if:

The cause of death is unknown
The deceased was not seen by the certifying doctor either after death or within 14 days before death
The death was violent or unnatural or suspicious
The death may be due to an accident
The death may be due to self-neglect or neglect by others
The death may be due to industrial disease or related to the deceased's employment
The death may be due to an abortion
The death occurred during an operation or before recovery from the effects of an anaesthetic
The death may be a suicide
The death occurred during or shortly after detention in police or prison custody

Table 3.2 Terms implying a mode of death rather than a cause of death

Asphyxia	Hepatorenal failure
Asthenia	Kidney failure
Brain failure	Liver failure
Cachexia	Renal failure
Cardiac arrest	Respiratory arrest
Cardiac failure	Shock
Coma	Syncope
Debility	Uraemia
Exhaustion	Vagal inhibition
Heart failure	Vasovagal attack
Hepatic failure	Ventricular failure

- Intermediate cause of death
  (b) Cerebral metastases
- Underlying cause of death
  (c) Squamous cell carcinoma of the left main bronchus

Occasionally, there are apparently two distinct conditions leading to death. If there is no way of choosing between them they should be entered on the same line and it should be indicated that they are joint causes of death.

Do not use terms that imply a mode of dying rather than a cause of death (Table 3.2).

Part II Any significant condition/disease that contributed to the death but which is not part of the sequence leading directly to death is recorded. Do not list all conditions present at the time of death. Do list any that may have hastened the death.

Example A diabetic patient died from an intracerebral haemorrhage caused by cerebral metastases from a primary malignant neoplasm of the left main bronchus.

This should be entered as follows:

- Disease or condition that led directly to death
  I (a) Intracerebral haemorrhage
- Intermediate cause of death
  (b) Cerebral metastases
- Underlying cause of death
  (c) Squamous cell carcinoma of the left main bronchus
- Other conditions contributing to death
  II. Diabetes mellitus

Employment-related death

- If you believe that the death may have been due to (or contributed to by) employment followed at any time by the deceased, you should indicate this by ticking the appropriate box on the front of the certificate and report the death to the coroner/procurator fiscal
- Signature of certifying doctor and name of the consultant
- Sign the certificate and add your qualifications, address and the date
- Print your name in block capitals also
- If the death occurred in hospital, the name of the consultant responsible for the care of the patient must also be recorded

● Finally, complete the Notice to Informant section and the counterfoil of the certificate

SUMMARY

OSCE examinations can include any practical aspect of day-to-day medical practice. Use textbooks of clinical skills and clinical skills labs to get an idea of the techniques and procedures.

Remember the cardinal rules

● Use lay language
● Introduce yourself
● Seek consent
● Follow the instructions
● Develop a rapport with the patient
● Clear your mind between stations.

Pharmacology and therapeutics 4

Pharmacology
- The study of the interaction between chemicals and the human body

Therapeutics
- The treatment of disease (any modality)

Pharmacodynamics
- The physiological and biochemical effects of a drug including their mechanism(s) of action

Pharmacokinetics
- The effect of physiological processes on drug concentrations and action

Cardinal features of therapeutics
- The right patient
- The right drug
- The right dose
- At an affordable cost

The right patient
- Clear diagnosis and/or clinical need (i.e. the drug will improve symptoms or outcome)
- Clear benefit in an asymptomatic/well patient (e.g. vaccination/ primary prevention of disease or contraception)
- Absence of a contraindication due to co-morbidity (Table 4.1) or drug interaction (Tables 4.2–4.4)

The right drug
- Tolerability (e.g. side-effects)
- Efficacy (improved symptoms/prognosis demonstrated in trial data)
- Safety (efficacy balanced against risks of therapy)
- Therapeutic index (Fig. 4.1)
- Compliance and patient preference

The right dose
- Careful prescribing
- Careful dispensing and patient instructions
- Monitoring: Table 4.4 (drug levels, toxicity, early detection of adverse effects)

Affordability
- Pharmacoeconomics (value for money)
- Marketing (using generic vs branded drugs)
- Assessment by independent review (e.g. National Institute for Health and Clinical Excellence, NICE)

Table 4.1 Common drug contraindications

Co-morbidity	Drugs to avoid	Effect
Asthma	Beta-blockers Adenosine	Bronchospasm
Hypertension	Non-steroidal anti-inflammatories	Increased hypertension via sodium retention
	COX-II inhibitors	
Parkinson's disease	Neuroleptics	Worsening symptoms
Respiratory failure	Opiates	Respiratory depression
Epilepsy	Tricyclic antidepressants	Reduced seizure threshold
	Anti-malarials	
	Anti-psychotics	
Atrioventricular block	Digoxin	Heart block
	Beta-blockers	
	Diltiazem	
Chronic liver disease	Warfarin	Increased sensitivity/ bleeding
Renovascular disease	ACE inhibitors	Reduced renal blood flow
	Angiotensin II receptor antagonists	

Table 4.2 Common pharmacokinetic drug interactions

Drug 1	Drug 2	Interaction
Warfarin	P450 inhibitors	Increased prothrombin time
	Aspirin	Increased bleeding time
Theophylline	P450 inhibitors	Arrhythmia
Iron	Calcium salts (e.g. milk, antacids)	Reduced iron absorption
Digoxin	Quinidine	Displacement of drug from protein binding → bradycardia
Lithium	Thiazides	Failure of excretion leading to seizures/ ataxia
	NSAIDs	
Oral contraceptive pill	Antibiotics	Failure of contraception
	Anti-epileptics	
Azathioprine	Allopurinol	Bone marrow suppression

Table 4.3 Common pharmacodynamic drug interactions

Drug 1	Drug 2	Interaction
Beta-blockers (Atenolol)	Verapamil	Bradycardia/asystole
	Diltiazem	
ACE inhibitors	Loop diuretics	Hypotension
Digoxin	Amiodarone	Heart block
	Verapamil	Heart block
	Diuretics	Hypokalaemia $\rightarrow$ toxicity
Beta$_2$ agonists (salbutamol)	Beta-blockers	Loss of effect/bronchospasm

Table 4.4 Drugs and the cytochrome P450 pathway

Drugs metabolized by the CyP450 pathway	Drugs that induce CyP450 activity	Drugs that inhibit CyP450
Warfarin	Phenytoin	Omeprazole
Amitriptyline	Carbamazepine	Diltiazem
Ciclosporin	Barbiturates	Erythromycin
Statins	Rifampicin	Sodium valproate
Phenytoin	Alcohol	Isoniazid
Losartan	Allopurinol	Quinolones
Sertraline	Protease inhibitors	Grapefruit juice
Aminophylline	St John's Wort	

$$\text{Therapeutic index} = \frac{\text{Lethal dose for 50\% of the population (LD}_{50}\text{)}}{\text{Effective dose for 50\% of the population (ED}_{50}\text{)}}$$

Fig. 4.1 Definition of the therapeutic index.

PHARMACOLOGY

Pharmacodynamics

Drug–receptor interactions

Biological effects of a drug will depend on several factors:
- Affinity – strength of binding to the target receptor
- Efficacy – effect by unit concentration
- Potency – dose of drug required for a given effect
- Dose response – effect plotted against dose
- Drug – receptor interactions
- Agonists – bind and activate receptor function
- Partial agonists – bind but cannot maximally activate a response
- Antagonists – block a receptor but no biological response – will inhibit physiological activation of the receptor

- Competitive antagonists – reversibly block so at high agonist concentrations their effect is reduced
- Irreversible agonists – only lose effect once new receptors are formed

Mechanisms of action

Direct physiochemical effect:
- Alteration of pH (e.g. sodium bicarbonate, antacids)
- Osmotic diuretics (mannitol)
- Osmotic laxatives (lactulose)

Receptor antagonism:
- Beta-blockers (atenolol)
- Angiotensin II receptor antagonists (losartan)
  Direct binding to target compound:
- Infliximab: antibody that binds to tumour necrosis factor and stops its activity

Receptor agonism:
- β_2 receptors (salbutamol)
- Epinephrine

Transmembrane channel blockade:
- Calcium channel blockers (amlodipine)
- Na^+/K^+ ATPase blocker (Digoxin)
- Neurotransmitter reuptake inhibitors (Sertraline)

Enzyme inhibitors:
- Cyclo-oxygenase inhibitors (aspirin/NSAIDs)
- HMG CoA reductase inhibitors (statins)

Purine analogues ($\rightarrow$ reduced DNA synthesis):
- Azathioprine

Antibacterials:
- Inhibition of bacterial cell wall formation (e.g. penicillins)
- Inhibition of bacterial genome replication (e.g. quinolones)
- Inhibition of bacterial RNA transcription (e.g. rifampicin)
- Inhibition of bacterial protein synthesis (e.g. aminoglycosides)
- Inhibition of folic acid metabolism (e.g. trimethoprim)

Hormones:
- Inhibition of hormone production (FSH/LH by the oral contraceptive pill)
- Increased secretion (insulin by sulphonylureas, e.g. gliclazide)
- Replacement (thyroxine, insulin)

Pharmacokinetics

Routes of administration

Oral/enteral
- Absorption via gastrointestinal tract
- Carried via portal vein via liver to peripheral circulation
- Therefore undergo first pass metabolism by liver
- Must be able to resist digestion (i.e. not protein based)
- May be altered by gut motility/presence or absence of food

Rectal/sublingual
- Allows delivery to site of action, e.g. mesalazine in ulcerative proctitis
- Rapid absorption
- Safe delivery in those who are nil-by-mouth
- Avoids first pass metabolism effect

Intravenous
- Direct administration into peripheral circulation. Peak plasma concentration achieved immediately

Intramuscular/subcutaneous
- Rapid delivery into circulation
- Formulation can delay absorption, e.g. depot injections

Topical
- Delivery to site of action (e.g. emollients for eczema, chloramphenicol eye drops)

Inhaled
- Direct action in pulmonary tissue (e.g. salbutamol)

Transdermal
- Absorption via skin
- Provides continuous, long duration therapy with predictable plasma drug levels
- e.g. nicotine replacement, fentanyl analgesia

Intrathecal
- Delivery directly into cerebrospinal fluid
- Allows bypassing of blood–brain barrier
- e.g. specific chemotherapies

Absorption

Depends on:
- Route of administration
- Degree of first pass metabolism
- Drugs that undergo significant first pass metabolism cannot be used orally
- Lipid solubility

Volume of distribution (V_D)

Determines final concentration of drug in target tissue and therefore dose effect

Depends on:
- Lipid solubility (ability to cross membranes into cells)
- Protein binding (protein bound drugs may not be detectable/active)
- Molecule size (ability to traverse endothelium into tissue fluid)

Can be measured:
- V_D <5 litre: drug retained in vascular space only
- V_D <15 litre: drug confined to extravascular space only
- V_D >15 litre: drug distributed throughout total body water

Metabolism

Drug metabolism may be required for:
- Activation of a prodrug → active form (e.g. valaciclovir → acyclovir)
- Termination of function of a drug
- Conversion to a hydrophilic compound to allow renal excretion

Phases of metabolism
  I. Transformation to a polar metabolite, e.g. p450 oxidation
  II. Conjugation, e.g. acetylation, methylation

Elimination

The majority of drugs and their metabolites are eliminated by the kidneys
- Phase I and II metabolism required to facilitate excretion rate of elimination depends on glomerular filtration rate and tubular reabsorption dose adjustments may be required in renal impairment

Biliary excretion:
- May be associated with enteral reabsorption (entero-hepatic circulation), e.g. metronidazole

Pharmacogenetics

Polymorphisms of metabolic enzymes can alter drug metabolism leading to:
- Reduced efficacy
- Increased toxicity, e.g. isoniazid acetylation, TPMT breakdown of azathioprine

Drug interactions

Important cause of morbidity due to iatrogenic injury:
- Pharmacokinetic: one drug alters the absorption, protein binding, metabolism or excretion of another (Table 4.2)
- Pharmacodynamic: The action of one drug alters the response to a second, e.g. enzyme inhibition (Tables 4.3, 4.4)
- Avoiding interactions:
  - Careful prescribing
  - Check for interactions (e.g. British National Formulary)
  - Avoid multiple drugs for the same indication where possible
  - Seek advice (e.g. pharmacist)

Drug monitoring (Table 4.5)

- Measurement of clinical effect or blood levels
- Assessment for side-effects/adverse effects
- Titration of dose to achieve therapeutic range/avoid sub-therapeutic or toxic doses
- Most important when the therapeutic index is small (Fig. 4.1)

Adverse drug reactions (ADRs)

Unforeseen event resulting from administration of a drug:
- Hypersensitivity – idiosyncratic/independent of dose (Table 4.6)
- Unexpected interaction – usually dose dependent (Tables 4.2–4.4)
- Side-effect – dose-dependent

Table 4.5 Drugs requiring monitoring

Drug	Monitoring	Toxicity/inadequate dose
Gentamicin	Peak and trough blood levels	Renal injury
Azathioprine	Full blood count and liver biochemistry	Bone marrow suppression (neutropenia) and liver injury
Anti-epileptics	Blood drug levels	Drowsiness/low seizure threshold
Tacrolimus	Blood levels	Bone marrow suppression
Lithium	Blood levels	Vomiting, ataxia, drowsiness, seizures

Table 4.6 Hypersensitivity reactions

Type	Pathology	Clinical signs	Example
I	Anaphylaxis: IgE mediated mast cell degranulation → histamine response	Tachycardia, oedema, shock, urticarial rash	Penicillin
II	Humoral: antibody synthesis against the drug	Haemolytic anaemia	Methyldopa
		Loss of efficacy	Infliximab
III	Antibody – antigen complex formation with reduced capillary blood flow	Digital ischaemia, lupus-like reaction	Hydralazine
IV	Delayed: cell-mediated memory response	Contact dermatitis	Topical antibiotics
V	Autoimmune	Target organ damage	Not induced by drugs

Long-term effects

- Predictable from mechanism of action, e.g. osteoporosis with corticosteroids
- Unpredictable, e.g. pulmonary fibrosis with amiodarone

Reporting

- Informs other doctors of the risks of a drug
- Provides information of risk of adverse events
- UK: Medicine and Healthcare products Regulatory Agency (MHRA)
- 'Yellow card' system from the BNF or www.MHRA.gov.uk

POISONING

Causes

- Deliberate self-harm (e.g. paracetamol)
- Substance misuse (e.g. opiates, amphetamines)
- Accidental (e.g. analgesics)
- Criminal
- Iatrogenic (drug errors, duplicate prescribing)

Treatment

- Immediate assessment: airway/breathing/circulation/conscious level
- Seek information (patient/relatives; ambulance crew):
  - What was taken?
  - How long ago?
  - Mixed or single drug overdose?
  - Taken with alcohol?

Table 4.7 Treatments for common poisons/overdoses

Poison	Antidote	Mechanism of action
Opiates	Naloxone	Opioid receptor antagonist
Benzodiazepines	Flumazenil	Receptor antagonist – use with care: can induce seizures
Paracetamol	Acetyl cysteine	Increases metabolism of drug
Methanol	Ethanol	Competes with metabolic pathway
Organophosphates	Atropine	Blocks effect of poison at cholinergic receptors

- Find out about the specific poison
  - ToxBase (www.toxbase.org)
  - Poisons unit help lines
  - Local guidelines
  - Senior advice
- If taken within the last 4 hours, consider treatments to reduce absorption
  - Gastric lavage within one hour (rarely used)
  - Activated charcoal
  - Induced vomiting (never use)
  - Whole bowel lavage
- Consider reversal agents/antidotes/antagonists (Table 4.7)

Management of specific drug overdoses

Paracetamol
- Used in UK in 45% of all deliberate self-harm related overdoses
- Toxic dose low (12 g/day or 150 mg/kg)
- Delayed toxicity, so may not present until late in clinical course

Mechanism of toxicity (Fig. 4.2)
- Saturation of glutathione metabolic pathway
- Accumulation of toxic metabolite
- Hepatic injury and necrosis

Clinical features
- Early: nonspecific nausea, vomiting, abdominal pain and malaise
- Late: 2 days–2 weeks: jaundice, coagulopathy, encephalopathy

Therapy (Fig. 4.3)
- Blood paracetamol levels
- Gastric lavage and charcoal in large amounts and within 4 hours
- If >24 g taken, treat straight away, DO NOT WAIT 4 HOURS
- If blood level on or above treatment line, give acetyl-cysteine (Table 4.8)

High risk groups
- Pre-existing glutathione depletion (AIDS, malnutrition, eating disorders)
- Chronic alcohol misuse

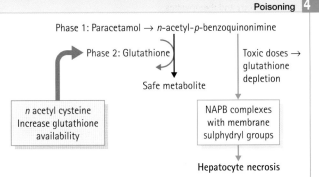

Phase 1: Paracetamol → *n*-acetyl-*p*-benzoquinonimine

Phase 2: Glutathione

Toxic doses → glutathione depletion

Safe metabolite

n acetyl cysteine Increase glutathione availability

NAPB complexes with membrane sulphydryl groups

Hepatocyte necrosis

Fig. 4.2 Normal and toxic metabolic pathways for paracetamol.

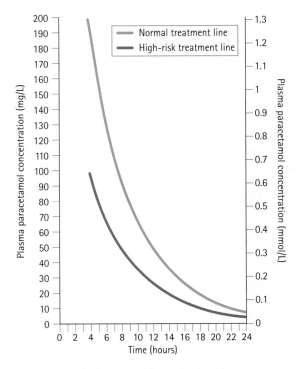

Fig. 4.3 Normogram for the treatment of paracetamol overdose.

Table 4.8 N-acetylcysteine (NAC) treatment regime

150 mg/kg NAC in 200 mL 5% dextrose over 15 minutes
50 mg/kg NAC in 500 mL 5% dextrose over 4 hours
100 mg/kg NAC in 1000 mL 5% dextrose over 16 hours

- CyP450 inducting drugs
- Staggered doses/inaccurate histories

Indicators of high risk of liver failure – consider referral to specialist unit

- ALT >1000 U/L
- Prothrombin time raised
- Worsening renal impairment
- Metabolic acidosis

Aspirin

Oral doses of:

- Less than 150 mg/kg – no toxicity to mild toxicity
- From 150–300 mg/kg – Mild-to-moderate toxicity
- From 301–500 mg/kg – Serious toxicity
- Greater than 500 mg/kg – Potentially lethal toxicity

Mechanism of toxicity

- Increased respiratory drive → respiratory alkalosis due to hyperventilation
- Combined metabolic acidosis (ketosis and lactic acidosis) with respiratory compensation

Clinical features

- Nausea and vomiting
- Tinnitus
- Hyperventilation
- Pyrexia, sweating, tachycardia
- Cerebral oedema → confusion, seizures, coma

Management

- Gastric lavage if within 12 hours as aspirin slows gastric emptying
- Activated charcoal
- Urine alkalinization
- If blood salicylate >700 mg/L consider haemodialysis

Tricyclic antidepressants

Clinical features

- Reduced level of consciousness
- Seizures
- Hyperreflexia and increased muscle tone
- Anticholinergic effects: dilated pupils, urinary retention, sinus tachycardia
- Ventricular arrhythmia/pulseless electrical activity, cardiac arrest

Management

- Gastric lavage and activated charcoal
- Assisted ventilation
- Cardiac monitoring
- Correction of acid-base imbalance
- Consider ITU care if airway compromised

Opiates

- Prescribed drugs: codeine/morphine
- Illegal drugs: heroin (diamorphine)

Clinical features

- Drowsiness
- Nausea and vomiting
- Respiratory depression
- Pinpoint pupils

Management

- Urine toxicology screen for other drugs
- Naloxone bolus (short-acting so may require repeated doses)
- Check for opiate patches on skin (inadvertent overdose)
- Monitor conscious level and respiratory rate

Alcohol

Common cause of reduced conscious level in emergency departments

Clinical features

- Associated with trauma/head injury
- Hypoglycaemia
- Respiratory depression
- Seizures
- Vomiting
- Aspiration pneumonitis

Management

- Supportive case: airway management and gastric lavage
- Monitor blood glucose and correct

PRESCRIBING

The following are requirements for a legal prescription:

- Written in ink
- Patient name
- Address or hospital identifier
- Date of birth
- Drug name (full spelling)
- Dose, frequency and route of administration
- Duration of course
- Prescriber's name, signature and date
  Consider:
- Generic vs trade names
- Generic drugs are just as safe and cheaper
- Trade names are sometimes useful for specific formulations (e.g. delayed release)
- Drug interactions (if in doubt check in the BNF at: http://bnf.org/bnf/index.htm)

Controlled drugs (Box 4.1)

- Hand written or produced by a secure computerized prescribing system
- Name, address and date of birth of the patient
- Name, preparation and strength of drug
- Total quantity to be dispensed in words and figures
- Dose and frequency

BOX 4.1. Controlled drug form	
Name:	John Smith
Address:	St Elsewhere's
	London
	AB1 2CD
Date of birth:	13.9.40
Prescription	
Morphine sulphate tablets (MST Continus) 20 mg three times daily to be taken orally 5 days' supply Total = 300 mg, three hundred milligrams	
Signature:	Date: 01.01.01
Name of prescriber:	Dr I Hope
	The Surgery
	West Street
	London AB2 3EF

Prescribing in specialist groups

Prescribing in the elderly

- Compliance reduced:
  - Multiple medications (poly-pharmacy)
  - Reduced cognitive function
- Change in volume of distribution:
  - Reduction in body mass
  - Reduced cardiac output
  - Changes in body composition
- Increased sensitivity to drug action:
  - Increased gastrointestinal and psychomotor effects of drugs
  - Reduced ability to regulate blood pressure → postural hypotension
  Therefore consider:
- Pragmatic prescribing – what is important and what is not
- Risk–benefit analysis: benefit of warfarin in AF vs risk of falls and haemorrhage
- Use scoring systems (e.g. CHADS2)
- Aim for once-a-day regimens
- Use Dosette boxes to improve compliance and avoid inadvertent overdose

Prescribing in pregnancy and breast-feeding

Medicine may:
- be teratogenic, e.g. ACE inhibitors, warfarin, anti-epileptics
- alter fetal growth
- alter physiology, e.g. NSAIDs → delayed closure of the ductus arteriosus
- alter maternal physiology, e.g. glucocorticoids → gestational diabetes
- have long-term risks to the child, e.g. diethylstilboestrol → vaginal carcinoma after puberty

Never assume a drug is safe – if in doubt do not prescribe.
Consider the benefits vs the risks of the drug for the individual and the pregnancy.
- Breast-feeding:
  - Doses in breast milk of most drugs are small
  - Risk–benefit should be discussed with the patient

ADDITIONAL RESOURCES

British National Formulary – www.bnf.org
Medicines and Healthcare products Regulatory Agency – www.MHRA.gov.uk
ToxBase – www.toxbase.org
National Institute for Health and Clinical Excellence – www.nice.org.uk
General Medical Council – www.gmc-uk.org

SELF-ASSESSMENT QUESTIONS

Multiple choice questions (true or false)

1. The following drugs exert their effect by binding to receptors:
    A. Aspirin
    B. Propranolol
    C. Nifedipine
    D. Cimetidine
    E. Omeprazole
2. The following drugs are receptor agonists:
    A. Salbutamol
    B. Atenolol
    C. Pilocarpine
    D. Phenylephrine
    E. Captopril
3. The following drugs undergo extensive first-pass metabolism:
    A. Glyceryl trinitrate
    B. Lidocaine (Lignocaine)
    C. Insulin
    D. Benzylpenicillin
    E. Probenecid
4. The following drugs induce P450 enzymes:
    A. Phenobarbital
    B. Rifampicin
    C. Cimetidine
    D. Paroxetine
    E. Carbamazepine
5. In paracetamol overdose:
    A. Paracetamol levels are essential in planning treatment
    B. Hepatic necrosis can occur up to 48 hours after ingestion
    C. N-acetylcysteine prevents paracetamol absorption from the stomach
    D. Rising INR is a poor prognostic indicator
    E. Co-ingestion of alcohol enhances paracetamol toxicity
6. In salicylate overdose:
    A. Aspirin delays gastric emptying
    B. Respiratory alkalosis occurs in conjunction with metabolic acidosis

C. Acidifying the urine enhances aspirin excretion by the kidney

D. Activated charcoal may be useful up to 12 hours after ingestion

E. N-acetylcysteine improves prognosis in large overdoses

Multiple choice questions (single best answer)

7. A 67-year-old man with longstanding ulcerative colitis, who was taking azathioprine, was seen with a clinical diagnosis of gout. Which one of the following is most likely to increase the risk of azathioprine toxicity?
   A. Allopurinol
   B. Bendroflumethiazide
   C. Colchicine
   D. Ibuprofen
   E. Paracetamol

8. A 34-year-old man was admitted with severe shortness of breath and facial oedema after eating shellfish. He was given adrenaline, hydrocortisone and chlorphenamine. Which one of the following best describes the mechanism of action of chlorphenamine?
   A. Direct receptor antagonist
   B. Enzyme inhibitor
   C. IgE receptor blocker
   D. Mast cell membrane stabilizer
   E. Trans-membrane channel blocker

9. A 56-year-old woman developed a raised, itchy, erythematous rash on starting a course of amoxicillin for a chest infection. Which one of the following best describes the underlying physiological process?
   A. Antibody – antigen complexes resulting in microvascular insufficiency
   B. Development of auto-immune dermatitis
   C. IgE mediated mast cell degranulation and histamine release
   D. IgG mediated intravascular haemolysis
   E. T lymphocyte cell mediated reaction

10. Which of the following physiological processes is most important for the excretion of a drug through the kidneys?
    A. Conjugation to increase water solubility
    B. Enterohepatic recirculation
    C. Oxidation to reduce polarity
    D. Protein binding to decrease tubular reabsorption
    E. Urinary alkalization

11. A 32-year-old woman was admitted following an overdose. She was nauseated with abdominal pain. On examination, she was drowsy, her pupils were dilated and she had a heart rate of 140 beats per minute. What is the most likely medication that she has taken?
    A. Aspirin
    B. Codeine
    C. Diazepam
    D. Imipramine
    E. Paracetamol

12. A 23-year-old man was admitted unconscious. On examination, he was unrousable, with a respiratory rate of 6 per minute and oxygen saturations of 87% on room air.

What is the most appropriate initial management?

A. Intravenous flumazenil
B. Intravenous naloxone
C. Oral activated charcoal
D. Placement of an oropharyngeal airway
E. Urine toxicology screen

Extended matching questions

Question 1 Theme: Pharmacology

A. Allopurinol
B. Amoxicillin
C. Atenolol
D. Glyceryl trinitrate
E. Imipramine
F. Methotrexate
G. Ranitidine
H. Rofecoxib
I. Salbutamol
J. Thyroxine
K. Verapamil

For each of the following questions, select the best answer from the list above:

I. A drug that acts as a trans-membrane channel blocker
II. A drug that causes bronchodilatation
III. A drug that inhibits an enzyme required for the metabolism of azathioprine
IV. A drug that can cause hypertension
V. A drug that undergoes extensive first pass metabolism
VI. A drug that acts at the cell nucleus
VII. A drug that can cause tachycardia and tremor

Radiology 5

Medical imaging remains a vital part of the diagnostic process. Diagnostic imaging is complemented by therapeutic procedures carried out by the radiologist. Interpretation of X-rays, CT and MRI scans, combined with the role of imaging in diagnosis and the risks of radiological procedures are important subjects in examinations.

Many radiological procedures involve exposure to ionizing radiation. They should only be used when indicated and will change the patient's management. Care must be taken in women of childbearing age in order to avoid exposing the fetus.

TYPES OF IMAGING

X-rays

- Utilize electromagnetic radiation
- Commonest form of medical imaging
- Image illustrates the variations in radiodensity of tissues to X-rays

Contrast studies

- Introduction of radio-opaque contrast
- Outlines hollow organs, e.g. barium swallow
- Water-soluble contrast substances allow
  - Examination of vasculature containing the agent, e.g. angiography
  - Excretion of the contrast agent, e.g. intravenous urogram

Computerized axial tomography (CT)

- Utilizes X-rays
- Integrates large quantities of data
- Allows computerized reconstruction of cross-sectional images

Ultrasound

- Utilizes high-frequency sound
- Measures reflection of sound waves. Non-invasive and no radiation exposure
  - Obstetric ultrasound
  - Renal, hepatic and pancreatic imaging
  - Doppler studies of blood vessels

Magnetic resonance imaging (MRI)

- Magnetic fields used to induce 'proton spin'
- No radiation exposure
- Data reconstruction allows detailed images
- Signal depends on water content of tissue

Nuclear medicine

- Use of isotopes in imaging
  - V̇/Q̇ scan for pulmonary embolus
  - Renal function studies
  - White cell scans for occult infection
  - Bone scans for malignancy
  - PET scans

THE CHEST X-RAY (FIG. 5.1)

Order of analysis

Basic details
- State name and age of the patient
- Date of the X-ray
- Antero-posterior (AP) or postero-anterior (PA) (describes the direction of travel of the X-rays)
- Check left and right markers

Rotation of film
- Look at medial ends of the clavicle
- Symmetry either side of spinous processes
- Sternum and vertebral column should be in line

Pneumothorax
- Collapse of lung → free air in the pleural space
  Simple (Fig. 5.2)
- Lung collapse
- No mediastinal shift
  Tension
- Mediastinal shift away from the side of the pneumothorax
- Usually due to penetrating chest wall injury (Fig. 5.3)
  Is there air under the diaphragm?
- Black line immediately under diaphragm (Fig. 5.4)

Expansion
- Count posterior ribs visible in the lung field
- Normal is 6–7

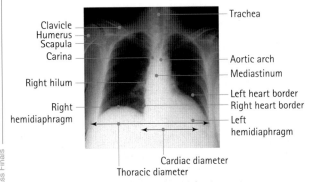

Fig. 5.1 The normal chest X-ray.

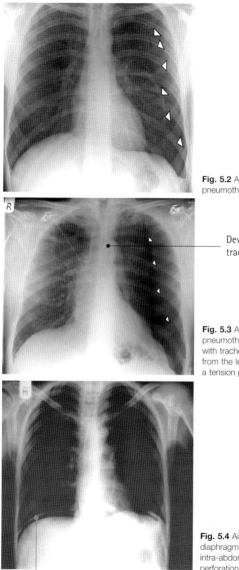

Fig. 5.2 A large left-sided pneumothorax is seen.

Deviated trachea

Fig. 5.3 A left-sided pneumothorax is visible, with tracheal shift away from the left, suggesting a tension pneumothorax.

Fig. 5.4 Air under the diaphragm indicates an intra-abdominal perforation.

Right hemidiaphragm (thin white line) with air (black shadow) beneath it

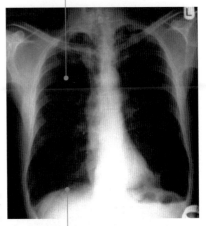

Dark hyperinflated lung fields

Fig. 5.5 Chronic obstructive pulmonary disease.

Flattened hemidiaphragm

Trachea
- Is the trachea deviated? Mediastinal shift
- Is the carina splayed? Right atrial enlargement

Hilar shadows
- Look for mass lesions

Diaphragm
- Flattening – over-expansion
- Calcification – asbestosis

Lung fields
- Look at lung markings
- Dark areas
  - Loss of vascular markings (PE, emphysema)
  - Hyperinflation (chronic obstructive pulmonary disease, COPD – Fig. 5.5)
- White shadows
  - Collapse (loss of air volume)
  - Consolidation (infection) (Figs 5.6–5.8)
  - Mass lesion
  - Fluid in pleural space – pleural effusion
  - Alveolar fluid – pulmonary oedema
  - Calcification
  - Check the lung apices – fibrosis suggests old tuberculosis

Cardiac shadow
- Look at heart size
  - PA film only
  - Normal <50% thoracic diameter
- Shape of cardiac outline

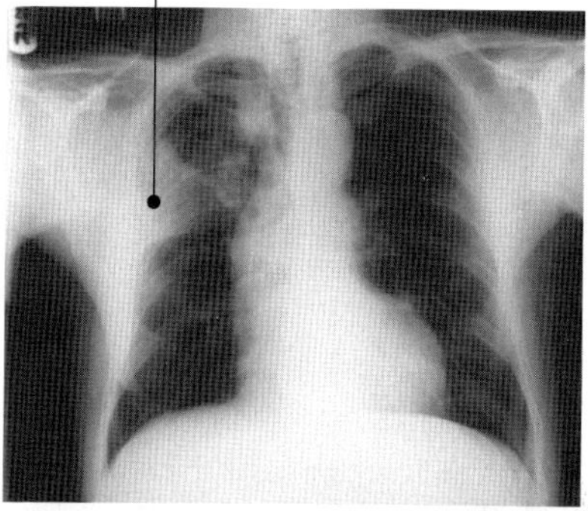

Collapsed right upper lobe

Fig. 5.6 Lobar collapse.

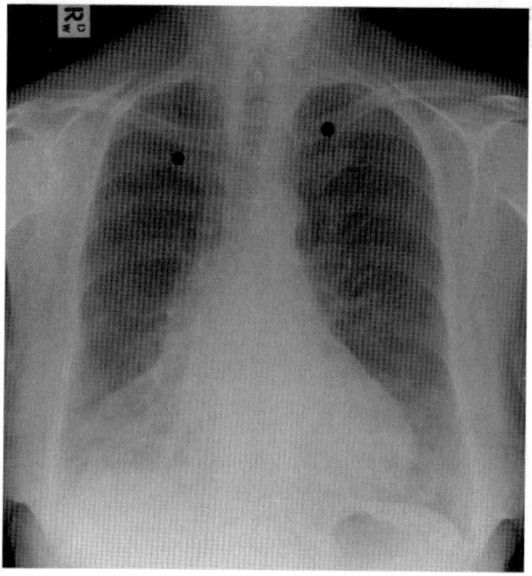

Fig. 5.7 There is shadowing adjacent to the right heart border suggesting a right middle lobe pneumonia.

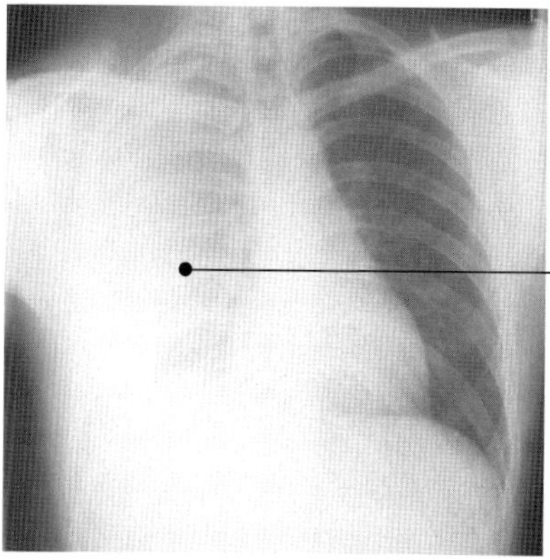

Right bronchopneumonia

Fig. 5.8 Right bronchopneumonia.

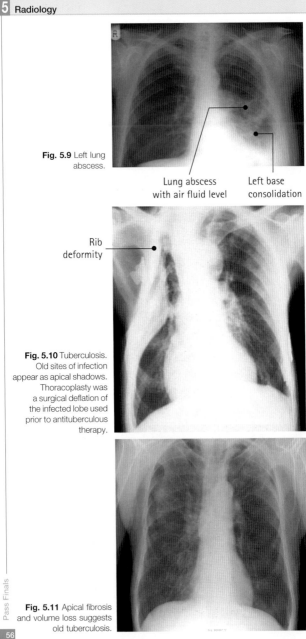

Fig. 5.9 Left lung abscess.

Lung abscess with air fluid level

Left base consolidation

Rib deformity

Fig. 5.10 Tuberculosis. Old sites of infection appear as apical shadows. Thoracoplasty was a surgical deflation of the infected lobe used prior to antituberculous therapy.

Fig. 5.11 Apical fibrosis and volume loss suggests old tuberculosis.

- Presence of mechanical valves
- Double right heart shadow – enlarged right atrium

Bones
- Look for rib fractures
- Bone lesions, e.g. metastases

Infections

Lobar pneumonia (Figs 5.6, 5.7)
- White patches of consolidation in lung field
- Collapse of lobe → loss of lung volume → Local structures may be moved, e.g
  - Elevated hemidiaphragm
  - Reduced rib spacing
- Bronchopneumonia (Fig. 5.8)
- Diffuse shadowing across more than one lobe

Lung abscess (Fig. 5.9)
- Circular lesion with air fluid level

Tuberculosis (Figs 5.10, 5.11)
- Apical shadowing or discrete lesion
- May show calcification
- Chest wall deformity due to thoracoplasty (removal of ribs)

Miliary shadows (Fig. 5.12)
- Miliary (blood-spread) tuberculosis
- Old chickenpox pneumonia
- Metastatic cancer, typically:
  - Renal
  - Prostatic
  - Breast
  - Bone
  - GI tract
  - Cervix
  - Ovary

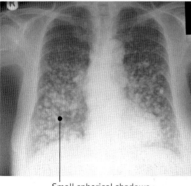

Small spherical shadows

Fig. 5.12 Miliary shadowing. This is classically seen after chickenpox pneumonia or miliary tuberculosis; however, it can also occur due to lung metastases.

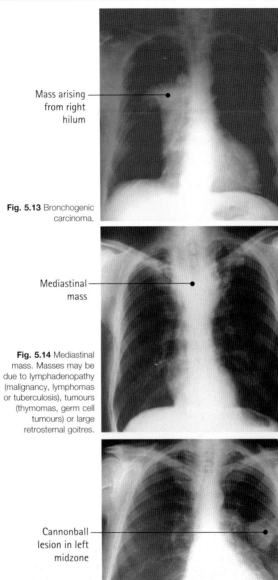

Mass arising from right hilum

Fig. 5.13 Bronchogenic carcinoma.

Mediastinal mass

Fig. 5.14 Mediastinal mass. Masses may be due to lymphadenopathy (malignancy, lymphomas or tuberculosis), tumours (thymomas, germ cell tumours) or large retrosternal goitres.

Cannonball lesion in left midzone

Fig. 5.15 A single pulmonary metastasis.

Neoplasms

Bronchogenic carcinoma (Fig. 5.13)
- Dense white shadows in lung field
- Mediastinal lymphadenopathy
- Hilar enlargement

Lymphoma (Fig. 5.14)
- Mediastinal masses

Metastases (Fig. 5.15)
- Cannonball lesions – discrete masses

Bony infiltration (Figs 5.16, 5.17)
- Mottling or radiolucent areas in bones

Cardiac lesions

Mechanical valves
- Visible metal valve ring or cage

Cardiac surgery (Fig. 5.18)
- Midline sternotomy wires

Mottled shadowing of humerus

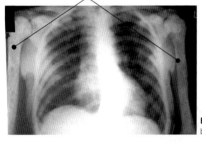

Fig. 5.16 Bony infiltration by tumour.

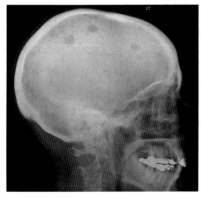

Fig. 5.17 Multiple lucent lesions in the skull suggestive of myeloma lytic lesions.

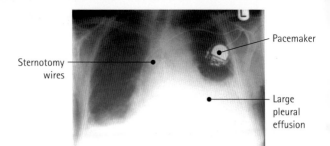

Fig. 5.18 Sternotomy wires from a previous coronary artery bypass graft are clearly visible. A large left pleural effusion can also be seen.

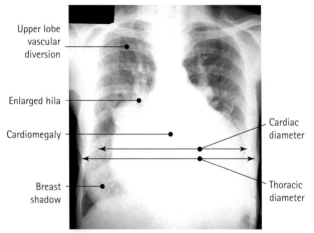

Fig. 5.19 Pulmonary oedema. The heart is enlarged, and the vascular engorgement is visible as increased upper zone vascular markings. The hila are also engorged.

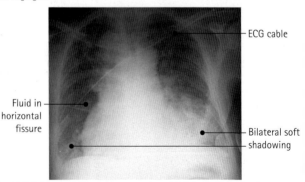

Fig. 5.20 Pulmonary oedema. There are bilateral fluffy basal shadows and fluid in the horizontal fissure.

Enlarged heart (Fig. 5.19)
- Cardiothoracic ratio >50% (PA film)
- Loss of atrial appendage shadow
- Atrial enlargement
  - Splayed carina
  - Double right heart border

Abnormal cardiac outline
- Boot-shaped heart – tetralogy of Fallot
- Globular heart – pericardial effusion

Pulmonary oedema (Figs 5.19, 5.20)
- Fluid in the horizontal fissure
- Kerley B lines (interstitial oedema)
- Upper lobe pulmonary vascular filling
- Peribronchiolar cuffing
- Enlarged heart
- Pleural effusions

Thoracic aortic aneurysm (Fig. 5.21)
- Dilated aortic arch

Pleural effusions

- Loss of costophrenic angle
- Dense white shadow with no lung markings

Unilateral (Fig. 5.22)
- Pneumonia
- Malignancy
- Pulmonary embolus
- Cardiac failure

Bilateral
- Cardiac failure
- Vasculitis, e.g. rheumatoid arthritis
- Hypoalbuminaemia

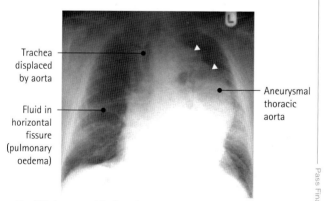

Trachea displaced by aorta

Fluid in horizontal fissure (pulmonary oedema)

Aneurysmal thoracic aorta

Fig. 5.21 Aneurysm of the thoracic aorta.

Fluid in
horizontal
fissure

Fluid in
pleural
space

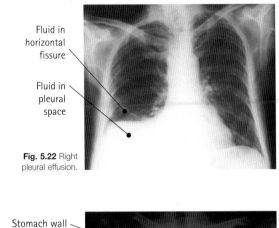

Fig. 5.22 Right
pleural effusion.

Stomach wall

Air fluid level

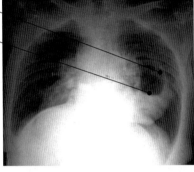

Fig. 5.23 Large hiatus
hernia. A hiatus hernia
may be seen as a hollow
viscus with an air fluid
level behind or to the left
of the heart.

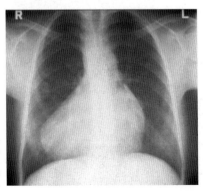

Fig. 5.24 Dextrocardia.
A right-sided cardiac
shadow, sometimes as
part of situs inversus.
Always check the side
markers on an X-ray.

Miscellaneous

Hiatus hernia (Fig. 5.23)
- Air fluid level in a viscus visible behind or left of the heart shadow

Dextrocardia (Fig. 5.24)
- A right-sided heart shadow may represent true dextrocardia or incorrectly placed side markers

THE PLAIN ABDOMINAL X-RAY (FIG. 5.25)

Order of analysis

Introduction
- Patient's name, age, date of X-ray
- Erect or supine

Bones
- Thoracic and lumbar spine

Gas shadows
- Gastric shadow – under left hemidiaphragm
- Small bowel loops – fold lines extend across the full width of the bowel
- Colonic shadow – haustral pattern does not extend across the full width of bowel

Organ shadows
- Liver (right upper quadrant)
- Gallbladder (if calcified gallstones present)
- Kidneys (and presence of calcification)
- Pancreatic calcification (chronic pancreatitis)

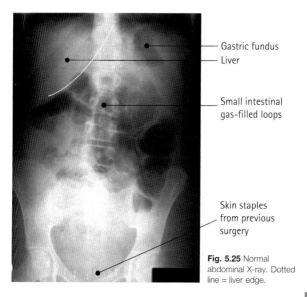

Gastric fundus
Liver

Small intestinal gas-filled loops

Skin staples from previous surgery

Fig. 5.25 Normal abdominal X-ray. Dotted line = liver edge.

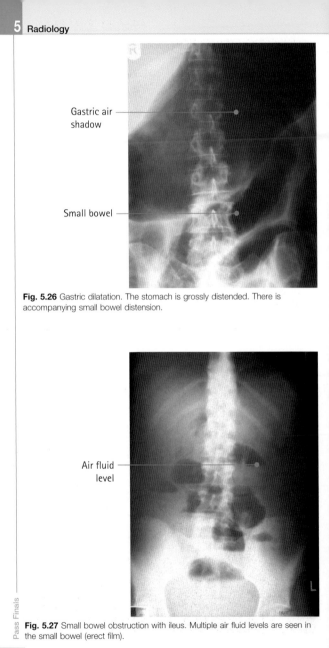

Gastric air
shadow

Small bowel

Fig. 5.26 Gastric dilatation. The stomach is grossly distended. There is accompanying small bowel distension.

Air fluid
level

Fig. 5.27 Small bowel obstruction with ileus. Multiple air fluid levels are seen in the small bowel (erect film).

Gastrointestinal abnormalities

Stomach
- Dilated stomach (Fig. 5.26)
  - Ileus
  - Pyloric stenosis
  - Diabetic gastroparesis

Small intestine
- Obstruction
  - Multiple air fluid levels (Fig. 5.27)
  - Dilatation (Fig. 5.28)
- Inflammation – separated bowel loops (due to thickened bowel wall)

Colon (Figs 5.29–5.32)
- Faeces – speckled appearance
- Toxic megacolon – dilated colon
- Volvulus – sigmoid dilatation (coffee bean sign)
- Colitis
  - Featureless colon
  - Ulceration
  - Mucosal islands

Liver
- Enlargement
- Gallstones
- Ascites – diffuse ground glass appearance

Pancreas
- Speckled calcification (chronic pancreatitis)

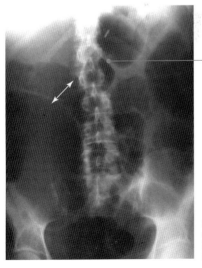

Small bowel, with folds extending across width of bowel

Fig. 5.28 Bowel distension due to obstruction. The loops are markedly dilated (arrow).

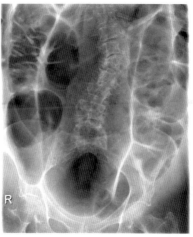

Fig. 5.29 The typical coffee bean shape shadow of a sigmoid volvulus on a plain film.

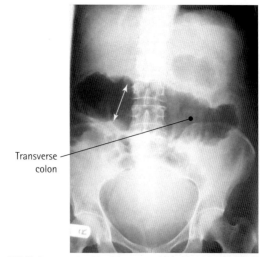

Transverse colon

Fig. 5.30 Toxic megacolon. The transverse colon is dilated (arrow). Classically, the transverse colon is the site of the dilatation. This is a medical emergency as there is a high risk of perforation and peritonitis.

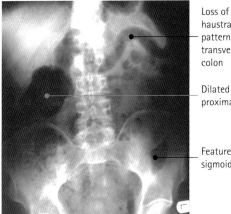

Loss of haustral pattern in transverse colon

Dilated proximal colon

Featureless sigmoid colon

Fig. 5.31 Ulcerative colitis. The colon is smooth and featureless.

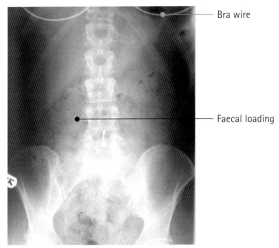

Bra wire

Faecal loading

Fig. 5.32 Constipation. Faeces appear as a speckled pattern in the colon.

Urinary tract

Kidneys (Fig. 5.33)
- Calcification
- Staghorn calculi
- Stone in ureter

Bladder
- Stones
- Urinary catheter

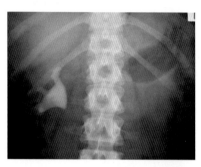

Fig. 5.33 Staghorn renal calculus.

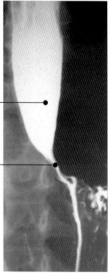

Dilated oesophagus

Narrowed lower oesophageal sphincter

Fig. 5.34 Achalasia. This barium swallow shows the classical rat's tail appearance of the distal oesophagus in achalasia.

CONTRAST STUDIES

Contrast (oral or rectal barium or intravenous water-soluble contrast) is used to define specific organs radiologically

Barium studies

Barium swallow
- Visualizes the pharynx and oesophagus
- Achalasia
  - Rat's tail appearance of narrowed lower oesophageal stricture (Fig. 5.34)
  - Dilated oesophagus, often with food debris
- Strictures
  - Benign – short and smooth
  - Malignant – long and ragged (Fig. 5.35)

Barium meal (rarely done now – gastroscopy has replaced)
- Visualizes the stomach and duodenum
- Ulcer – discrete collections of barium
- Cancers – filling defects

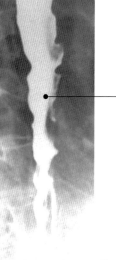

— Long irregular maligant stricture

Fig. 5.35 Barium swallow showing a malignant oesophageal stricture.

Barium follow-through (Fig. 5.36)
- Visualizes small bowel
- Strictures ⎫
- Inflammation ⎬ Crohn's disease
- Tumours ⎭
- Diverticulae – Meckel's diverticulum

Barium enema (Figs 5.37–5.39) (rarely done now – colonoscopy has replaced)
- Visualizes colon
- Malignancy – apple-core lesions
- Diverticular disease
- Inflammatory colitis
- Polyps

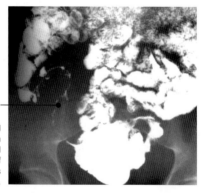

Stricture ——

Fig. 5.36 Barium meal and follow-through showing a terminal ileal stricture (the string sign of Kantor) in Crohn's disease.

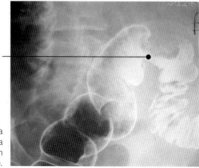

Stricture ——

Fig. 5.37 Barium enema of a colonic carcinoma demonstrating an 'apple-core' stricture.

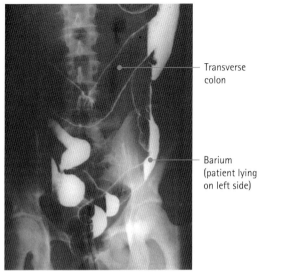

Transverse
colon

Barium
(patient lying
on left side)

Fig. 5.38 Barium enema in ulcerative colitis. The colon is featureless with a loss of the normal haustral pattern.

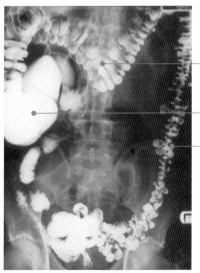

Normal
transverse
colon

Caecum

Diverticulae
with stricturing
in ascending
colon

Fig. 5.39 Diverticular disease on a barium enema.

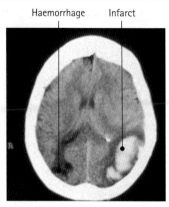

Fig. 5.40 Ischaemic and haemorrhagic stroke. Fresh blood appears white; infarcts appear dark.

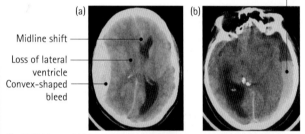

Fig. 5.41 Intracranial bleeds. (a) Extradural haematoma. (b) Subdural haematoma.

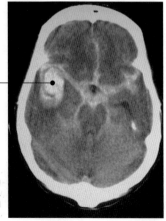

Fig. 5.42 Subarachnoid haemorrhage. Fresh blood appears white and is seen in the cortex and fissures.

COMPUTED AXIAL TOMOGRAPHY (CT)

Computerized axial tomography (CT or CAT scans) utilize computer-generated images captured using an array of X-ray beams. They have a high radiation dose. Intravenous contrast can be given to enhance vascular lesions. Oral contrast can be given to enhance the bowel

CT scans of the head

Cerebrovascular accidents (Fig. 5.40)
- Ischaemic strokes may not be apparent for 48 hours; they appear as dark areas
- Haemorrhagic strokes appear as white areas

Intracranial bleeds (Figs 5.41, 5.42)
- Acutely blood appears white
- Extradural haemorrhages are biconvex
- Subdural haemorrhages are crescent-shaped
- Intracerebral bleeds are within the substance of the brain
- Subarachnoid bleeds appear as white areas in the ventricular system of the brain

Mass lesions (Fig. 5.43)
- Malignancies (primary or secondary)
- Local oedema appears black
- Look for midline shift

CT scans of the body (Figs 5.44–5.47)

CT scans of the body are useful for a very wide range of diseases. Staging of malignancy and location of occult malignancy are common uses. Variations in the scanning protocol allow for specific organs to be optimally imaged:
- CT pneumocolon for colonic cancer and polyps
- Pancreatic protocol for pancreatic tumours and pancreatitis
- CT KUB for urinary tract stones
- CT pulmonary angiogram for pulmonary embolus

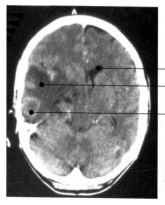

— Left lateral ventricle

— Oedema

— Enhancing mass

Fig. 5.43 Intracerebral mass lesion (contrast-enhanced CT of the head). There is an enhancing mass with surrounding oedema and obliteration of the right lateral ventricle with midline shift.

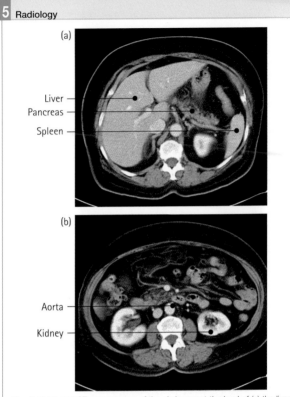

(a)

Liver
Pancreas
Spleen

(b)

Aorta
Kidney

Fig. 5.44 Normal CT appearances of the abdomen at the level of (a) the liver and (b) the kidneys.

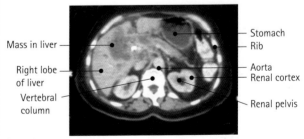

Mass in liver

Right lobe
of liver

Vertebral
column

Stomach
Rib

Aorta
Renal cortex

Renal pelvis

Fig. 5.45 CT of the abdomen. There is a mass lesion in the liver.

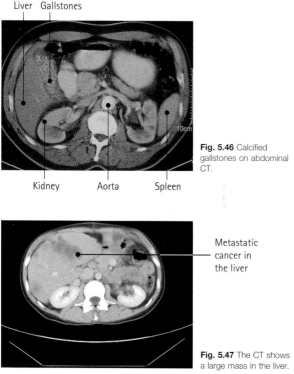

Liver Gallstones

Fig. 5.46 Calcified gallstones on abdominal CT.

Kidney Aorta Spleen

Metastatic cancer in the liver

Fig. 5.47 The CT shows a large mass in the liver.

ULTRASOUND

Ultrasound utilizes sound waves and their reflections in order to image structures. It is safe, quick and non-invasive. Boundaries between solids and fluids give strong signals, making ultrasound useful for identifying collections such as abscesses and pleural effusions

Liver, pancreas and biliary tree (Fig. 5.48)

- Mass lesions in the liver
- Stones in the biliary tree
- Fatty change
- Biliary obstruction
- Carcinoma of the pancreas

Renal ultrasound

- Renal masses
- Hydronephrosis
- Renal stones
- Congenital renal abnormalities

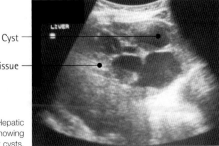

Cyst

Liver tissue

Fig. 5.48 Hepatic ultrasound showing liver cysts.

(a)

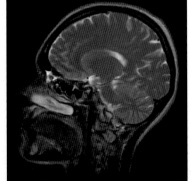

(b)

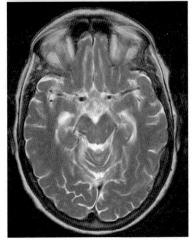

Fig. 5.49 (a) Saggital and (b) coronal sections through a normal brain on MRI.

Vascular tree

- Doppler ultrasound of leg veins for deep vein thrombosis
- Carotid Dopplers for stenosis in cerebrovascular disease

MAGNETIC RESONANCE IMAGING (MRI)

MRI provides high-resolution imaging of internal structures based on the water content of the tissue. It is useful for accurate localization of pathology and its relationship to surrounding structures, notably in the central nervous system.

- Head (Fig. 5.49) and spinal cord to look for neurological disease
- Bones and joints to look for orthopaedic problems
- Small bowel – has replaced barium follow through in many centres
- Pelvis to stage malignancies, e.g. rectum or gynae
- Liver – to characterize mass lesions
- MRCP – to examine the biliary tree

INTRAVENOUS CONTRAST STUDIES

Angiograms

- Outline vascular tree (Fig. 5.50)
- Coronary arteries for ischaemic heart disease
- Renal arteries for hypertension
- Cerebral arteries for subarachnoid haemorrhage

Digital subtraction angiography

- The digitized image prior to contrast is electronically subtracted from that with contrast, leaving just the contrast-outlined vascular bed
- Removes any overlying anatomical features

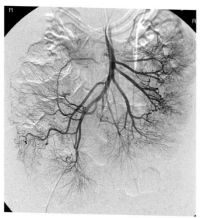

Fig. 5.50 Normal mesenteric angiogram.

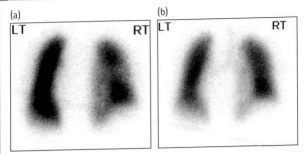

(a)   (b)

LT   RT   LT   RT

Fig. 5.51 A V̇/Q̇ scan. The perfusion scan (a) shows a left mid-zone defect not seen on the ventilation scan (b), suggesting a pulmonary embolus.

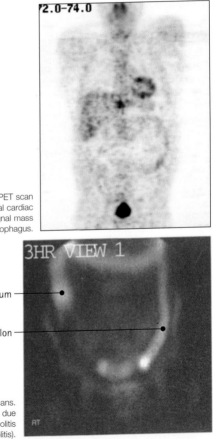

`2.0-74.0`

Fig. 5.52 A PET scan demonstrating normal cardiac activity and a high signal mass in the lower oesophagus.

3HR VIEW 1

Caecum —

Sigmoid colon —

RT

Fig. 5.53 White cell scans. The colon is outlined due to an acute pancolitis (ulcerative colitis).

Urograms

- Intravenous contrast excreted by kidneys
- Outlines the collecting ducts, renal pelvis, ureters and bladder
- Detects:
  - Non-functioning kidney
  - Hydronephrosis
  - Tumours
  - Calculi

NUCLEAR MEDICINE

Isotopes can be detected with photosensitive films or a gamma camera. The isotope is incorporated into a molecule designed to be picked up by a specific organ or excreted by the liver or kidney. Alternatively, blood cells can be labelled.

V/Q scans (Fig. 5.51)

- Ventilation and perfusion scans of lung fields
- A well ventilated area with no perfusion suggests a pulmonary embolus

PET (Fig. 5.52)

- Positron emission tomography
- Utilizes labelled glucose to identify tissues with a high metabolic rate
- Used in cancer detection and stage assessment

Red cell scan

- The patient's erythrocytes are labelled and re-injected
- May detect a site of occult blood loss

White cell scan (Fig. 5.53)

- Labelled leucocytes are injected
- Localize at site of infection or inflammation, e.g. abscesses

Bone scan (Fig. 5.54)

- Shows sites of high bone turnover, e.g. bone metastases

Renal function scans

[^{99}Tc]DTPA scans
- Technetium diethylenetriaminepenta-acetic acid
- Measures glomerular filtration
- Each kidney measured separately

[^{99}Tc]DMSA scans
- Tc-labelled dimercaptosuccinic acid
- Measure renal tubular function

Captopril scans (Fig. 5.55)

- DTPA scan with captopril given
- May reveal renal artery stenosis
- Indicated by a delay in peak signal

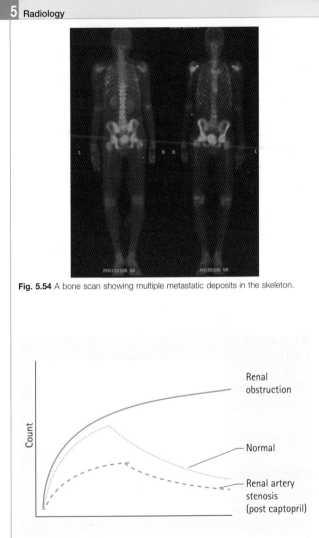

Fig. 5.54 A bone scan showing multiple metastatic deposits in the skeleton.

Fig. 5.55 Renal scintigraphy. The strength of signal over the kidney is measured. A normal kidney reaches a peak signal at 10–12 minutes. With an obstructed kidney the count reaches a plateau rather than reducing, as the technetium does not pass into the bladder. Renal artery stenosis results in a delay in reaching a signal peak, with a lower peak. This is most marked after captopril is given.

INTERVENTIONAL RADIOLOGY

Interventional radiology allows therapeutic and diagnostic procedures to be carried out without the need for general anaesthetic and in a less invasive way than surgery, although haemorrhage and perforation of a viscus or a blood vessel are important risks. Vascular procedures carry the risk of arterial spasm or occlusion and therefore tissue ischaemia.

Directed biopsy

- Masses can be biopsied under CT or ultrasound control rather than requiring an open procedure under general anaesthetic

Vascular procedures

- Angioplasty of arterial stenosis
- Insertion of filters to prevent embolism
- Insertion of coils into berry aneurysms to prevent subarachnoid haemorrhage

Biliary stenting

- Insertion of a stent to overcome obstruction of the biliary tree, e.g. in cholangiocarcinoma
- Percutaneous transhepatic cholangiography (PTCA)

Drain insertion

- Nephrostomies to relieve hydronephrosis
- Insertion of drains into abscesses

SELF-ASSESSMENT QUESTIONS

Multiple choice questions (true or false)

1. The following are accepted risks of CT-guided biopsy:
   A. Haemorrhage
   B. Secondary tumours along the path of the biopsy needle
   C. Radiation mucositis
   D. Intestinal perforation
   E. Abscess formation
2. The following are true of CT scans of the head:
   A. A CT scan carried out within 24 hours of an ischaemic stroke is often normal
   B. Fresh blood appears dark on an unenhanced CT scan
   C. Acoustic neuromas are seen as masses arising from the pituitary fossa
   D. Oedema around mass lesions appears black
   E. Intravenous contrast is useful in the diagnosis of intracerebral mass lesions

Multiple choice questions (single best answer)

3. A 32-year-old man was admitted with severe colicky abdominal and loin pain and haematuria. Which of the following would be the most useful diagnostic test?
   A. Plain abdominal X-ray
   B. Ultrasound of the abdomen
   C. CT KUB

D. MR cholangiogram

E. Barium follow-through

4. A 54-year-old woman with a long history of alcohol misuse was seen following a fall. She was drowsy and incoherent. Which one of the following would be most appropriate?

A. Plain skull X-ray

B. CT brain

C. Ultrasound of the portal vein

D. CT pancreas

E. Plain chest X-ray

5. A 76-year-old man was referred with deteriorating renal function on blood tests following the prescription of lisinopril. Which of the following would be most appropriate to confirm the diagnosis of renal artery stenosis?

A. CT KUB

B. Ultrasound of the renal tract

C. Captopril renogram

D. Renal angiogram

E. MRI both kidneys

6. A 16-year-old asthmatic man was admitted with worsening shortness of breath and chest pain. Which one of the following indicates a tension pneumothorax?

A. Visible pleural shadow

B. Loss of peripheral lung markings

C. Tracheal shift towards the affected lung

D. Tracheal shift away from the affected lung

E. Visible air-fluid level

7. A 43-year-old woman was admitted with abdominal pain and vomiting. An erect chest X-ray demonstrates air under both hemidiaphragms. Which one of the following may result in this sign?

A. Liver haematoma

B. Splenic rupture

C. Duodenal ulcer

D. Acute pancreatitis

E. Ectopic tubal pregnancy

8. A 76-year-old man is admitted with back pain and pain in his left thigh. He has had previous treatment for a renal cell carcinoma. Which of the following tests would be appropriate in his further investigation?

A. Plain X-rays of the thoracic and lumbar spine

B. Nucleotide bone scan

C. CT scan of the abdomen

D. Venogram of the left leg

E. MRI scan of the spine

Extended matching questions

Question 1 Theme: Radiology

A. Plain PA chest X-ray

B. Plain AP chest X-ray

C. Plain abdominal X-ray

D. Plain skull X-ray

E. CT head

F. High resolution CT scan of the chest

G. CT pulmonary angiogram

H. CT abdomen
I. CT chest abdomen and pelvis
J. Whole body PET scan
K. Ultrasound of the upper abdomen

For each of the following questions, select the best answer from the list above:

I. Which investigation would give the most accurate assessment of cardiac size?
II. Which investigation is most useful in assessing the stage of an oesophageal tumour?
III. Which investigation is most useful to determine the nature of liver cysts?
IV. Which investigation is most useful to detect multiple myeloma?

Clinical chemistry 6

Throughout this chapter, the following simple abbreviations will be used:
- Sodium – Na^+
- Potassium – K^+

FLUID AND ELECTROLYTE BALANCE

Water – Total body water

- 50–60% of lean body weight ♂
- 45–50% of lean body weight ♀
- In a 70 kg male total body water is 42 litres
  - 28 litres intracellular
  - 9.4 litres interstitial
  - 4.6 litres plasma

Distribution of water

- Osmotic pressure is the primary determinant of water distribution between compartments
- In each compartment the following are responsible for osmotic pressure
  - Intracellular compartment – K^+
  - Extracellular fluid compartment – Na^+
  - Vascular compartment – proteins

Distribution of 1 litre of standard intravenous replacement fluids

- 5% glucose distributes equally across all three compartments
- 0.9% saline remains in the extracellular compartment
- Colloid stays in the vascular compartment

Normal fluid and electrolyte requirements

- Normal daily fluid requirement is 2–3 litres with 100 mmol Na^+ and 70 mmol K^+ which allows for urinary, faecal and insensible loss

Sodium content of standard intravenous replacement fluids

- 1 litre of 0.9% (physiological) saline contains 150 mmol Na^+
- 1 litre of 5% glucose contains no Na^+
- 1 litre of glucose saline contains 30 mmol Na^+

An example of a standard 24-hour fluid regime in a fasting patient

- 1 litre 0.9% saline
- +2 litres 5% glucose
- Each with 20 mmol KCl added
  All patients need assessment of volume status and recent electrolyte results before i.v. fluids can be safely prescribed.

When to decrease the above fluid regime

- Elderly patients – require less volume, particularly if in heart failure
- Acute kidney injury – replace fluids as the previous day's urine output + 500 mL (remember these patients are often hyperkalaemic and may not require KCl supplements)
- Heart failure – reduce the volume
- Drugs – can alter water and electrolyte excretion, e.g. ACE inhibitors induce K^+ retention

When to increase the above fluid regime

- Dehydration
- Shock
- Increased GI losses, diarrhoea, vomiting, NG aspiration – replace nasogastric losses with KCl supplemented 0.9% saline
- Increased insensible losses – fever/burns
- Pancreatitis
- Drugs – can alter water and electrolyte losses, e.g. diuretics increase Na^+ and water loss

Regulation of extracellular fluid volume (Fig. 6.1)

- Extracellular fluid volume is regulated by Na^+ excretion from the kidneys, which is dependent on the circulating blood volume
- Circulating volume is determined by neurohumoral mechanisms via
  - Volume receptors
  - Catecholamines
  - Atrial natriuretic peptide
  - Renin/angiotensin/aldosterone

Regulation of water homeostasis

- Water homeostasis is affected by thirst and the concentrating and diluting functions of the kidney via the effects of antidiuretic hormone (ADH)

Increased extracellular volume

Aetiology
- Heart failure
- Hypoalbuminaemia, e.g. nephrotic syndrome
- Cirrhosis
- Renal sodium retention
  - Acute nephritis
  - Chronic kidney disease
  - Oestrogens
  - Mineralocorticoids
  - NSAIDs

Clinical features
- Peripheral oedema
- Pulmonary oedema
- Pleural effusion
- Ascites
- Raised jugular venous pressure
- Raised blood pressure
- Third heart sound

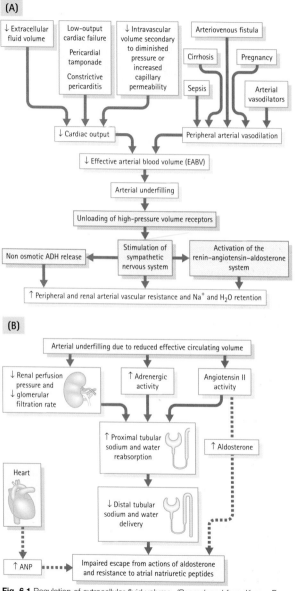

Fig. 6.1 Regulation of extracellular fluid volume. *(Reproduced from Kumar P, Clark M. Kumar and Clark's Clinical Medicine, 8th edn. Edinburgh: Elsevier; 2012, with permission from Elsevier.)*

Management
- Diuretics
- Treat underlying cause where possible

Decreased extracellular volume

Aetiology
- Haemorrhage
- Burns
  - Dehydration secondary to GI losses
  - Vomiting
  - Diarrhoea
  - Ileostomy
  - Ileus
- Renal losses
  - Polyuria
  - Diuretics
- Reduced renal tubular Na⁺ conservation
  - Reflux nephropathy
  - Papillary necrosis – NSAIDs, diabetes mellitus, sickle cell disease

Clinical features
- Postural hypotension – a fall in BP from lying to standing (normally the blood pressure rises on standing). May be due to reduced circulating volume, altered autonomic function or prolonged bed rest (Table 6.1)
- Low jugular venous pressure
- Peripheral vasoconstriction (cold skin and empty veins in the peripheries)
- Tachycardia
- Hypotension

Management
- Replacement of what is missing
  - Fluid/electrolytes lost (orally or intravenously)
  - Red cells
  - Plasma
- Treat underlying cause

Table 6.1 Causes of postural hypotension

Hypovolaemia
Autonomic failure
    Diabetes mellitus
    Shy–Drager syndrome
    Systemic amyloidosis
Drugs altering autonomic function
    Ganglion blockers
    Tricyclic antidepressants
Drugs altering peripheral vasoconstriction
    Nitrates
    Calcium channel blockers
    α-blockers
Prolonged bed rest

Sodium

- Disorders of Na^+ concentration are caused by disturbance of water balance
- In all disorders of Na^+ concentration, treatment should aim for slow changes in Na^+ concentrations to avoid precipitating cerebral oedema
- Plasma and urine osmolality are often useful measures to investigate the cause of altered sodium concentrations
- Plasma osmolality can be estimated as:
  $2[Na^+]+[urea]+[glucose]$

Hyponatraemia

- May be associated with euvolaemia, hypovolaemia or hypervolaemia

Hyponatraemia with normal extracellular volume (euvolaemia)

Aetiology
- Abnormal ADH release
  - Syndrome of inappropriate antidiuretic hormone (ADH) (see Ch. 13)
  - Adrenal insufficiency, e.g. Addison's disease
  - Hypothyroidism
  - Vagal neuropathy
  - Stress
  - Osmotically active substances causing ADH release, e.g. glucose, mannitol, alcohol, sickle cell syndrome
- Psychiatric illness
  - Psychogenic polydipsia
  - Tricyclic antidepressants
- Drugs
  - Desmopressin
  - Tolbutamide/chlorpropamide

Clinical features
- Euvolaemia
- Signs of underlying cause

Management
- Treat underlying cause
- Sometimes water restriction

Salt-deficient hyponatraemia (hypovolaemic)

Aetiology
- GI losses
  - Vomiting
  - Diarrhoea
  - Haemorrhage
- Renal losses
  - Osmotic diuresis (e.g. hyperglycaemia)
  - Diuretics
  - Adrenocortical insufficiency
  - Tubulo-interstitial renal disease
  - Unilateral renal artery stenosis
  - Recovery phase of acute tubular necrosis

Clinical features
- Hypovolaemia (see above)

Management
- Replace lost fluid/electrolytes
- Treat underlying cause

Hyponatraemia due to water excess (hypervolaemic)

Aetiology
- Heart failure
- Liver failure
- Oliguric renal failure
- Hypoalbuminaemia
- Excess fluids (iatrogenic)

Clinical features
- Volume overload (see above)
- If severe, can cause drowsiness, convulsions and coma
- Signs of underlying disease

Management
- Fluid restriction
- Treat underlying cause

Pseudohyponatraemia

- Rarely hyperlipidaemia or hyperproteinaemia produces a spuriously low measured Na^+ concentration
- Plasma osmolality is normal

Hypernatraemia

- Hypernatraemia nearly always indicates water deficiency
- In normal individuals with an intact thirst axis and free access to water, hypernatraemia is rare
- Thirst is frequently deficient in elderly patients, which makes them more prone to hypernatraemia

Aetiology
- Inadequate water intake PLUS
- ADH deficiency
  - Diabetes insipidus
- Insensitivity to ADH (nephrogenic diabetes insipidus)
  - Drugs (e.g. lithium, tetracyclines, amphotericin B)
  - Acute tubular necrosis
- Osmotic diuresis
  - Hyperosmolar diabetic coma
  - Total parenteral nutrition

Clinical features
- Volume depletion (see above)
- Confusion/convulsions
- Fever
- Features of underlying cause

Investigations
- Plasma osmolality will be high
- A low urine osmolality indicates diabetes insipidus

Management
- Replace fluid
- Treat underlying cause (Table 6.2)

Potassium

Serum K$^+$ concentrations are determined by:
- Uptake of K$^+$ into cells (Fig. 6.2)
- Renal excretion (controlled by aldosterone)
- Extrarenal losses, e.g. gastrointestinal

Table 6.2 Average concentrations and potential daily losses of water and electrolytes from the gut

	Na$^+$ mmol/L	K$^+$ mmol/L	Cl$^-$ mmol/L	Volume (mL in 24 hours)
Stomach	50	10	110	2500
Small intestine Recent ileostomy	120	5	110	1500
Adapted ileostomy	50	4	25	500
Bile	140	5	105	500
Pancreatic juice	140	5	60	2000
Diarrhoea	130	10–30	95	1000–2000+

(Reproduced from Kumar P, Clark M. Kumar and Clark's Clinical Medicine, 8th edn. Edinburgh: Elsevier; 2012, with permission from Elsevier.)

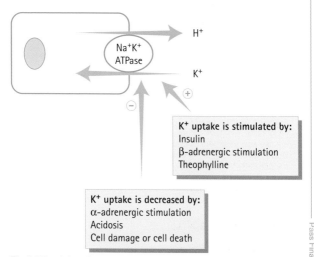

K$^+$ uptake is stimulated by:
Insulin
β-adrenergic stimulation
Theophylline

K$^+$ uptake is decreased by:
α-adrenergic stimulation
Acidosis
Cell damage or cell death

Fig. 6.2 Regulation of uptake of potassium into cells.

Hypokalaemia

Aetiology
See Table 6.3.

Clinical features
- If severe, muscle weakness
- Cardiac arrhythmias in abnormal hearts
- Potentiation of digoxin toxicity

Management
- Give supplements
- Potassium-sparing drugs
- Treat underlying cause

Table 6.3 Causes of hypokalaemia

Increased renal excretion
    Diuretics – thiazide and loop
Increased aldosterone secretion
    Liver failure
    Heart failure
    Nephrotic syndrome
    Cushing syndrome
    Conn syndrome
    Adrenocorticotropic hormone (ACTH) producing tumours
Exogenous mineralocorticoid
    Corticosteroids
    Carbenoxolone
    Liquorice
Renal disease
    Renal tubular acidosis types 1 and 2
    Renal tubular damage
    Acute leukaemia
    Cytotoxics
    Nephrotoxic drugs, e.g. gentamicin
    Release of urinary tract obstruction
Severe dietary deficiency
Redistribution into cells
    β-adrenergic stimulation
    Acute myocardial infarct
    β-agonists, e.g. salbutamol
    Insulin, e.g. treatment of diabetic ketoacidosis
    Correction of vitamin B_{12} deficiency
    Alkalosis
GI losses
    Vomiting
    Diarrhoea
    Purgative abuse
    Villous adenoma
    Ileostomy
    Fistulae
    Ileus/intestinal obstruction

Hyperkalaemia

Aetiology
See Table 6.3.

Clinical features
- Cardiac arrhythmias
- Hypotension/bradycardia if severe
- Kussmaul breathing (associated acidosis)
- Widened QRS/tented T waves on ECG

Management
- See page 352 (Box 14.2) for emergency treatment
- Calcium resonium – exchange resin given orally or rectally
- Dialysis
- Treat cause

Calcium

Disorders of calcium metabolism are discussed in Chapter 11 (p. 263)

Magnesium

- Serum magnesium concentrations are determined by uptake in the small bowel and renal excretion
- Disordered magnesium concentrations occur in association with other electrolyte imbalance

Hypomagnesaemia

Aetiology
See Table 6.4.

Clinical features
- Inability to correct hypokalaemia
- Irritability
- Tremor
- Ataxia
- Carpopedal spasm
- Hyperreflexia
- Confusion/hallucinations
- Convulsions
- ECG shows prolonged QT interval, flat T waves

Management
- Give supplements
- Treat underlying cause

Hypermagnesaemia

Aetiology
See Table 6.5.

Clinical features
- Lethargy
- Muscle weakness
- Hyporeflexia
- Narcosis
- Respiratory paralysis
- Cardiac conduction defects

Table 6.4 Causes of hyperkalaemia

Decreased excretion
    Renal failure
    Drugs
        Spironolactone
        Amiloride
        ACE inhibitors
        NSAIDs
        Ciclosporin
        Heparin
    Aldosterone deficiency
    Renal tubular acidosis type 4
    Addison's disease
    Increased release from cells
    Acidosis
    Diabetic ketoacidosis
    Rhabdomyolysis and tissue damage (surgery, burns)
    Tumour lysis
    Succinylcholine
    Digoxin poisoning
    Vigorous exercise
Increased extraneous load
    Potassium chloride administration
    Blood transfusion
Spurious
    Increased *in vitro* release (either from abnormal cells, e.g.
    leukaemia, or as a result of difficult phlebotomy, 'haemolysed
    sample')

Management
- Calcium gluconate, dextrose and insulin
- Dialysis
- Remove cause

Phosphate

- The regulation of phosphate concentrations is closely linked to that of calcium

Hypophosphataemia

Aetiology
See Table 6.6.

Clinical features
- Diaphragmatic muscle weakness
- Convulsions

Management
- If mild, rarely requires treatment
- If severe, give i.v. replacement slowly

Table 6.5 Causes of hypo/hypermagnesaemia

Hypomagnesaemia
  Decreased magnesium absorption
    Malabsorption
    Malnutrition
    Alcohol excess
  Increased renal excretion
    Drugs
      Diuretics – loop and thiazide
      Digoxin
    Diabetic ketoacidosis
    Bartter syndrome
    Alcohol excess
    Hypercalciuria
    Drug toxicity
      Amphotericin
      Aminoglycosides
      Cisplatin
      Ciclosporin
  GI losses
    Prolonged nasogastric suction
    Excessive purgatives
    GI/biliary fistulae
    Severe diarrhoea
    Acute pancreatitis
Hypermagnesaemia
  Impaired renal excretion
    Chronic kidney disease
    Acute kidney injury
  Increased magnesium intake
    Purgatives
    Antacids

Hyperphosphataemia

Aetiology
See Table 6.6.
- Common in patients with chronic kidney disease

Management
- If acute, rarely requires treatment
- If chronic, give gut phosphate binders or dialyse

ACID–BASE DISORDERS

Acid–base balance is tightly buffered. The bicarbonate–carbonic acid buffer pair is the most clinically relevant due to variability of excretion of CO_2 by the lungs and bicarbonate and hydrogen ions by the kidneys

$$H^+ + HCO_3^- \leftrightarrow H_2CO_3 \xleftrightarrow{\text{Carbonic anhydrase}} CO_2 + H_2O$$

Table 6.6 Causes of hypo/hyperphosphataemia

Hypophosphataemia
  Redistribution
    Respiratory alkalosis
    Treatment of diabetic ketoacidosis
    Carbohydrate administration after starvation (re-feeding syndrome)
    Post-parathyroidectomy
  Renal losses
    Hyperparathyroidism, renal tubular defects, diuretics
  Decreased intake/absorption
    Dietary
    Malabsorption
    Vomiting
    Gut phosphate binders, e.g. aluminium hydroxide
    Vitamin D deficiency
    Alcohol withdrawal
Hyperphosphataemia
  Chronic kidney disease
  Tumour lysis
  Rhabdomyolysis
  Old blood sample

- Acid–base disturbance may be caused by:
  - Abnormal carbon dioxide removal in the lungs (respiratory alkalosis/acidosis)
  - Abnormalities of the regulation of bicarbonate and other buffers in the blood (metabolic alkalosis/acidosis)
- Arterial blood gas analysis provides information on:
  - pH
  - Bicarbonate concentrations
  - Partial pressures of oxygen and carbon dioxide

Respiratory acidosis

- Caused by retention of carbon dioxide
- Renal retention of bicarbonate may partly compensate (see Ch. 8)

Respiratory alkalosis

- Caused by increased removal of carbon dioxide as a result of hyperventilation (see Ch. 8)

Metabolic acidosis

- Caused by accumulation of acid
- Demonstrated by a fall in plasma bicarbonate
- Arises from:
  - Acid administration
  - Acid generation
  - Impaired acid excretion by kidneys
  - Bicarbonate losses from GI tract

- Anion gap (unmeasured anions) helps differentiate the causes
  Anion gap $= ([Na^+] + [K^+]) - ([HCO_3^-] + [Cl^-])$
- Normal anion gap $= 10–18 \text{ mmol/L}^{-1}$
- Note that albumin is a major unmeasured anion; a fall in albumin will reduce the anion gap

Metabolic acidosis with a normal anion gap

- Suggests that either hydrochloric acid is being generated or bicarbonate is being lost
- In all cases plasma bicarbonate is low and plasma chloride high

Aetiology

- Increased GI bicarbonate losses
  - Diarrhoea
  - Ileostomy
- Increased renal bicarbonate losses
  - Acetozolamide
  - Proximal (type 2) renal tubular acidosis
  - Hyperparathyroidism
  - Renal tubular damage – heavy metal poisoning, paraproteins, drugs
- Decreased renal hydrogen ion losses
  - Distal (type 1) renal tubular acidosis
  - Type 4 renal tubular acidosis

Metabolic acidosis with a high anion gap

- Suggests presence of unmeasured endogenous or exogenous anions

Aetiology

- Renal failure
- Lactic acidosis
- Ketoacidosis
- Exogenous acid such as salicylate (aspirin)

Metabolic alkalosis

- Causes
  - Chloride depletion – gastric losses, diuretics, diarrhoea, cystic fibrosis
  - Potassium depletion – mineralocorticoid excess, Conn syndrome, thiazide/loop diuretics
  - Exogenous alkalis, e.g. antacids plus one of the above

CARDIAC MARKERS

Biochemical markers of myocyte death can be used to stratify risk in acute coronary syndromes.

Cardiac troponin (troponin T and I)

Cardiac microfilament proteins which are sensitive markers for cardiac injury

- Not detectable in normal people
- Released early (2–4 hours) after injury and persist for up to 7 days
- If negative then repeat 9–12 hours after admission
- When elevated in patients presenting with chest pain can be very useful for determining prognosis

Creatine kinase (CK)

Sources
- Heart, skeletal muscle and brain (MM/MB/BB isoforms)

Raised in
- Myocardial infarction
- Muscle dystrophies
- Polymyositis
- Pulmonary embolus
- Postoperative period
- Myocarditis
- Muscle trauma, e.g. fits, injections, exercise

Aspartate aminotransferase (AST)

Sources
- Heart, liver, muscle and kidney

Raised in
- Myocardial infarction
- Liver disease (hepatitis of any cause)
- Haemolytic anaemia
- Muscle trauma, e.g. fits, injections, exercise

Lowered in
- Renal failure

Lactate dehydrogenase (LDH)

Sources
- All cells release LDH when damaged

Raised in
- Myocardial infarction
- Tissue necrosis of any cause
- Liver disease
- Kidney disease
- Haematological diseases, e.g. lymphoma haemolysis
- Muscle trauma, e.g. fits, injections, exercise

LIVER BIOCHEMISTRY

Liver function tests in the blood can be divided into three groups. Note that in severe disease, the first two groups can both be elevated and that drugs can induce liver enzymes (see Ch. 4)

- Tests suggesting *bile duct obstruction (intra- or extra-hepatic)*
  - Bilirubin
  - Alkaline phosphatase
  - γ-glutamyltranspeptidase
- Tests suggesting *disease of hepatocytes*
  - Aminotransferases ALT and AST
- Tests of liver *synthetic function*
  - Albumin
  - Prothrombin time

Further information is given in Chapter 10.

Bilirubin

Sources
- Mainly haemoglobin destruction

Raised in
- Bile duct obstruction of any cause
- Hepatitis of any cause
- Haemolytic anaemia
- Gilbert syndrome

Alkaline phosphatase

Sources
- Bile ducts, bone and placenta
- If source is the liver:
  - γ-glutamyl transpeptidase is elevated
- If source is bone:
  - γ-glutamyl transpeptidase is not elevated
  - Calcium/phosphate may be abnormal

Raised in
- Bile duct obstruction of any cause
- Liver malignancy/space-occupying lesion
- Bony metastases
- Hepatitis of any cause
- Osteomalacia
- Paget's disease of bone
- Haematological malignancy, e.g. lymphoma
- Heart failure (liver congestion)
- Also normally higher in children and pregnancy

Lowered in
- Hypothyroidism

Gamma glutamyl transpeptidase (γ-GT)

Sources
- Bile ducts and kidney

Raised in
- Alcohol excess
- Bile duct obstruction of any cause including malignancy/space-occupying lesion
- Hepatitis of any cause if severe
- Renal carcinoma
- Induction by drugs

Alanine aminotransferase (ALT)

Sources
- Liver and heart

Raised in
- Hepatitis of any cause
- Bile duct obstruction of any cause

TESTS OF RENAL FUNCTION

Urea and creatinine are dependent on glomerular filtration rate (GFR). They do not rise above normal range until GFR is reduced by 50–60%

Urea

- Plasma urea varies with protein intake, tissue catabolism and renal excretion

Raised in
- Renal disease of any cause
- Dehydration
- Upper GI bleeding
- Shock – infection, trauma (increased catabolism)
- Cardiac failure

Lowered in
- Liver failure
- Starvation, low protein diet
- Pregnancy
- Overhydration

Creatinine (and eGFR)

Levels alter with age, gender and muscle mass
- Retention of creatinine indicates glomerular insufficiency

Raised in
- Renal disease of any cause
- Old age

Lowered in
- Muscle-wasting
- Pregnancy

Urate

- End-product of protein metabolism
- Excreted by kidneys

Raised in
- Gout
- Eclampsia
- Leukaemia/myeloma/lymphoma
- Renal insufficiency
- Thiazide diuretic therapy

Lowered in
- Allopurinol therapy
- Acute hepatitis of any cause
- Salicylate therapy

ACUTE PHASE REACTANTS

- Nonspecific tests for inflammation/infection
- Include:
  - Erythrocyte sedimentation rate (ESR)
  - C-reactive protein (CRP)

SELF-ASSESSMENT QUESTIONS

Multiple choice questions (single best answer)

1. Persistent vomiting may result in:
   A. Respiratory acidosis
   B. Peripheral oedema
   C. Metabolic acidosis
   D. Hypokalaemia
   E. Hypercalcaemia
2. Hyperkalaemia may be a result of the use of which of the following diuretics:
   A. Furosemide
   B. Bendroflumethiazide
   C. Spironolactone
   D. Metolazone
   E. Bumetanide
3. Which of the following statements are correct for standard i.v. fluid solutions:
   A. 0.9% saline distributes to all three fluid compartments
   B. 5% dextrose remains in the vascular compartment
   C. Colloid is used in hypovolaemia
   D. 0.9% saline is indicated in most cases of hyponatraemia
   E. Hypertonic saline from 0.9% is useful i.v. fluid replacement therapy in patients with chronic liver disease
4. Which of these is a cause of a metabolic acidosis with a normal anion gap:
   A. Sepsis
   B. Diabetic ketoacidosis
   C. Aspirin overdose
   D. Acute kidney injury
   E. Type 4 renal tubular acidosis
5. Which of these is a cause of a metabolic acidosis with a high anion gap:
   A. Diabetic ketoacidosis
   B. Type 4 renal tubular acidosis
   C. Diarrhoea
   D. Lead poisoning
   E. Hyperparathyroidism
6. In which of the following situations is the pH likely to be lower than normal:
   A. Vomiting
   B. Hypokalaemia
   C. Conn syndrome
   D. Hyperventilating
   E. Hyperparathyroidism
7. An elevated troponin I occurs in the following circumstance:
   A. 12 hours after the onset of pain in an acute coronary syndrome
   B. Day 2 after hip replacement
   C. Following a tonic-clonic seizure
   D. Heart failure
   E. Rhabdomyolysis
8. Serum bilirubin would be normal in patients with:
   A. Gilbert syndrome
   B. A gallstone obstructing the common bile duct

C. Gallstones in the gallbladder

D. Autoimmune haemolytic anaemia

E. Acute fulminant hepatitis A

9. A low blood urea would be expected in:

A. Pregnancy

B. Upper GI bleeding

C. Cardiac failure

D. Acute kidney injury

E. Dehydration

Extended matching questions

Question 1 Theme: Abnormal blood test results

A. Shock

B. Cardiac failure

C. Cardiac failure treated with loop diuretics

D. Pneumonia

E. Renal failure

F. Nephrotic syndrome

G. Renal tubular acidosis

H. Diarrhoea

I. High ileostomy volumes

For each of the following questions, select the best answer from the list above:

I. An 84-year-old female presents with confusion and ankle oedema. Blood results show the following: Na^+ 132, K^+ 2.8, Urea 9.8, Creat 128. What is the most likely diagnosis?

II. A 37-year-old patient with Crohn's disease presents with malaise. Blood tests reveal the following: Na^+ 132, K^+ 2.8, Urea 10, Creat 60, Mg^{2+} 0.54 (low), Cl^- 105, pH 7.3, Bicarbonate 15. What is the most likely diagnosis?

III. A 56-year-old male presents with fever and malaise. Blood tests reveal the following: Na^+ 124, K^+ 4.5, Urea 7.6, Creat 98, pH 7.54, PO_2 8.2, PCO_2 3.2. What is the most likely diagnosis?

Question 2 Theme: Acid-base disturbance

A. Acute kidney injury

B. Acute liver failure

C. Aspirin overdose

D. Recurrent vomiting

E. Renal tubular acidosis

F. Diabetic ketoacidosis

G. Respiratory alkalosis

H. Type II respiratory failure

For each of the following questions, select the best answer from the list above:

I. A 64-year-old female presents with confusion and breathlessness. Blood gas analysis shows the following: pH 7.3, PCO_2 9.6, PO_2 4.5, Bicarbonate 28. What is the most likely diagnosis?

II. A 37-year-old patient with diabetes presents with a history of vomiting and confusion. Blood gas analysis shows the following: pH 7.15, PCO_2 2.5, PO_2 12.5, Bicarbonate 10. What is the most likely diagnosis?

III. An 18-year-old male is found collapsed at home. There is no history available. Blood tests reveal the following: pH 7.25, PCO_2 3.6, PO_2 13.5, Bicarbonate 8, Na^+ 135, K^+ 4, Cl^- 101. What is the most likely diagnosis?

Question 3 Theme: Abnormal blood test results

A. Acute coronary syndrome
B. Cardiac failure
C. Polymyositis
D. Hodgkin's lymphoma
E. Haemolytic anaemia
F. Nephrotic syndrome
G. Renal tubular acidosis

For each of the following questions, select the best answer from the list above:

I. A 74-year-old man presents with chest pains which he has had for 48 hours. Blood results show elevation of CK, AST and troponin I. What is the most likely diagnosis?

II. A 37-year-old patient presents with malaise. He has noticed a lump in his neck ever since he had an upper respiratory tract infection 2 weeks ago. Blood tests reveal the following: Haemoglobin 123 g/L, CK 70 U/L, LDH 637 U/L, troponin I not detected. What is the most likely diagnosis?

III. A 21-year-old male student presents with yellowness of the skin. He has recently been diagnosed with glandular fever. Blood tests reveal the following: Bilirubin 95 μmol, ALT 24 U/L, AST 31 U/L, haemoglobin 89 g/L. What is the most likely diagnosis?

Infectious diseases 7

Infectious disease remains the most common cause of morbidity and mortality worldwide. In order for an infectious agent to propagate within the population, there must be a reservoir of infection and a mode of transmission. Thus, avoidance of infection starts with reduction of the reservoir and limiting or avoiding the transmission of an organism.

System-specific infections are discussed in the appropriate chapters.

DIAGNOSIS OF INFECTIOUS DISEASE

History

- Exposure to the causative agent
- Travel to a high-risk area or environmental exposure
- Contact with an infected individual
- Occupation and leisure activity history
- Animal exposure
- Sexual history
- Parenteral drug use
- Blood transfusion
- Vaccination history

Examination

- Presence of a fever (Table 7.1)
- Rashes
- Lymphadenopathy
- Hepatosplenomegaly
- Evidence of septic shock (hypotension, tachycardia, peripheral vasodilatation)
- Delirium (confusion, hallucination)

Investigations

Full blood count and blood film
- Neutrophilia suggests bacterial infection
- Lymphocytosis suggests viral infection
- Lymphopenia may suggest HIV infection
- Neutropenia may suggest viral infection
- Eosinophilia suggests parasitic infection

Thrombocytopenia
- Malaria or disseminated intravascular coagulation

Cell fragments – haemolysis
- Parasites on blood film, e.g. malaria

Blood culture
- Aerobic and anaerobic bottles
- Follow sterile procedure
- May require repeated samples

Table 7.1 Causes of fever (pyrexia) of unknown origin (F(P)UO)

Infections (20–40%)	Immune (15–20%)
Abscess	Drugs
Tuberculosis	Autoimmune rheumatic disease
Urinary infection	Sarcoidosis
Biliary infection	Other (10–25%)
Endocarditis	Thyrotoxicosis
Epstein–Barr or	Ulcerative colitis
cytomegalovirus	Crohn's disease
Toxoplasmosis/Brucellosis/	Familial Mediterranean Fever
Lyme disease	Factitious
Primary HIV infection	5–25% remain undiagnosed
Malignancy (10–30%)	
Lymphomas	
Leukaemia	
Solid tumours, e.g. renal cell,	
hepatocellular	

Liver function
- Elevated transferases liver enzymes in viral hepatitis

Microscopy, culture and sensitivity
- Can be performed on stool, urine, CSF, sputum, ascitic fluid, pleural fluid, joint aspirates
- Provides organism identification and antibiotic sensitivity

Immunological diagnosis
- Presence of antibodies against specific antigens
- Presence of specific antigens due to their reaction with a known antibody

Genetic diagnosis
- Detection of genome of organism, e.g. hepatitis C virus RNA
- Assessment of 'viral load' or replication, e.g. HIV, Hepatitis B

Histological examination
- Pathology of specific infections on tissue biopsy

Imaging
- Localization of an infection, e.g. by ultrasound or CT scanning
- Labelled white cell scanning localizes the source of an infection

TREATMENT OF INFECTIOUS DISEASE

Antibacterial drugs (Fig. 7.1)

β-lactams

Penicillins
- Block cell wall growth
- Group 1: parenteral formulations
  - e.g. Benzylpenicillin
- Group 2: oral penicillin
  - e.g. Phenoxymethylpenicillin (penicillin V)
- Group 3: β-lactamase-stable penicillins
  - e.g. Flucloxacillin

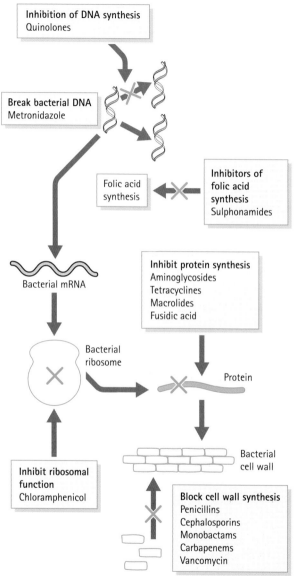

Fig. 7.1 Mechanism of action of antibacterial drugs.

- Group 4: extended spectrum
  - e.g. Amoxicillin, ampicillin
- Group 5: β-lactamase-resistant penicillin
  - e.g. Temocillin

Cephalosporins
- Inhibit cell wall synthesis
- Penicillinase-resistant
- Broader antibacterial range
- 10% of patients with penicillin allergy will have a reaction to cephalosporins

First generation
- Gram-positive cocci and Gram-negative
  - Cefalexin, cefradrine

Second generation
- Gram-negative infections
  - Cefuroxime, cefaclor

Third generation
- Gram-negative infections
  - Ceftazidime, ceftriaxone, doripenem, ertapenem

Fourth and fifth generation now available

Monobactams
- Aztreonam

Carbapenems
- Imipenem, meropenem, doripenem, ertapenem

Aminoglycosides
- Inhibit bacterial protein synthesis
- Gram negatives, e.g. *Pseudomonas*
- Gentamicin, neomycin
- *Note*: Renal and ototoxicity, therefore serum levels need monitoring

Tetracyclines
- Inhibit bacterial protein synthesis
- Atypical pneumonias, acne
- Tetracycline, doxycycline, tigecycline
- *Note*: Contraindicated in children and during pregnancy as they cause permanently stained teeth

Macrolides
- Inhibit bacterial protein synthesis
- Useful in atypical pneumonia
- Erythromycin, clarithromycin, azithromycin
- Gram-negative infection

Chloramphenicol
- Inhibits bacterial ribosome function
- Conjunctivitis (local therapy)

Fusidic acid
- Inhibits bacterial protein synthesis
- *Staphylococcus aureus* osteomyelitis

Sulphonamides
- Inhibit bacterial folic acid synthesis
- Used with trimethoprim in urinary tract and *Pneumocystis jiroveci* infection

Quinolones
- Inhibit DNA synthesis
- Gram-negative infections
- Ciprofloxacin, moxifloxacin

Nitroimidazoles
- Break bacterial DNA
- Anaerobic infections
- Metronidazole

Glycopeptides
- Inhibit cell wall synthesis
- Gram-positive bacteria
- Vancomycin, teicoplanin

Side-effects of antibacterials

- Sensitivity: rash/anaphylaxis
- Organism resistance, e.g. MRSA/VRE
- Disruption of normal gut flora → antibiotic related diarrhoea or pseudomembranous colitis

Antifungal drugs

Polyenes
- Disrupt fungal membranes
  - Amphotericin B – systemic disease
  - Nystatin – oral and enteric *Candida*

Azoles
- Broad-spectrum antifungals
  - Clotrimazole – ringworm
  - Ketoconazole – candidiasis

Triazoles
  - Fluconazole – penetrates CSF
  - Itraconazole

Others
  - Terbinafine
  - Griseofulvin
  - Echinocandins

Side-effects of antifungals

- Itraconazole – fulminant hepatic failure and hepatic dysfunction
- Heart failure – avoid prescribing with calcium channel blockers

Antiviral drugs

Aciclovir
- Terminates viral DNA synthesis
- *Herpes simplex* and *varicella zoster* virus

Ganciclovir
- Cytomegalovirus infection

Amantadine
- Influenza virus

Interferons
- Hepatitis B and C
- Pegylated formulations are more effective and require less frequent dosing

Ribavirin
- Combination therapy (with interferon) for chronic hepatitis C

Protease inhibitors

- e.g. bocepravir for hepatitis C

Antiretrovirals

See page 122.

Nucleoside and nucleotide analogues

- e.g. Lamivudine, tenofovir, used in combination therapy, e.g. for hepatitis B

VACCINATION (TABLE 7.2)

Passive

- Antibody raised against the infecting organism, e.g. tetanus immunoglobulin, diphtheria, rabies

Active

- Immunogenic antigen induces antibody production

Live attenuated vaccines
- Measles, mumps, rubella
- BCG

Inactivated (killed) vaccines
- Hepatitis A
- Pertussis (whooping cough)
- *Haemophilus influenzae b*
- Meningococcus A and C
- Pneumococcus
- Influenza
- Polio

Table 7.2 UK Vaccination schedule
2, 3 and 4 months Diphtheria, pertussis and tetanus *Haemophilus influenzae b* Oral polio Meningococcus gp C Tuberculosis (BCG) for infants at high risk
13 months Measles Mumps } MMR Rubella
2, 14 and 12-13 months Pneumococcal
By school entry Diphtheria, pertussis, tetanus MMR and oral polio
13–18 years Diphtheria, tetanus and oral polio (plus human papilloma vaccine for girls)

Toxoids
- Tetanus
- Diphtheria

Recombinant vaccines
- Hepatitis B

BACTERIAL INFECTION

Gram-positive cocci

Staphylococcus
- *Staph. aureus*, epidermidis, saprophyticus (Fig. 7.2)
- Skin: cellulitis, impetigo, necrotizing fasciitis
- Lungs: pneumonia, abscesses
- Heart: endocarditis
- CNS: meningitis, abscesses
- Bones: osteomyelitis

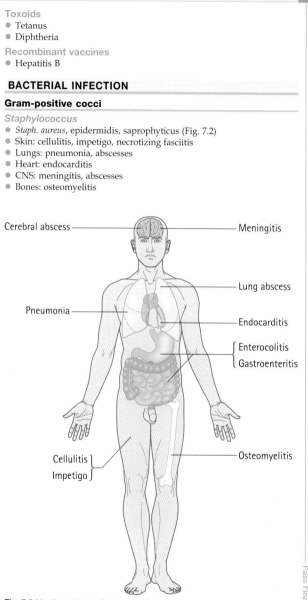

Fig. 7.2 Manifestations of *Staphylococcal* infection.

- Gut: enterocolitis
- *Staph. aureus* produces a toxin, which may cause:
  - Food poisoning
  - Toxic shock syndrome
  - Scalded skin syndrome

Management
- Much community-acquired infection is penicillin-sensitive
- However, hospital spread of methicillin-resistant *Staph. aureus* (MRSA) is increasing

Streptococcus
- Majority of infections are due to β-haemolytic *Strep. pyogenes*
- Skin: impetigo, erysipelas
- Mouth: pharyngitis, tonsillitis
- Lungs: pneumonia – *Strep. pneumoniae*
- Other: endocarditis – *Strep. viridans*, scarlet fever, rheumatic fever

Management
- Majority are sensitive to penicillins

Gram-negative cocci

Neisseria
- *Neisseria meningitidis* → meningitis and septicaemia
- *Neisseria gonorrhoeae* → gonorrhoea

Management
- Penicillin or cefotaxime

Gram-positive bacilli

Corynebacterium
- *C. diphtheriae*
- Toxin-producing forms → diphtheria
- Nasal discharge
- Pharyngeal inflammation
- Laryngeal inflammation → husky voice
- → Respiratory obstruction
- Myocarditis
- Neurological manifestations – cranial nerve palsies, polyneuropathy

Management
- Antitoxin + penicillin

Listeria
- *L. monocytogenes*
- → Abortions, meningitis or septicaemia

Management
- Ampicillin and gentamicin

Clostridium
- *C. botulinum, C. difficile* (see Ch. 10)
- *C. tetani* → tetanus
  - Infects puncture wounds and bites
  - Neurotoxin production
  - → Neuromuscular blockade, lockjaw, muscle spasm, autonomic neuropathy

Management
- Antitoxin, penicillin, ITU care

B. anthracis (Bacillus group)
- Anthrax
- → Erythematous skin lesion that ulcerates
- → Black central eschar
- Pulmonary and GI tract involvement

Management
- Penicillin

B. cereus (Bacillus group)
- → Toxin mediated food poisoning

Gram-negative bacilli

Brucella
- *B. abortus, melitensis, suis*
- Endotoxin → headache, fever, weakness
- Lymphadenopathy, hepatosplenomegaly
- Arthritis, encephalitis and endocarditis
- Contracted from non-pasteurized milk

Management
- Doxycycline

Bordetella
- *B. pertussis* – whooping cough
- Childhood disease
- Catarrhal phase – rhinorrhoea and conjunctivitis
- Paroxysmal phase – coughing attacks

Management
- Erythromycin in catarrhal phase

Haemophilus
- *H. influenzae*, *ducreyi*, *parainfluenzae*
- Increased risk of infection post-splenectomy
- Pneumonia, bronchitis
- Meningitis (*H. influenzae b*)
- Epiglottitis

Management
- Cefotaxime, cefuroxime

Prevention
- HiB vaccine

Cholera
- *Vibrio cholerae* (see Ch. 10)

Enterobacteria

- *Escherichia coli*
- *Salmonella*
- *Campylobacter* ⎫ (see Ch. 10)
- *Shigella*
- *Helicobacter*
- *Yersinia*

MYCOBACTERIAL DISEASE

Mycobacterium tuberculosis

- Acid-fast aerobic bacillus (Fig. 7.3)
- Droplet spread
- → Caseating granuloma
  - Lung
  - Adrenals
  - Terminal ileum
  - Lymph nodes
- → Cough, fever, weight loss, night sweats
- Immunosuppression → haematogenous spread (miliary TB)

Complications
- TB meningitis
- TB peritonitis

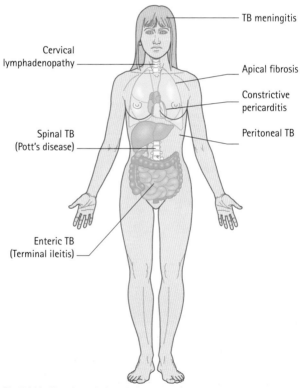

TB meningitis

Cervical lymphadenopathy

Apical fibrosis

Constrictive pericarditis

Spinal TB (Pott's disease)

Peritoneal TB

Enteric TB (Terminal ileitis)

Fig. 7.3 Manifestations of tuberculosis.

- Arthritis and osteomyelitis
- Constrictive pericarditis

Investigations
- Imaging – X-ray/CT scan of the chest
- Microbiology – Ziehl–Neelson staining of sputum
- Bronchoscopy and washings
- Biopsy of solid lesions
- CSF examination in meningitis
- Early morning urine

Management
- Combination therapy (Table 7.3)

Contact tracing
- X-ray and tuberculin testing in close contacts

Immunization
- Bacille Calmette-Guérin (BCG)
- Bovine strain of TB with very low virulence after tuberculin testing

Mycobacterium leprae

- Leprosy (Hansen's disease)
- Immune response determines disease type (there are two ends of a clinical spectrum)

Tuberculoid
- High cell-mediated immunity
- Hypopigmented skin patches
- Loss of sensation over patch
- Tender thickened nerves

Lepromatous
- Macules, papules or nodules in the skin
- Laryngitis and hoarse voice
- Collapse of nasal cartilage
- Leonine face

Investigations
- Impossible to culture organism
- Diagnosis is basically clinical

Management
- Dapsone, rifampicin and clofazimine for 2 years

Table 7.3 Drug regimens for tuberculosis

Pulmonary TB
  Rifampicin and isoniazid for 6 months, pyrazinamide and
    ethambutol for the first 2 months
TB meningitis and pericarditis
  Rifampicin and isoniazid for 12 months, with pyrazinamide and
    ethambutol for the first 2 months and glucocorticoids
Drug resistance and HIV
  Start standard therapy as above but alter based on sensitivities
    and known prevalence of resistance loner therapy and other
    agents e.g. quinolones may be needed

SPIROCHAETES

Syphilis

- *Treponema pallidum*

Primary syphilis (10–90 days post-infection)
- Painless ulcer (chancre) at infection site

Secondary syphilis (4–10 weeks)
- Lymphadenopathy
- Rash – papules or pustules
- Warty skin lesions (condylomata lata)
- Oral 'snail track' ulcers

Tertiary syphilis
- Granulomatous lesions
- Skin, bones, liver
- Aortic dilatation and valve regurgitation

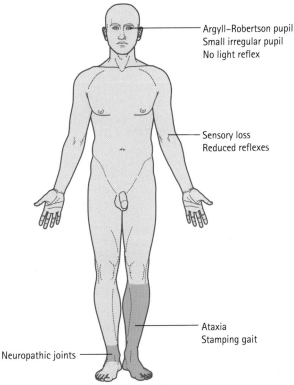

Argyll–Robertson pupil
Small irregular pupil
No light reflex

Sensory loss
Reduced reflexes

Ataxia
Stamping gait

Neuropathic joints

Fig. 7.4 Some manifestations of tertiary syphilis.

- Neurosyphilis – meningitis, cerebral gumma
- Tabes dorsalis – dorsal root demyelination (Fig. 7.4)

Congenital syphilis
- Hutchinson's (notched) teeth
- Sabre tibia
- Long bone abnormalities
- Loss of nasal bridge

Management
- Procaine penicillin

Leptospirosis (Weil's disease)

- *Leptospira interrogeais*
- Contact with animal reservoirs (rat's urine)
- Headache, fever, myalgia
- Conjunctival suffusion
- Hepatosplenomegaly and lymphadenopathy

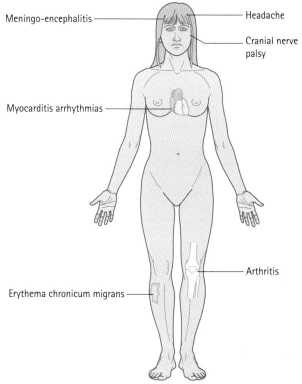

Meningo-encephalitis

Headache

Cranial nerve palsy

Myocarditis arrhythmias

Erythema chronicum migrans

Arthritis

Fig. 7.5 Manifestations of Lyme disease.

- May progress to:
  - Jaundice
  - Haemolytic anaemia
  - Renal failure

Investigations
- IgM antibodies
- *Leptospira* cultured in blood

Management
- Penicillins
- Erythromycin

Lyme disease (Fig. 7.5)

- *Borrelia burgdorferi*
- Carried by ixodid ticks (from deer and sheep)
- Erythema chronicum migrans
- Headache, fever and malaise
- Meningoencephalitis
- Cranial nerve palsies
- Cardiac arrhythmias, myocarditis
- Arthritis

Investigations
- IgM antibodies against organism

Management
- Amoxicillin/penicillin

VIRAL INFECTIONS

- Viral hepatitis is discussed in Chapter 10

DNA viruses: Adenoviruses

- Croup
- Gastroenteritis
- Mesenteric adenitis in children

α-Herpesvirus

Herpes simplex-1 (HSV-1)
- Stomatitis (primary infection)
- Cold sores
- Erythema multiforme

Herpes simplex-2 (HSV-2)
- Genital herpes

Varicella zoster virus (VZV)
- Chickenpox (primary infection)
- Shingles (see Ch. 12)

β-Herpesvirus

Cytomegalovirus (CMV)
- Retinitis
- Pneumonitis } in immunocompromised
- Gastrointestinal ulcers

Human herpes viruses 6 and 7
- Roseola infantum (children)

γ-Herpesvirus

Epstein–Barr virus (EBV)
- Infectious mononucleosis
- Burkitt's lymphoma
- Nasopharyngeal carcinoma
- Gastric carcinoma

Human herpes virus 8
- Kaposi's sarcoma

Erythrovirus B19

- Erythema infectiosum in children (fifth disease/slapped cheek syndrome)
- Aplastic crisis in sickle cell disease
- Anaemia, leucopenia and thrombocytopenia

Poxvirus

- Smallpox (now eradicated worldwide)
- Molluscum contagiosum

RNA viruses/PicoRNAviruses

Poliovirus
- Poliomyelitis
- 95% asymptomatic
- 0.1% suffer paralytic poliomyelitis
- Asymmetric paralysis
- No sensory involvement

Coxsackievirus
- Hand, foot and mouth disease (vesicular rash)
- Meningitis and encephalitis
- Myocarditis and pericarditis

Togaviruses

Rubella (German measles)
- Conjunctivitis
- Lymphadenopathy
- Macular pink/red rash
- Fetal infection → cardiac defect, cataracts, mental retardation and deafness

Flaviviruses

Yellow fever
- Mosquito spread
- Africa and Asia
- High fever
- Bradycardia
- Jaundice
- Clotting abnormalities → bleeding

Dengue
- Spread by biting arthropod *A. aegypti* which lives in standing water in inner cities
- South America, Africa and Asia

- High fever, malaise, headache, flushing, retrobulbar pain, backache
- Lymphadenopathy, petechiae on palate and skin rashes
- Haemorrhagic capillary leak syndrome
- Antibody testing for diagnosis
- Treatment is supportive

Orthomyxovirus

Influenza
- Type A → epidemics and pandemics
- Type B → localized outbreaks
- Type C → rarely produces disease

Paramyxovirus

Measles (rubeola)
- Incubation 8–14 days
- Malaise, fever, cough
- Koplik's spots in the mouth
- Erythematous rash
- Complications
  - Pneumonia
  - Myocarditis
  - Encephalomyelitis
  - Subacute sclerosing panencephalitis

Mumps
- Incubation 18 days
- Fever, headache, anorexia
- Parotid gland swelling ± submandibular involvement
- Epididymo-orchitis after puberty

Rhabdovirus

Rabies
- Contracted in animal bites
- Anxiety, agitation, hydrophobia and aerophobia
- Hyperreflexia and muscle spasm
- Death at 10–14 days
- No effective treatment

HUMAN IMMUNODEFICIENCY VIRUS (HIV) AND ACQUIRED IMMUNE DEFICIENCY SYNDROME (AIDS)

Epidemiology
- Young adults and children in developing world – heterosexual and vertical spread, breast-feeding
- Sexual intercourse (vaginal and anal)
- Blood spread (shared needles, transfusions)

HIV (Fig. 7.6)
- Two subtypes:
  - **HIV1** Europe/America and South-East Asia
  - **HIV2** Africa
- Retrovirus (reverse transcriptase allows DNA synthesis from RNA)
- Binds to CD4 lymphocyte surface marker
- Enters lymphocyte → viral synthesis

Clinical features
- Seroconversion illness 2 weeks after infection
- Fever, lymphadenopathy, headache

Investigations
- IgG against gp120
- IgG against p24
- Viral p24 antigen
- Viral culture
- Viral load (RNA copies/mL)

Clinical latency
- Median time of 10 years until clinical presentation of AIDS

Effects of HIV infection

- Infections due to low CD4 lymphocyte count
- Diagnosis based on low CD4 count and the presence of an AIDS-defining illness

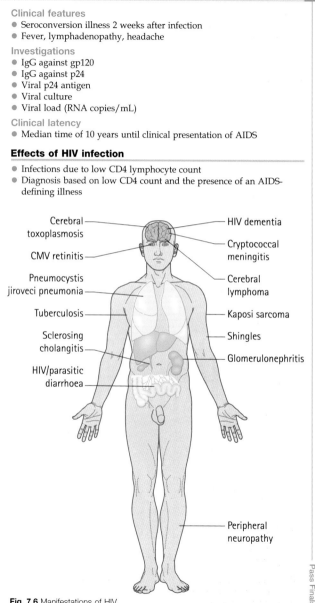

Fig. 7.6 Manifestations of HIV.

Neurological disease

- HIV-related dementia
- Distal sensory polyneuropathy
- Autonomic neuropathy
- Progressive multifocal leucoencephalopathy
- Cryptococcal meningitis
- Cerebral lymphoma
- Cerebral toxoplasma

Eye disease

- CMV retinitis

Mucocutaneous disease

- Kaposi's sarcoma
- Molluscum contagiosum
- Shingles
- Oral hairy leucoplakia (tongue)
- Oral/oesophageal candidiasis
- Squamous cell carcinomas

Haematological disease

- Low CD4 (<200)
- Anaemia
- Neutropenia
- Isolated thrombocytopenia

Gastrointestinal disease

- Weight loss
- HIV-related diarrhoea
  - *Cryptosporidium*
  - *Microsporidium*
  - HIV enteropathy
  - CMV colitis
  - Bacterial infection
  - *Mycobacterium*
- Sclerosing cholangitis
- Oesophageal candidiasis

Renal disease

- HIV associated nephropathy
- Focal glomerulonephritis

Respiratory disease

- Pneumonia
- *Pneumocystis jiroveci* pneumonia (PCP)

Disease monitoring

- CD4 lymphocyte count
- HIV viral load (HIV RNA)

Management (Table 7.4)

Antiretroviral drugs

- HAART: highly active antiretroviral therapy–combination therapy that significantly reduces viral load and improves survival
- Nucleoside analogues, e.g. zidovudine/abacavir/lamivudine/ didanosine/tenofovir
- Protease inhibitors, e.g. ritonavir/saquinavir/indinavir

Table 7.4 Post-exposure prophylaxis

Post-needlestick injury
 Blood from patient and injured person
Then 4 weeks of
 Tenofovir and emtrictiabine with polinavir and ritinavir

- Non-nucleoside reverse transcriptase inhibitors (only active against HIV1), e.g. nevirapine/efavirenz
- HIV cell fusion inhibitors, e.g. enfuvirtide

Complications of antiretroviral therapy
- Lipodystrophy syndrome (insulin resistance/dyslipidaemia/fat redistribution)

Early management of opportunistic infections
- Screening for infection, e.g. ophthalmoscopy for CMV retinitis

Prevention of infection

- Safe sex practices
- Needle exchanges
- Screening of blood transfusions

FUNGAL DISEASE

Candidiasis

- *Candida albicans*
- Vaginal and oral thrush
- Oesophagitis
- Increased in the immunocompromised, e.g. antibiotics, steroids and in the elderly

Diagnosis
- Microscopy
- Clinical appearance

Management
- Nystatin for oral lesions
- Fluconazole/Amphotericin B

Histoplasmosis

- *Histoplasma capsulatum*
- TB-like disease
- Pulmonary focus
- Erythema nodosum and multiforme
- Treat with ketoconazole/itraconazole/amphotericin B

Aspergillosis

Bronchopulmonary allergic aspergillosis
- Mimics asthma
- Bronchiectasis and eosinophilia

Aspergilloma
- Fungus ball in cavity in lung
- Often in old TB focus

Invasive aspergillosis
- Immunocompromised patients
- Pneumonia
- Meningitis and intracerebral abscess

PROTOZOAL DISEASE

Leishmaniasis

Visceral leishmaniasis (*kala-azar*)
- Fever, cough, diarrhoea
- Pigmented rough skin
- Splenomegaly (often massive)
- Hypersplenism → pancytopenia
- Hepatomegaly

Cutaneous leishmaniasis
- Transmitted by sandfly
- Multiple painless nodules → ulceration

Trypanosomiasis

Sleeping sickness (African disease)
- Tsetse fly transmission
- Meningoencephalitis
- Apathy and somnolence

Chagas disease (American disease)
- Lymphadenopathy
- Hepatosplenomegaly
- Conjunctivitis
- GI motility disturbance
- Neurological complications

Toxoplasmosis

- *Toxoplasma gondii*
- Transmission by cats
- Lymphadenopathy
- Neck stiffness and headache
- Acute febrile illness

Malaria

Epidemiology
- 500 million people worldwide
- Hot humid countries

Aetiology
- *Plasmodium – vivax, ovale, falciparum, malariae*
- Transmitted by ♀ *Anopheles* mosquito

Clinical features
- High fever
- Splenomegaly
- *Vivax, ovale* and *malariae* → milder chronic disease
- *Falciparum* → more serious acute disease:
- Blackwater fever: haemolysis → black urine
- Cerebral malaria: convulsions, coma

Table 7.5 Prevention of malaria
Avoid insect bites
Repellents
Impregnated mosquito nets
Chemoprophylaxis
Seek advice prior to travel due to changes in resistance patterns

- Severe malaria: 1% erythrocytes infected (*falciparum* malaria)
  → Cerebral, renal and GI involvement
  - Risk of splenic rupture
  - Renal failure
  - Haemolysis and thrombocytopenia
  - Hypoglycaemia and acidosis

Investigations
- Thick and thin blood film shows parasites and allows identification
- Quantification of percentage of infected red cells
- Blood count, liver function tests, urea and electrolytes for complications

Management
- Falciparum: first line treatment is i.v. artesunate; if not available use i.v. quinine if severe malaria
- Other species: chloroquine

Prevention
See Table 7.5.

NEMATODE, TREMATODE AND CESTODE INFECTIONS

Nematodes *Filariasis*

- Lymphangitis and elephantiasis

Toxocara

- Transmitted by dogs and cats
- Abdominal pain and hepatomegaly

Intestinal infections

See Chapter 10.

Trematodes *Schistosomiasis (Bilharzia)*

S. japonicum/mansoni
- Intestinal ulceration and fibrosis
- Granulomatous hepatitis
- Hepatosplenomegaly
- Portal hypertension

S. haematobium
- Dysuria and haematuria
- Bladder carcinoma

Cestodes

- Tapeworms

SEXUALLY TRANSMITTED DISEASES

Gonorrhoea

- *Neisseria gonorrhoeae*
- ♂ Urethritis and urethral discharge
- ♀ 50% asymptomatic
- Dysuria and vaginal discharge
- Conjunctival infection in the newborn
- Arthritis and rash in systemic disease

Investigations
- Nucleic acid amplification tests (NAATs) on urine. Microscopy and culture of urethral or vaginal swabs

Management
- Ceftriaxone and azithromycin

Chlamydia

- *Chlamydia trachomatis*
- ♂ Urethritis with discharge
- ♀ Acute salpingitis → subfertility
- Ophthalmic trachoma → blindness
- Reiter syndrome – oral ulcers, arthritis, conjunctivitis, urethritis

Investigations
- Nucleic acid amplification tests (NAATs) on urine. Serology (IgM) or antigen detection

Table 7.6 Diseases notifiable under the Health Protection (notification) Regulations 2010

Acute encephalitis	Malaria
Acute infectious hepatitis	Measles
Acute meningitis	Meningococcal septicaemia
Acute poliomyelitis	Mumps
Anthrax	Plague
Botulism	Rabies
Brucellosis	Rubella
Cholera	SARS
Diphtheria	Scarlet fever
Enteric fever (typhoid or paratyphoid fever)	Smallpox
Food poisoning	Tetanus
Haemolytic uraemic syndrome (HUS)	Tuberculosis
Infectious bloody diarrhoea	Typhus
Invasive group A streptococcal disease	Viral haemorrhagic fever (VHF)
Legionnaires' Disease	Whooping cough
Leprosy	Yellow fever

Management
- Doxycycline or azithromycin

Syphilis

See Spirochaetes, above.

HIV

See Viral infections, above.

Human papilloma virus (HPV)

- Sexual transmission
- Results in cervical dysplasia
- Cervical carcinoma
- Vaccine available

NOTIFIABLE DISEASES

See Table 7.6

SELF-ASSESSMENT QUESTIONS

Multiple choice questions (true or false)

1. The following diseases are paired with their correct mode of transmission:
   A. Leishmaniasis – sandfly bites
   B. Hepatitis A – intravenous drug use
   C. *Giardiasis* – faecal–oral spread
   D. *Taenia solium* – infected meat products
   E. *Neisseria gonorrhoeae* – sexual intercourse
2. The following antibiotics act by disrupting bacterial cell wall synthesis:
   A. Amoxicillin
   B. Metronidazole
   C. Cefuroxime
   D. Ciprofloxacin
   E. Gentamicin
3. The following are live attenuated vaccines:
   A. Oral polio vaccine
   B. Tetanus
   C. Bacille Calmette–Guérin (BCG)
   D. *Haemophilus influenzae b*
   E. Hepatitis B vaccine
4. The following are recognized side-effects of the named antibiotic:
   A. Ampicillin – rash in infectious mononucleosis
   B. Gentamicin – renal toxicity
   C. Flucloxacillin – ototoxicity
   D. Sulphonamides – erythema multiforme
   E. Fusidic acid – seronegative arthropathy
5. The following may result in atypical lymphocytes on a blood film:
   A. Epstein–Barr virus
   B. Cytomegalovirus
   C. Influenza A
   D. Toxoplasmosis
   E. Salmonellosis

6. The following are manifestations of staphylococcal disease:
   A. Osteomyelitis
   B. Scarlet fever
   C. Impetigo
   D. Infective endocarditis
   E. Cerebral abscesses

7. The following are true of *Mycobacterium tuberculosis*:
   A. It may cause a terminal ileitis
   B. Tuberculous meningitis results in a low protein and glucose in CSF
   C. Pyrazinamide is useful in eradicating organisms in macrophages
   D. Infection may cause lupus vulgaris
   E. Miliary infection results from haematogenous spread

8. The following organisms release a neurotoxin:
   A. *Clostridium botulinum*
   B. *Clostridium difficile*
   C. *Clostridium tetani*
   D. *Corynebacterium diphtheriae*
   E. *Yersinia*

9. The following belong to the herpesvirus family:
   A. Cytomegalovirus
   B. Epstein–Barr virus
   C. Coxsackievirus
   D. Varicella zoster virus
   E. Rhabdovirus

10. The following are of use in chronic viral hepatitis:
    A. Lamivudine
    B. Azathioprine
    C. Ribavirin
    D. Interferon-α
    E. Zidovudine

11. In the following diseases animal vectors constitute an important mode of transmission:
    A. Yellow fever (togavirus)
    B. Fifth disease (parvovirus B19)
    C. Rabies (rhabdovirus)
    D. Hand, foot and mouth disease (paramyxovirus)
    E. Molluscum contagiosum (pox virus)

12. The following are recognized complications of the named infection:
    A. Measles virus – subacute sclerosing panencephalitis
    B. Rabies – aerophobia
    C. Varicella – pneumonia
    D. Cytomegalovirus – retinitis
    E. Parvovirus B19 – aplastic anaemia

13. The following are causes of abnormal liver function tests in HIV infection:
    A. Zidovudine
    B. Lamivudine
    C. Sclerosing cholangitis
    D. Cytomegalovirus infection
    E. *Mycobacterium avium intracellulare*

14. The following drugs are paired with the appropriate mechanism of action:
    A. Ritonavir – protease inhibitor
    B. Zidovudine – nucleoside analogue
    C. Nevirapine – viral RNA inhibitor
    D. Lamivudine – inhibition of cell wall synthesis
    E. Saquinavir – protease inhibitor
15. The following increase the risk of systemic candidiasis:
    A. Diabetes mellitus
    B. Oral prednisolone
    C. Chronic kidney disease
    D. Acute viral hepatitis
    E. Intravenous cephalosporin therapy
16. The following are not features of falciparum malaria:
    A. Thrombocytopenia
    B. Intravascular haemolysis
    C. Bronchospasm
    D. Hyposplenism
    E. Hypoglycaemia
17. The following are indicators of severe malaria:
    A. Fever >38°C
    B. Parasitaemia >2%
    C. Dark urine
    D. Glucose-6-phosphate deficiency
    E. Convulsions
18. The following may cause conjunctivitis in the newborn babies of infected mothers:
    A. Syphilis
    B. Chlamydia
    C. Gonorrhoea
    D. HIV
    E. Rubella
19. The following are true of syphilis infection:
    A. Acute infection usually presents as a painless ulcer
    B. A rash involving the palms of the hands suggests a secondary streptococcal infection
    C. Neurological signs may be due to intracerebral abscesses
    D. Syphilis meningitis may complicate tertiary syphilis
    E. Congenital infection results in an internuclear ophthalmoplegia
20. The following may result in oral ulceration:
    A. Syphilis
    B. Ulcerative colitis
    C. Behçet syndrome
    D. Mumps infection
    E. *Toxoplasma gondii*

Multiple choice questions (single best answer)

21. The following are true of sexually transmitted disease:
    A. The incidence of nonspecific urethritis is falling
    B. Gonorrhoea infection is asymptomatic in 90% of infections in males
    C. Chlamydia is an important cause of male infertility
    D. Gonorrhoea may result in a pustular rash
    E. Reactive arthritis is not associated with chlamydia infection

22. Which one of the following is true of HIV infection:
    A. *Pneumocystis jiroveci* pneumonia is an AIDS-defining illness
    B. The CD4-positive lymphocyte count is a poor marker of immune status
    C. The median duration of infection prior to the development of AIDS is 2 years
    D. HIV dementia is due to a parvovirus infection
    E. Kaposi's sarcoma is an indication of adenovirus infection

23. Which one of the following causes an acute hepatitic illness:
    A. Rhabdovirus
    B. Parvovirus B19
    C. Togaviruses
    D. Dane particle
    E. Epstein–Barr virus

24. Which one of the following is a Gram-positive organism?
    A. *Staphylococcus aureus*
    B. *Escherichia coli*
    C. *Helicobacter pylori*
    D. *Salmonella typhi*
    E. *Giardia lamblia*

25. A 23-year-old man presents with a cough, with rust-coloured sputum, peri-oral *Herpes Simplex* and findings of left lower lobe consolidation on chest X-ray. What is the most likely cause of his pneumonia?
    A. *Staph. aureus*
    B. *Strep. pneumoniae*
    C. *H. influenzae*
    D. *Pneumocystis jiroveci* pneumonia
    E. *M. tuberculosis*

26. A 76-year-old man presents with a fever, shortness of breath and a cough. On examination he has a pansystolic murmur that radiates to the axilla. On testing he has microscopic haematuria. What is the most likely diagnosis?
    A. Interstitial glomerulonephritis
    B. Pyelonephritis
    C. Bacterial endocarditis
    D. Cordae tendonae rupture
    E. Mycoplasma pneumonia

27. A 43-year-old woman was referred with weight loss, sweats and a fever. Investigations revealed lymphopenia. A CD4 lymphocyte count was recorded as <100. What is the most likely underlying cause?
    A. Parvovirus B19
    B. Epstein–Barr virus
    C. Human immunodeficiency virus
    D. Human papilloma virus
    E. Cytomegalovirus

28. A 67-year-old man is being treated with steroids and antibiotics for an infective exacerbation of chronic obstructive pulmonary disease. He reports pain and difficulty in swallowing. What is the most likely diagnosis?
    A. Peptic oesophageal stricture
    B. *Helicobacter pylori* induced ulceration
    C. Oesophageal cytomegalovirus

    D. Oesophageal candidiasis
    E. Eosinophilic oesophagitis
29. A 14-year-old boy presents with a 3-day history of a non-productive
    cough, followed by the appearance of multiple erythematous spots
    on the torso, arms and legs. On examination he has white spots on
    the buccal mucosa. What is the most likely cause?
    A. Chicken pox
    B. Rubella
    C. Erythema infectiosum
    D. Scarlet fever
    E. Measles

Extended matching questions

Question 1 Theme: Fever of unknown origin
  A. Acute bronchopulmonary aspergillosis
  B. *Pneumocystis jiroveci*
  C. Staphylococcal pulmonary abscess
  D. Aspergilloma
  E. *Mycobacterium tuberculosis*
  F. Falciparum malaria
  G. Leishmaniasis
  H. Liver abscess
  I. Acute hepatitis A
  J. *Streptococcus pneumoniae* pneumonia
  K. *Mycoplasma* pneumonia
  L. Schistosomiasis

For each of the following questions, select the best answer from the list above:
  I. A 42-year-old Ugandan woman with known HIV infection and a
    CD4 lymphocyte count of 86 is admitted with a cough, haemoptysis,
    weight loss and cervical lymphadenopathy. A chest X-ray reveals
    diffuse apical shadowing of the left lung. What is the most likely
    diagnosis?
  II. An 18-year-old man is admitted with a cough with rust-coloured
    sputum, anorexia, a temperature of 38.6°C and marked shortness of
    breath. On examination he is noted to have perioral herpes and
    coarse crackles at the right upper zone with some bronchial
    breathing. What is the most likely diagnosis?
  III. A 28-year-old woman is admitted with a fever and jaundice. She has
    recently returned from India after visiting her family. She has a
    moderately enlarged liver and spleen. On full blood count she is
    noted to have a platelet count of 76. What is the most likely
    diagnosis?

Question 2 Theme: Investigation of pyrexia
  A. Full blood count
  B. Thick and thin blood film
  C. Urea and electrolytes
  D. Liver function tests
  E. Serum calcium
  F. Blood glucose
  G. Blood cultures
  H. Urine microscopy and culture
  I. Sputum culture

J. Chest X-ray

K. Abdominal X-ray

L. Ultrasound of the liver

M. CT scan of the head

N. CT scan of the liver and pancreas

O. Endoscopic retrograde cholangiopancreatogram

For each of the following questions, select the best answer from the list above:

I. A 57-year-old woman is admitted with right upper quadrant pain, jaundice and a fever. On examination, she is tender in the right hypochondrium. What single investigation would be most useful in reaching a diagnosis?

II. A 28-year-old man returns from a trip to Kenya. He has a fever and is jaundiced. He has moderate splenomegaly. What single investigation would you choose to make the diagnosis?

III. A 76-year-old man develops a fever and cough with white frothy sputum a week after a mitral valve replacement. On examination he has fine crackles in both lung bases and a pansystolic murmur. Which investigation will be of most use in guiding treatment?

STRUCTURE AND FUNCTION

The structure of the respiratory system facilitates its role in extracting oxygen from the environment and disposing of waste gases (primarily carbon dioxide):

- The lungs provide a large surface area for gas exchange
- The alveolar walls present minimal resistance to gas exchange
- Efficient gas transfer is facilitated by matching ventilation to perfusion in the pulmonary capillary bed
- Host defences protect against inhaled gases, dusts and infectious agents

SMOKING

Cigarette smoke contains polycyclic aromatic hydrocarbons and nitrosamines which are potent carcinogens and mutagens. Smoking also causes release of enzymes from neutrophils and macrophages which destroy elastin leading to lung damage. Smoking is addictive. The dangers of smoking and the effects on the lungs are listed in Tables 8.1 and 8.2.

EXAMINING THE RESPIRATORY SYSTEM

Examination should contain all of the following and be done in roughly this order:

Look for:

- Clues around the bed
  - Oxygen
  - Inhalers
  - Nebulizers
  - Peak flow meter

Expose the chest

- Maintain the dignity of the patient. Act professionally
- Look for:
  - Cyanosis
  - Breathlessness/use of accessory muscles
  - Weight loss
  - Chest wall scars or deformity
  - Prominent veins on the chest wall (suggesting superior vena cava (SVC) obstruction)

Hands

- Flapping tremor of CO_2 retention – hold arms outstretched with wrists fully extended and fingers splayed and watch for movements of fingertips

Table 8.1 The dangers of cigarette smoking

General
　　Lung cancer
　　COPD
　　Carcinoma of the oesophagus
　　Ischaemic heart disease
　　Peripheral vascular disease
　　Bladder cancer
　　An increase in abnormal spermatozoa
　　Memory problems
Maternal smoking
　　Decreased infant birth weight
　　Increased fetal and neonatal mortality
　　Increase in asthma
Passive smoking
　　Risk of asthma, pneumonia and bronchitis in infants of smoking
　　　parents
　　An increase in cough and breathlessness in smokers and
　　　non-smokers with CPOD and asthma
　　Increased cancer risk

Table 8.2 The effects of cigarette smoking on the lungs

Large airways
　　Increase in submucosal gland volume
　　Increase in number of goblet cells
　　Chronic inflammation
　　Metaplasia and dysplasia of the surface epithelium
Small airways
　　Increase in number and distribution of goblet cells
　　Airway inflammation and fibrosis
　　Epithelial metaplasia/dysplasia
　　Carcinoma
Parenchyma
　　Proximal acinar scarring
　　Increase in alveolar macrophage numbers
　　Emphysema (pan- and centri-acinar)

- Clubbing (Table 8.3)
- Peripheral cyanosis
- Nicotine staining

Face

- Anaemia
- Central cyanosis

Neck

- Examine JVP (remember a fixed distended JVP suggests SVC obstruction)
- Check for lymphadenopathy

Table 8.3 Some common causes of finger clubbing

Respiratory
    Lung cancer
    Fibrosis, e.g. idiopathic pulmonary fibrosis
    Chronic lung sepsis
    Bronchiectasis
    Lung abscess
    Empyema
    Mesothelioma
Cardiovascular
    Cyanotic heart disease
    Infective endocarditis
    Atrial myxoma
Gastrointestinal
    Cirrhosis
    Inflammatory bowel disease (IBD)
Others
    Congenital

Thorax (Table 8.4)

- Locate tracheal position and apex beat
- Check for lymphadenopathy (axilla)

Assess chest expansion

Anterior

- Place hands on upper aspect of chest either side of sternum
- Ask patient to breathe in and out and watch your thumbs move laterally
- Do they move symmetrically?
- Repeat with your hands over lateral lower aspect of chest

Posterior

- Place hands over lateral lower aspect of chest and repeat the above

Percussion

- Compare left with right anteriorly and posteriorly
- Don't forget apices and under arms

Listen to breath sounds

- Use diaphragm of stethoscope and again compare left with right
- Listen for added sounds (wheeze, crackles) (Table 8.5)

Check for vocal resonance and fremitus

- Ask patient to say 99 and listen with stethoscope (resonance) or palpate (vocal fremitus)

Measure peak flow

- See Chapter 3, page 26
- Normal values
  - 40-year-old – 175 cm tall ♂ = 620 L/min
  - 40-year-old – 155 cm tall ♀ = 460 L/min

Table 8.4 Physical signs of respiratory disease

Pathology	Chest wall movement	Tracheal deviation	Percussion note	Breath sounds	Vocal resonance	Added sounds
Consolidation (pneumonia)	Reduced on affected side	None	Dull	Bronchial	Increased	Crackles
Collapse (major bronchus)	Reduced on affected side	Towards lesion	Dull	Diminished/absent	Reduced/absent	None
Fibrosis (generalized)	Reduced	None	Normal	Vesicular	Increased	Crackles
Pleural effusion (>500 mL)	Reduced	Away if massive	Stony dull	Diminished/absent	Reduced/absent	None
Pneumothorax (large)	Reduced	Away from lesion	Normal or hyper-resonant	Diminished/absent	Reduced/absent	None
Chronic obstructive pulmonary disease (COPD)	Reduced	None	Normal	Prolonged expiration	Normal	Expiratory wheeze
Asthma	Reduced	None	Normal	Prolonged expiration	Normal	Expiratory wheeze Crackles

Table 8.5 Abnormal and additional breath sounds

Pathogenic process	Description of breath sounds	Auscultatory features
Airways obstruction	Wheezes	High-pitched end-expiratory 'squeaking' noises
		Monophonic = single airway obstruction
		Polyphonic = many small airways obstruction
Consolidation	Bronchial breathing	Breath sounds in inspiration are the same as expiratory phase (similar to breath sounds heard over trachea)
Fibrosis	Fine crackles	Short-lived end-inspiratory high-pitched added sounds 'like bubbles popping'
Fluid in alveoli (pulmonary oedema)		
Pleural inflammation	Pleural rub	Localized creaking/groaning added sounds

INVESTIGATIONS IN LUNG DISEASE

Imaging

- Chest X-ray (see Ch. 5)
- CT scan of the chest
  - Mass lesions
  - Interstitial lung disease
  - Bronchiectasis
  - Pulmonary embolism
- Ventilation perfusion (V/Q) scan
  - Diagnosis of pulmonary embolus
- PET (positron emission topography) scanning
  - Assessment of lymph node involvement and metastases in lung cancer

Endoscopy

- Bronchoscopy
  - Allows direct visualization of bronchi
  - Biopsies and cytology

MEASURING RESPIRATORY FUNCTION

Peak flow rate

↓ in airflow limitation (used to monitor the condition and its treatment)

Blood gas analysis (Table 8.6)

- Arterial blood sample (usually radial artery) measures partial pressure of O_2 and CO_2
- Essential to manage acute severe asthma and respiratory failure

Table 8.6 Abnormalities of blood gases in respiratory failure

	P_aO_2	P_aCO_2	pH	HCO_3
Type I				
e.g. Severe asthma, pneumonia, acute respiratory distress syndrome (ARDS)	↓	↓ or →	↓ or →	→ or ↓
Type II				
e.g. COPD, CNS depression (opiates), respiratory muscle weakness	↓	↑	↓	↑

Pulse oximetry

- Measures the difference in absorption of light by oxyhaemoglobin and deoxyhaemoglobin
- Used to assess and monitor arterial oxygen saturation

Spirometry

- Involves a maximum inspiration then forced expiration into a spirometer. Measures FEV1 and FVC
- Forced expiratory volume in 1 second (FEV_1) = volume of air expired in first second
- Forced vital capacity (FVC) = maximum volume of air expired
- The FEV_1:FVC ratio (normal >75) ↓ in airflow limitation, e.g. asthma
- Both FEV1 and FVC ↓ in restrictive diseases, e.g. fibrosis

Transfer factor

- Measures transfer of gas across the alveolar–capillary membrane
- Decreased in alveolar disease/loss
  - Idiopathic pulmonary fibrosis
  - Sarcoidosis
  - Asbestosis
  - Emphysema
- Increased in pulmonary haemorrhage

SAMPLING PLEURAL TISSUE

Pleural biopsy

- Pleural lesions
  - Malignancy
  - Tuberculosis

Pleural aspirate

- Removing pleural effusion fluid
- Microscopy and culture in infection
- Protein content (transudate vs exudates)
- Cytology (malignancy)
- LDH

PULMONARY INFECTION

Pneumonia

- Lung infections are classified by site (e.g. lobar pneumonia or bronchopneumonia) or by aetiology

Aetiology (Table 8.7)
- Bacterial
- Viral
- Opportunistic organisms
- Chemical (e.g. aspiration of vomit)
- Radiotherapy
- Allergic mechanisms

Clinical features (Table 8.8)
- Cough
- ± Purulent sputum
- Fever
- Pleuritic chest pain
- Breathlessness

Table 8.7 Aetiology of pneumonia in the UK		
Infecting agent	(%)	Clinical circumstance
Streptococcus pneumoniae	>50	Community pneumonia patients usually previously fit
Mycoplasma pneumoniae		
Influenza A		
Haemophilus influenzae	5	Pre-existing lung disease, e.g. COPD
Staphylococcus aureus	2	Children/i.v. drug users/flu outbreaks
Chlamydia pneumoniae	5	Community-acquired in institutions/families
Legionella pneumophila		
Chlamydia psittaci	3	Contact with birds (not inevitable)
Pseudomonas aeruginosa	<1	Cystic fibrosis
Pneumocystis carinii	<1	AIDS/lymphomas/leukaemias/use of immunosuppressant drugs
Actinomyces israelii		
Nocardia asteroides		
Cytomegalovirus		
Tuberculosis		
Aspergillus fumigatus		
Anaerobic organisms	<1	Inhalation pneumonia/alcohol excess/postoperative
None isolated	20	

Table 8.8 CURB 65 score for community acquired pneumonia

Each of the following scores 1:

Confusion (MTS <9, new disorientation in time/person/place
Urea >7 mmol/L
Respiratory rate =30/minute
Blood pressure (SBP <90 mmHg or DBP = 60 mmHg)
Age >65 years
    Score 0 or 1: Mortality low – could go home
    Score 2: Mortality intermediate – admit to hospital
    Score 3–5: Mortality high – consider HDU/ITU care

Specific features
Strep. pneumoniae
- Rust-coloured sputum
- Peri-oral HSV

Mycoplasma
- White cell count normal, cold agglutinins occur in 50%
- Extra-pulmonary complications, e.g. rash, myocarditis, pericarditis, haemolytic anaemia, myalgia, neurological abnormalities, abnormal liver function, diarrhoea

Staphylococcus aureus
- Abscesses – in lung and elsewhere

Coxiella burnetii
- Multiple lesions on chest X-ray

Investigations
- Chest X-ray
- Arterial blood gases or oxygen saturation
- Blood/sputum culture
- Microbiological: urine for pneumococcal or legionella antigen, serology in atypical cases

Management
- Antibiotics choice depends on severity and may vary according to local protocols (Table 8.8)
  - Mild: amoxicillin 500 mg three times a day (or clarithromycin if allergic)
  - Moderate: i.v. amoxicillin 500 mg three times a day and clarithromycin 500 mg twice a day
  - Severe: i.v. cefuroxime 1.5 g four times a day and clarithromycin 500 mg twice a day
  - Adjust as appropriate if particular organism suspected or known
- Oxygen
- Correct/prevent dehydration

Complications
- Respiratory failure
  - Type 1 – low P_aO_2, low/normal P_aCO_2
- Lung abscess
  - Particularly aspiration pneumonia, staphylococcal or *Klebsiella* infection, bronchial obstruction (cancer or foreign body)
- Empyema
  - Pus in the pleural space

Prognosis

- Overall 5% mortality for hospital inpatients
- >25% mortality for *Staph. aureus* pneumonia
- 50% mortality for severe community acquired pneumonia (Table 8.8)

Tuberculosis

- Caseating granulomatous infection due to *Mycobacterium* tuberculosis in the lung
- TB is a notifiable disease and contact tracing is important

Patients at risk

- Those from endemic areas
- Immunosuppressed patients
- HIV, steroids, malignancy
- Alcoholics/homeless people/people living in overcrowded conditions

Clinical features

- See Figure 8.1
- May be none
- Malaise and lethargy
- Anorexia/weight loss
- Fever
- Cough
- Haemoptysis
- Signs of
  - Pleural effusion
  - Pneumonia
  - Fibrosis

Investigations

- Chest X-ray
  - Affects upper zones particularly
  - ± Calcification
  - ± Cavitation
- Sputum microscopy (Ziehl–Neelsen stain) and culture
- Lung tissue microscopy and culture: bronchoscopy and washings or lung/pleural biopsies
- IGRA interferon gamma release assay: blood test which detects latent TB

Management

- 6 months of combination of antibiotics, usually
  - Rifampicin and isoniazid
  - + Pyrazinamide for first 2 months +
  - Add ethambutol if risk of drug resistance is increased
- Compliance is vital
- Multi-resistant TB occurs particularly in HIV, and may require more antibiotics (according to sensitivities) over a longer period

Side-effects of anti-TB drugs

Rifampicin

- Liver dysfunction
- Discoloration of body fluids
- Reduced effectiveness of oral contraceptives and other drugs

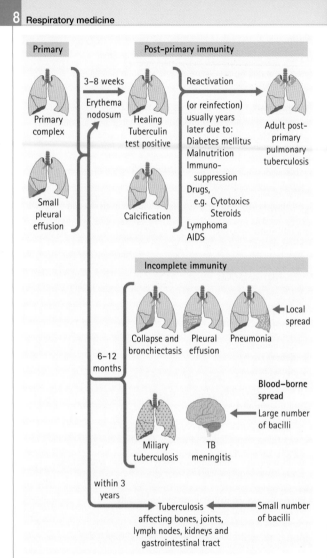

Fig. 8.1 Manifestations of primary and post-primary tuberculosis.

Isoniazid
- High doses cause polyneuropathy
- Pyridoxine is added to prevent this

Pyrazinamide
- Liver dysfunction

Ethambutol
- Retrobulbar neuritis (patients need ophthalmology monitoring)

Streptomycin
- Vestibular nerve damage

Other mycobacteria

M. kansasii
- COPD and working in dusty conditions (e.g. miners)

M. avium intracellulare (MAI)
- Immunosuppressed patients, e.g. HIV

PULMONARY MALIGNANCY

Bronchial carcinoma

- Malignant tumour of bronchial tree

Epidemiology
- Most common malignancy 1.3 million cases per year worldwide
- Third most common cause of death in UK
- $\male > \female$ (3:1)

Cell types
- Small cell (20–30%)
- Non-small cell
  - Squamous (40%)
  - Large cell (25%)
  - Adenocarcinoma (10%)
  - Bronchoalveolar cell (1–2%)

Aetiology
- Smoking (including passive)
- Asbestos

Clinical features
Symptoms See Table 8.9.

Table 8.9 Frequency of common presenting symptoms of bronchial carcinoma

Symptom	Frequency (%)
Cough	41
Chest pain	22
Cough and pain	15
Haemoptysis	7
Chest infection	<5
Others (malaise, breathlessness, etc.)	<5

Signs
- Often none
- Clubbing
- Supraclavicular nodes (small cell)
- Signs of:
  - Pleural effusion or lung collapse
  - Chronic lung disease (e.g. asbestosis)

Spread of bronchial carcinoma
Direct
- Pleural effusion
- Erosion of ribs and involvement of chest wall structures in apical tumours (Pancoast's tumour)
- Sympathetic ganglion (Horner syndrome – small pupil and ptosis)
- Recurrent laryngeal nerve palsy with unilateral vocal cord paralysis (hoarseness, bovine cough)
- Phrenic nerve palsy
- Oesophagus (dysphagia)
- Pericardial effusion
- SVC obstruction (headache, facial congestion, fixed distended veins)

Metastatic
- Bones (spinal cord compression can complicate)
- Liver
- Brain
- Adrenal glands (usually asymptomatic)

Non-metastatic extrapulmonary manifestations
- Weight loss
- Ectopic adrenocorticotropic hormone (ACTH), e.g. small cell
- Neurological, e.g. myasthenic (Eaton Lambert) syndrome
- Hypertrophic pulmonary osteoarthropathy (HPOA)

Investigations
- Chest X-ray
  CT scan and PET scanning for staging
- Bronchoscopy biopsy (proximal lesions) or percutaneous biopsy (peripheral lesions)

Management
- Multidisciplinary team approach

Surgery
- Only 5–10% of cases suitable
- For non-small cell

Radiotherapy
- Particularly for squamous cell
- Can be useful for symptom control
- Used for SVC obstruction

Chemotherapy
- Combination chemotherapy
  - Particularly useful for small cell
  - Also used for non-small cell

Prognosis
- 70% 5-year survival for those with local disease undergoing surgery
- Overall 20% at 1 year, 6–8% survival at 5 years

OBSTRUCTIVE LUNG DISEASE

Asthma

- Chronic inflammatory disease of the airways
- Three components
  - Reversible airflow limitation
  - Airway hyper-responsiveness to stimuli
  - Inflammation of the bronchi

Epidemiology

- Prevalence increasing, up to 15% population in UK

Aetiology and precipitating factors

- Atopy and allergy
- Increased airway responsiveness
- Cold air, exercise, pollution
- Occupational, e.g. isocyanates (paint-sprayers)
- Drugs, e.g. NSAIDs, beta-blockers

Clinical features

Episodes of:
- Cough
- Wheeze
- Breathlessness
- Chest tightness

Investigations

- Lung function tests
- Peak flow charts
- Skin testing of allergies

Management (Table 8.10)

- Self-management plan
- Avoid precipitants
- Stepwise drug treatments
- β_2-agonists (short- and long-acting)
- Antimuscarinics
- Anti-inflammatories, e.g. sodium cromoglycate
- Corticosteroids (inhaled or oral)
- Leukotriene antagonists (selected cases)

Chronic obstructive pulmonary disease (COPD)

- Progressive airflow limitation that is not fully reversible

Aetiology

- Smoking accounts for 90% of cases
  - 10–20% of heavy smokers develop COPD
- Rarely, α_1-antitrypsin deficiency

Clinical features

- Cough and sputum
- Wheeze
- Breathlessness
- Exacerbating factors
  - Upper respiratory tract infection
  - Cold/foggy weather
  - Pollution

Table 8.10 Acute severe asthma

Clinical features
  Inability to complete a sentence in one breath
  Respiratory rate > 25/min
  Tachycardia >110 beats/min
  Peak flow <50% of predicted normal or best
Life-threatening features
  Silent chest, cyanosis or feeble respiratory effort
  Exhaustion, confusion or coma
  Bradycardia or hypotension
  Peak flow <30% of predicted normal or best
Very severe life-threatening features
  A high P_aCO_2 >6 kPa
  A very low P_aO_2 <8 kPa despite oxygen
  A low and falling arterial pH
Management
  Reassure the patient and monitor pulse oximetry and arterial blood
    gases
  Give oxygen 40–60%
  Nebulized β_2 agonist, e.g. salbutamol 5 mg and repeat if no
    improvement otherwise use 4-hourly
  Add nebulized anti-muscarinics, e.g. ipratropium bromide 0.5 mg
  Give i.v. steroids, e.g. hydrocortisone 200 mg i.v. every 4 hours
  Exclude pneumothorax on chest X-ray
  If no improvement, consider i.v. infusion of magnesium sulphate or
    salbutamol and ventilation
  Urgent referral to ITU

- Tachypnoea with prolonged expiration
- Use of accessory muscles
- Intercostal muscle recession on inspiration
- Pursed lips on expiration
- Reduced chest expansion
- Hyperinflation
- Cyanosis
- Signs of respiratory failure:
  - CO_2 retention (bounding pulse, peripheral vasodilatation, tremor,
    confusion, coma)
- Signs of cor pulmonale
  - Right ventricular failure (oedema, hepatomegaly ↑ JVP)

Investigations
- Spirometry: FEV1:FVC ratio <70%
- Chest X-ray
- ECG (P pulmonale, right branch bundle block, right ventricular
  hypertrophy)
- α_1-antitrypsin level (in non-smokers)

Management
- Stop smoking
- Flu and pneumococcal vaccines
- β_2-agonists
- Antimuscarinics, e.g. tiotropium

- Corticosteroids
- Prompt antibiotics if infection present
- Assisted ventilation with bilevel positive airway pressure ventilatory support – (BiPAP)
- Home oxygen (if meets recognized criteria for benefit)

Surgery
- Lung volume reduction in carefully selected patients

Prognosis
- 50% of patients with severe breathlessness die within 5 years
- Stopping smoking improves prognosis

Obstructive sleep apnoea

- Occurs in patients who are overweight
- 30% have other correctable factors, e.g. ENT problems, drugs (sedatives), alcohol, acromegaly

Clinical features
- Snoring/nocturnal choking
- Daytime sleepiness
- Unrefreshed or restless sleep
- Morning headaches or 'drunkenness'
- Reduced libido
- Ankle swelling

Investigations
- Sleep study (measure oximetry, abdominal/thoracic movement and EEG during sleep)

Management
- Weight loss, ENT surgery, or correction of other factors listed above
- CPAP ventilation at night

Bronchiectasis

- Abnormal and permanently dilated airways

Aetiology
See Table 8.11.

Clinical features
- Cough and excessive sputum
- Recurrent chest infections
- Halitosis
- Haemoptysis
- Clubbing
- Coarse crackles in affected areas

Investigations
- Chest X-ray
- High-resolution CT of the lung
- Sputum examination
- Sinus X-rays
- Immunoglobulins
- Sweat electrolytes for cystic fibrosis

Management
- Postural drainage
- Antibiotics

> **Table 8.11** Causes of bronchiectasis
>
> Congenital
>   Deficiency of bronchial wall elements
>   Pulmonary sequestration
> Mechanical bronchial obstruction
>   Intrinsic
>   Extrinsic
> Postinfective bronchial damage
>   Bacterial and viral pneumonia, including pertussis, measles and
>   aspiration pneumonia
> Granuloma and fibrosis
>   Tuberculosis, sarcoidosis and fibrosing alveolitis
> Immunological over-response
>   Allergic bronchopulmonary aspergillosis
>   Post-lung transplant
> Immune deficiency
> Mucociliary clearance defects
>   Genetic
>   Primary ciliary dyskinesia (Kartagener syndrome with
>   dextrocardia and situs inversus)
>   Cystic fibrosis
>   Acquired
>   Young syndrome – azoospermia, sinusitis

- Bronchodilators if airflow limitation
- Steroids
- Heart/lung transplant

Cystic fibrosis

- Autosomal recessive disorder of the cystic fibrosis transmembrane
  conductance regulator (CFTR) which induces low salt and chloride
  excretion into airways leading to increased viscosity of airway
  secretions

Clinical features

Respiratory

- Recurrent chest infections
- Clubbing
- Sinusitis
- Haemoptysis
- Nasal polyps
- Spontaneous pneumothorax
- Respiratory failure
- Right ventricular failure

Gastrointestinal

- Steatorrhoea (pancreatic insufficiency)
- Meconium ileus
- Gallstones
- Cirrhosis

Investigations

- Sweat electrolyte test
- DNA analysis for genotype

Management

- Vaccinations (influenza, pneumococcus)
- Antibiotics
- Pancreatic/nutritional supplements
- Inhaled antibiotics, corticosteroids and recombinant human DNase
- CFTR gene therapy
- Lung transplant

Prognosis

- Median survival 40 years

OCCUPATIONAL LUNG DISEASE

Exposure to dusts, gases, vapours and fumes at work can lead to:

- Acute bronchitis and pulmonary oedema from irritants, e.g. SO_2, chlorine
- Pulmonary fibrosis due to mineral dust, e.g. coal
- Occupational asthma
- Hypersensitivity pneumonitis
- Bronchial carcinoma due to industrial agents, e.g. asbestos, radon

Coal-worker's pneumoconiosis

- Patients may qualify for industrial injuries benefit

Aetiology

- Deposition of dust particles in small airways

Investigations

- Chest X-ray – fine micronodular shadowing
- Spirometry – mixed restrictive and obstructive pattern with reduced gas transfer

Complications

- Progressive massive fibrosis
  - Large round masses in upper lobes ± necrotic centres
  - May be associated with rheumatoid factor and antinuclear factor
  - Respiratory failure

Asbestosis

- Ubiquitous use of asbestos put many at risk
- Particular problems with roofers, shipyard workers, those making gas masks in the Second World War

Aetiology

- Deposition of inhaled blue fibres in airways
- Synergistic effect of smoking

Clinical features

- Breathlessness
- Cough
- Chest pain

Investigations
- Chest X-ray
  - Fine reticulonodular shadowing
  - Honeycomb lung
  - Pleural plaques/effusion
- Spirometry – restrictive $\pm \downarrow$ gas transfer

Diseases caused by asbestos
- Pleural plaques
- Pleural effusion
- Bilateral diffuse pleural thickening*
- Mesothelioma* occurs 20–40 years after exposure to asbestos dust
- Asbestosis (restrictive fibrotic lung disease)*
- Carcinoma of the bronchus*

PULMONARY INFLAMMATION AND FIBROSIS

Sarcoidosis

- A multisystem granulomatous disorder presenting usually as
  - Bilateral hilar lymphadenopathy
  - Pulmonary infiltration
  - Skin/eye lesions

Epidemiology
- 19 in 100 000
- ♀ > ♂
- More severe in blacks than whites

Aetiology
- Unknown

Clinical features (Table 8.12)
- Commonly presents in third or fourth decade

Extrapulmonary features
- Skin
  - Erythema nodosum
  - Lupus pernio
- Eye
  - Uveitis
  - Conjunctivitis
  - Keratoconjunctivitis sicca

Table 8.12 Presenting symptoms of sarcoid	
Presentation	(%)
Respiratory symptoms/abnormal chest X-ray	50
Fatigue or weight loss	5
Peripheral lymphadenopathy	5
Fever	4
Normal chest X-ray	20

*Patients eligible for industrial injuries benefit

- Face
  - Parotitis
  - Facial nerve palsy
- Metabolic
  - Hypercalcaemia (10%)
- CNS
  - Meningoencephalitis
  - Spinal cord disease
  - Myopathy
  - Polyneuropathy
- Gastrointestinal
  - Hepatosplenomegaly
- Cardiovascular
  - Cardiomyopathy

Investigations
- Chest X-ray
- CT chest
- Blood tests
  - FBC (normocytic anaemia)
  - $\uparrow$ ESR
  - $\uparrow$ Ca^{++}
  - $\uparrow$ Serum angiotensin-converting enzyme (ACE)
- Transbronchial biopsy
- Spirometry
  - Restrictive defect
  - $\downarrow$ Gas transfer

Management
- Steroids

Pulmonary involvement in systemic diseases

Rheumatoid arthritis (Fig. 8.2)
- Rheumatoid factor always present
- Lung features may precede arthropathy

Systemic lupus erythematosus
- Pleurisy/pleural effusion

Systemic sclerosis
- Pulmonary fibrosis/honeycomb lung

Granulomatosis with polyangiitis (Wegener's granulomatosis)
- Granulomatous vasculitis of small arteries
- Rhinorrhoea
- Nasal ulceration
- Nodular masses (± cavitation)
- Migratory pulmonary infiltrates
- Associated with antineutrophil cytoplasmic antibodies (ANCA)
- Treated with cyclophosphamide

Churg–Strauss syndrome
- Systemic vasculitis
- Asthma
- Rhinitis
- Eosinophilia

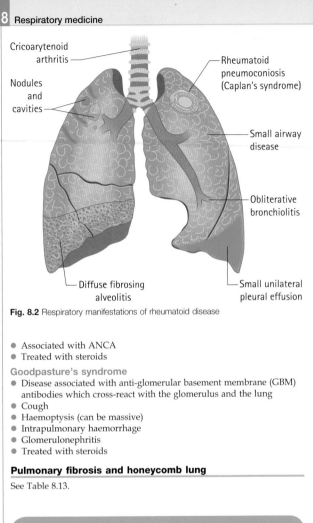

Fig. 8.2 Respiratory manifestations of rheumatoid disease

Labels on figure:
- Cricoarytenoid arthritis
- Nodules and cavities
- Rheumatoid pneumoconiosis (Caplan's syndrome)
- Small airway disease
- Obliterative bronchiolitis
- Diffuse fibrosing alveolitis
- Small unilateral pleural effusion

- Associated with ANCA
- Treated with steroids

Goodpasture's syndrome
- Disease associated with anti-glomerular basement membrane (GBM) antibodies which cross-react with the glomerulus and the lung
- Cough
- Haemoptysis (can be massive)
- Intrapulmonary haemorrhage
- Glomerulonephritis
- Treated with steroids

Pulmonary fibrosis and honeycomb lung

See Table 8.13.

Table 8.13 The main causes of honeycomb lung

Localized	Diffuse
Systemic sclerosis	Idiopathic pulmonary fibrosis
Sarcoidosis	Rheumatoid lung
Tuberculosis	Langerhans' cell histiocytosis
Asbestosis	Tuberous sclerosis
Berylliosis	Neurofibromatosis

Cryptogenic fibrosing alveolitis (also known as usual interstitial pneumonia (UIP)) and idiopathic pulmonary fibrosis

Clinical features
- Breathlessness
- Cyanosis
- Clubbing
- Bilateral fine inspiratory crackles
- Signs of:
  - Respiratory failure
  - Pulmonary hypertension
  - Right heart failure

Disease associations
- Autoimmune diseases

Investigations
- Chest X-ray – reticulonodular shadowing
- High-resolution CT
- Spirometry
  - Restrictive pattern with ↓ gas transfer
- Bronchoalveolar lavage – hypercellular
- Transbronchial biopsy

Management
- Oxygen
- Steroids
- Immunosuppressants, e.g. azathioprine
- Single lung transplant

Complications
- Respiratory failure

Prognosis
- Median survival 5 years

Hypersensitivity pneumonitis

Aetiology
- Inhalation of microbe spores e.g. farmer's lung, bird fancier's lung

Clinical features
- Fever
- Malaise
- Breathlessness
- Cough
- Tachypnoea
- Coarse inspiratory crackles
- Wheeze

Investigations
- Chest X-ray – fluffy nodular shadowing
- Precipitating antibodies (e.g. pigeon protein)
- Spirometry
  - Restrictive pattern with ↓, gas transfer
- Bronchoalveolar lavage – hypercellular

Management
- Avoid precipitant
- Steroids

PNEUMOTHORAX

- Air in the pleural space leading to lung deflation

Aetiology
- Spontaneous
- Chest trauma
- Intubation and ventilation

Clinical features
- See Table 8.4
- Pleuritic chest pain
- Breathlessness

Specific features
- Spontaneous pneumothorax: young patients: ♂ > ♀ 6:1, often tall and thin
- >40 years usually associated with COPD
- Rarely caused by asthma, carcinoma, lung abscess, severe pulmonary fibrosis
- If severe can present as tension pneumothorax (mediastinal shift and respiratory compromise)

Investigations
- Chest X-ray

Management
- Simple aspiration (second intercostal space mid-clavicular line)
- Intercostal drain if recurs after aspiration
- Surgery for recurrent pneumothorax

Complications
- Bronchopleural fistula

CARBON MONOXIDE POISONING

- Carbon monoxide combines readily with haemoglobin and prevents the formation of oxyhaemoglobin

Aetiology
- Gas appliances with poor ventilation

Clinical features
- Mental impairment
- Nausea and vomiting
- Headache
- Hallucinations
- Fits
- Drowsiness and coma
- Mild–moderate toxicity
  - Tachycardia
  - Tachypnoea
- Severe toxicity
  - Hypotension
  - Bradycardia
  - Myocardial damage
  - Respiratory distress

Investigations
- Blood carboxyhaemoglobin level

Management
- Remove the source
- High-flow oxygen
- Hyperbaric oxygen if:
  - Coma
  - Carboxyhaemoglobin level >10%

SELF-ASSESSMENT QUESTIONS

Multiple choice questions (single best answer)

1. Clubbing is seen in:
   A. Mesothelioma
   B. Asthma
   C. COPD
   D. Diverticular disease
   E. Pneumonia
2. The clinical findings of a pleural effusion are:
   A. Hyper-resonant percussion note
   B. Stony dull percussion note
   C. Increased tactile vocal fremitus
   D. Increased vocal resonance
   E. Tracheal deviation even with small effusions
3. In asthma:
   A. Peak flow rate is low during exacerbations
   B. Patients always have reduced air entry on chest auscultation
   C. FEV_1:FVC ratio is normal
   D. FVC is low
   E. JVP is elevated
4. In pneumonia:
   A. *Strep. pneumoniae* is an unusual cause
   B. *Haemophilus influenzae* pneumonia usually occurs in patients with normal lungs
   C. Pneumonia is only caused by bacteria
   D. *Pneumocystis carinii* pneumonia occurs in patients who are immunosuppressed
   E. Extrapulmonary abscesses do not occur in *Staph. aureus* pneumonia
5. In pneumonia:
   A. *Coxiella Burnetti* is associated with contact with birds
   B. Cold agglutinins are rare in *Mycoplasma* pneumonia
   C. Patients with *Staph. aureus* pneumonia have a good prognosis
   D. *Mycobacterium kansasii* usually presents in young adults
   E. *Staph. aureus* is associated with recent influenza infection
6. Tuberculosis:
   A. Treatment is with combination antibiotics
   B. Prevalence is reducing
   C. Mycobacteria are identified by haematoxylin and eosin stain
   D. Pneumonia usually affects the lower zones of the lungs
   E. Treatment with isoniazid causes eye problems

7. Lung cancer:
   A. Is the most common cause of malignancy-related death in the UK
   B. Most commonly is an adenocarcinoma
   C. Never occurs in non-smokers
   D. Patients usually present with haemoptysis
   E. Patients always have clinical signs

8. In lung cancer:
   A. A Pancoast's tumour presents with pain in the chest
   B. Recurrent laryngeal nerve palsy is not a result of direct tumour spread
   C. Horner syndrome is associated with ptosis and a dilated pupil
   D. Spread to bone is uncommon
   E. Dermatomyositis may occur

9. In the treatment of lung cancer:
   A. Surgery is appropriate for most patients
   B. Radiotherapy is used for SVC obstruction
   C. Chemotherapy is most successful in adenocarcinoma
   D. A 20% 5-year survival is the norm for those with local disease only
   E. Radiotherapy is not used for palliation

10. In asthma:
    A. Airway hyper-responsiveness is a major feature
    B. Exacerbations are not precipitated by particular weather conditions
    C. Attacks can be precipitated by use of paracetamol
    D. Peak flow is elevated during exacerbations
    E. Intravenous magnesium sulphate is used for mild cases

11. In COPD:
    A. A common cause is α_1-antitrypsin deficiency
    B. Disease occurs in smokers
    C. A small volume pulse suggests CO_2 retention
    D. Stopping smoking will not improve prognosis in severe cases
    E. Home oxygen is used in patients with P_aO_2 <12 kPa

12. Obstructive sleep apnoea:
    A. Is treated with inhaled steroids
    B. Can present with morning headaches
    C. Commonly affects people with a low body mass index
    D. ENT assessment is rarely necessary
    E. Is treated with single lung transplant

13. Pneumothorax:
    A. Can be a complication of mechanical ventilation
    B. Leads to a dull percussion note on the affected side
    C. Is usually treated with chest drain insertion
    D. Always requires chest drain insertion
    E. Usually presents with haemoptysis

14. In cryptogenic fibrosing alveolitis:
    A. Coarse crackles are heard on auscultation
    B. Spirometry shows a reduced FVC
    C. There is a good prognosis
    D. Clubbing is not a clinical feature
    E. There is an association with Crohn's disease

15. Regarding occupational lung disease:
    A. In coal-worker's pneumoconiosis large round opacities are usually seen on the chest X-ray

B. Patients may qualify for industrial injury benefits
C. Mesothelioma usually occurs 5–10 years after exposure to asbestos fibres
D. The risk of lung cancer is not increased
E. Cigarette smoking in patients exposed to asbestosis only slightly increases the risk of bronchial adenocarcinoma

Extended matching questions

Question 1 Theme: Breathlessness
A. Adenocarcinoma of the lung
B. Asthma
C. Chronic obstructive pulmonary disease
D. Extrinsic allergic alveolitis
E. Cryptogenic fibrosing alveolitis
F. Mesothelioma
G. Heart failure
H. Iron deficiency anaemia
I. Pneumothorax

For each of the following questions, select the best answer from the list above:

I. A 23-year-old female has intermittent episodes of breathlessness and cough. She has a past history of eczema and her FEV_1:FVC ratio is reduced. What is the most likely diagnosis?

II. A 50-year-old male smoker who works on a farm presents with progressive increasing breathlessness and weight loss over 6 months. He has finger clubbing. What is the most likely diagnosis?

III. An 80-year-old female presents with episodes of breathlessness on exertion. She takes ibuprofen for joint pains and nifedipine for hypertension. She has normal pulmonary function tests and the PA chest X-ray is also normal. What is the most likely cause of her symptoms?

Question 2 Theme: Pneumonia
A. *Streptococcus pneumoniae*
B. *Mycobacterium tuberculosis*
C. *Haemophilus influenzae*
D. *Mycoplasma pneumoniae*
E. *Pneumocystis carinii*
F. *Staphylococcus aureus*
G. *Chlamydia psittaci*
H. *Legionella pneumophila*
I. *Coxiella burnetii*
J. *Influenza A*

For each of the following questions, select the best answer from the list above:

I. A 28-year old female who has previously been well and takes the oral contraceptive pill presents with a fever and a cough productive of rust-coloured sputum. A chest X-ray reveals a right middle lobe pneumonia. What is the most likely microbiological causal agent?

II. A 50-year-old male who is known to have HIV with a low CD4 count presents with a history of fever and breathlessness. The chest X-ray looks normal and there are few clinical findings apart from marked hypoxia. What is the most likely microbiological causal agent?

III. An 80-year-old female presents with fever and cough. She lives in an old people's home where there has recently been a flu outbreak. A chest X-ray shows right lower zone shadowing with an area suggesting a cavity. What is the most likely microbiological causal agent?

Question 3 Theme: Abnormal chest X-rays

A. Sarcoid
B. Goodpasture syndrome
C. Cryptogenic fibrosing alveolitis
D. Pneumothorax
E. Pneumocystis pneumonia
F. Extrinsic allergic alveolitis
G. Cystic fibrosis
H. Mesothelioma
I. Asbestosis
J. Tuberculosis

For each of the following questions, select the best answer from the list above:

I. A 20-year old student who has previously been well, takes a summer job on a local farm when she is travelling. Since she started working on the farm she has had a fever and malaise each afternoon but feels well again each morning. A chest X-ray shows fluffy nodular shadowing. What is the most likely diagnosis?

II. A 34-year-old female from South Africa who has been in the UK for 20 years saw her GP, with a troublesome cough. Her GP arranged a chest X-ray which has shown bilateral hilar lymphadenopathy. What is the most likely diagnosis?

III. An 82-year-old man presents with chest pain and cough. He lives in the East End of London and was exposed to asbestos during the war years. He has previously been told his chest X-ray is abnormal but not to be concerned. He completed a 4-week course of steroids for some arthralgia symptoms 1 week previously. A chest X-ray shows pleural plaques and a pleural effusion. What is the most likely diagnosis?

EXAMINING THE CARDIOVASCULAR SYSTEM

Position the patient:
- Position the patient at 30°–45° to the horizontal with the chest and upper body exposed. Remember to maintain the dignity of the patient.

General inspection

- Central cyanosis
- Cough or breathlessness
- Peripheral oedema
- Respiratory rate: 12–18 breaths per minute in adults
- Paraphernalia around the bed: ECGs/monitors/oxygen

Hands

- Peripheral cyanosis
- Nicotine stains
- Clubbing: congenital cyanotic heart disease, infective endocarditis
- Peripheral signs of infective endocarditis
  - Splinter haemorrhages and nail fold infarcts
  - Osler's nodes: painful red raised lesions
  - Janeway lesions: small, non-tender red lesions on the palms

Face

- Central cyanosis: blue lips and tongue
- Malar flush: red flush on cheeks ± bridge of nose in mitral valve disease
- Pallor
- High arched palate – Marfan's associated with aortic regurgitation

Chest

- Scars: sternotomy, pacemaker, mitral valvotomy
- Visible pulsations: ventricular heaves or apex beat

Radial pulse

- Heart rate – measure for at least 30 seconds

Rate
- Record the rate as beats per minute (be exact)
- Palpate both radial pulses (radio-radial delay – coarctation of the aorta or dissecting aortic aneurysm)
- Palpate radial and femoral pulse (radio-femoral delay – coarctation of the aorta)

Rhythm
- Irregular:
  - Atrial fibrillation (irregularly irregular – absolutely no pattern)
  - Multiple ventricular ectopics
  - Missed beats (heart block)

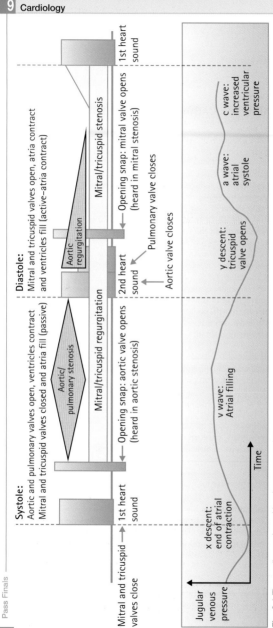

Systole:
Aortic and pulmonary valves open, ventricles contract
Mitral and tricuspid valves closed and atria fill (passive)

Diastole:
Mitral and tricuspid valves open, atria contract and ventricles fill (active–atria contract)

Mitral and tricuspid valves close → 1st heart sound

Aortic/pulmonary stenosis

Mitral/tricuspid regurgitation

Opening snap: aortic valve opens (heard in aortic stenosis)

2nd heart sound

Aortic valve closes

Pulmonary valve closes

Opening snap: mitral valve opens (heard in mitral stenosis)

Mitral/tricuspid stenosis

Aortic regurgitation

1st heart sound

Jugular venous pressure

x descent: end of atrial contraction

v wave: Atrial filling

y descent: tricuspid valve opens

a wave: atrial systole

c wave: increased ventricular pressure

Time

Fig. 9.1 The cardiac cycle and jugular venous pulse.

Character

(Table 9.1, Box 9.1)

Blood pressure

(Box 9.2)

Carotid pulse

- Feel each carotid artery separately
- Use fingertips along the line of the carotid

Jugular venous pulse (JVP)

See Fig. 9.1, Tables 9.2 and 9.3 and Box 9.3.

Table 9.1 The radial pulse	
Character of radial pulse	**Cause**
Low volume	Low BP
Low volume and slow rising	Aortic stenosis
Collapsing pulse	Aortic regurgitation
Pulsus alternans	Variable volume due to cardiac failure
Pulsus paradoxus	Volume reduces on inspiration in acute asthma
Pericardial effusion after asthma	

BOX 9.1. Collapsing pulse

- Raise the arm above the level of the heart
- Palpate radial or brachial pulse
- *Normal*: The pulse is felt normally at the radial pulse, diminishing a little as the arm is raised
- *Abnormal* (Waterhammer): Strong tapping pulse hitting the fingers at the radial artery

BOX 9.2. Blood pressure

- Use an appropriately sized cuff
- Apply the cuff 25 mm above the antecubital fossa and palpate brachial artery. Inflate cuff until pulsation not palpable, place the diaphragm of the stethoscope over the artery, then deflate at a rate of 2–5 mmHg/second
- When a sound is heard with each pulse (Korotkoff 1) this is the systolic pressure
- The point at which the sound disappears (Korotkoff 5) represents the diastolic pressure
- Record each to the nearest 2 mmHg

Table 9.2 Features which differentiate the jugular venous pulse from the carotid pulse

Jugular venous pulse	Carotid pulse
Double impulse	Single impulse
Falls on sitting and inspiration	No change with sitting and inspiration
Impalpable	Palpable
Fills from above if the internal jugular vein is occluded by light pressure at the base of the neck	Does not fill from above
Hepatojugular reflux – if pressure is put on the abdomen it increases venous return from the liver and the JVP becomes more prominent	No hepatojugular reflex
Obliterated by light pressure	Not obliterated by light pressure

Table 9.3 Causes of an abnormal jugular venous pressure

Right ventricular failure
Fluid overload
Tricuspid regurgitation (large V wave)
Pericardial effusion or restrictive pericarditis
Complete heart block (giant a waves (cannon wave) due to atrial
    contraction against a closed tricuspid valve)
Superior vena caval obstruction (non-pulsatile)

BOX 9.3. Jugular venous pulse

- With the patient at 45° turn the face to the left to relax the neck strap muscles
- Assess the internal jugular venous pulsation
- The height of the JVP is measured vertically from the sternal angle. Use a ruler or finger breadths to measure the height accurately
- The upper limit of normal is 4 cm

Apex beat (Table 9.4)

- Position in terms of intercostal space and mid-clavicular line
  - Normal: 5th IC space, midclavicular line
- Record the most lateral and inferior position of palpable beat

Reasons for failure to locate the apex beat
- Fat or muscular chest wall
- Left pneumothorax or pleural effusion
- Emphysema
- Pericardial effusion
- Dextrocardia

Table 9.4 The apex beat

Quality	Haemodynamics	Causes
Hyperdynamic (thrusting)	Volume overload	Aortic regurgitation Mitral regurgitation
Sustained (heaving)	Pressure overload	Aortic stenosis Hypertension
Tapping	Palpable first heart sound	Mitral stenosis
Dyskinetic segment		Left ventricular aneurysm

Precordium (Fig. 9.2)

- Palpate over each valvular area with the palm of the hand for thrills (palpable murmurs)
- Right ventricular hypertrophy may cause a sustained impulse (heave) at the left sternal edge
- Thrills – palpable heart murmurs (usually aortic stenosis)

Auscultation (Fig. 9.2 and Table 9.5)

- Listen with both the bell and the diaphragm to each valvular area
- Time any abnormal sounds with the carotid pulse

Heart sounds (Fig. 9.1)

S_1 Closure of mitral and tricuspid valves at the onset of systole

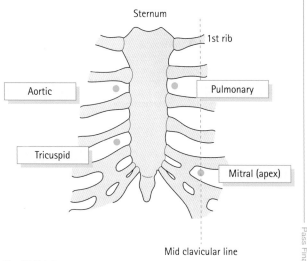

Fig. 9.2 Valvular areas.

Table 9.5 Cardiac auscultation

High-pitched sounds (diaphragm)
  S_1 and S_2
  Opening snap
  Ejection murmurs
  Early diastolic murmur of aortic regurgitation
Low-pitched sounds (bell)
  S_3 and S_4
  Mid-diastolic murmur of mitral stenosis

S_2 Closure of the aortic and pulmonary valves at the end of systole
- Aortic and pulmonary elements that may be separate:
  - Split S_2 normal in inspiration
  - Wide split S_2 in right bundle branch block and pulmonary stenosis
- Change in volume:
  - Loud S_2 in aortic stenosis
  - Obliterated S_2 in mitral regurgitation

S_3
- Occurs in early diastole and is due to rapid ventricular filling
- Normal in young people, or if the left ventricle is stiff
- Volume overload in mitral regurgitation, cardiac failure

S_4
- Occurs in late diastole due to ventricular filling in atrial systole
- Always abnormal due to reduced ventricular distensibility, e.g. aortic stenosis, acute myocardial infarction (MI)

Prosthetic valve sounds
- Mechanical valves make loud heart sounds often audible without a stethoscope
- Audible on closure:
  - Metallic aortic valve loudest at S_2
  - Metallic mitral valve loudest at S_1

Mitral valve
- Listen in the left axilla for radiation of mitral murmurs
- Turn the patient on to the left side and listen to the apex and axilla again in held expiration to accentuate quiet murmurs, e.g. mid-diastolic murmur of mitral stenosis
- If you suspect a mitral stenosis murmur, accentuate it with exercise (e.g. sit-ups)

Aortic valve
- Listen at the left sternal edge: sit the patient forward in held expiration to accentuate the early diastolic murmur of aortic regurgitation
- Listen for radiation of aortic murmurs to the carotids with the diaphragm followed by the bell for carotid bruits

Common murmurs
- Regurgitation murmurs occur when a closed valve leaks
- Stenosis murmurs occur when an open valve has a reduced luminal area
- Record grade of murmur (Table 9.6)

Table 9.6 Grades of cardiac murmur

Grade	Description
0	Not present
1	Barely audible. May be apparent is you are pre-warned that it is present and have 'tuned-in')
2	Quietly audible
3	Moderately well heard
4	Heard and thrill present
5	Loud, even if stethoscope partly off chest, with a thrill
6	Audible even if stethoscope is off the chest, with a thrill

Lung bases

- Sit the patient forward and listen at the lung bases for fine inspiratory crackles indicating pulmonary oedema

Abdomen

- Liver enlargement in right ventricular failure
- Pulsation of liver in tricuspid regurgitation
- Hepato-jugular reflux: pressure on the liver raises the height of the JVP
- Abdominal aortic aneurysm
- Aortic and renal bruits (auscultate in the midline and mid clavicular lines in the subcostal region)

Peripheral pulses

- Palpate:
  - Arm: Radial/brachial
  - Neck: Carotids (and listen for bruits)
  - Leg: Femoral/popliteal/posterior tibial (posterior to medial malleolus at the ankle) and dorsalis pedis (anterior aspect of the foot)

Peripheral oedema

- Check for dependent pitting oedema at ankles and sacrum

INVESTIGATIONS IN CARDIOLOGY

Chest X-ray (see Ch. 5)

- Heart size and shape
- Lung fields
  - Rib-notching in coarctation of aorta

Electrocardiography (Fig. 9.3 and Box 9.4)

- The electrocardiogram (ECG) is a recording of the electrical activity of the heart
- It is the vector sum of all the depolarization and repolarization potentials of all the myocardial cells

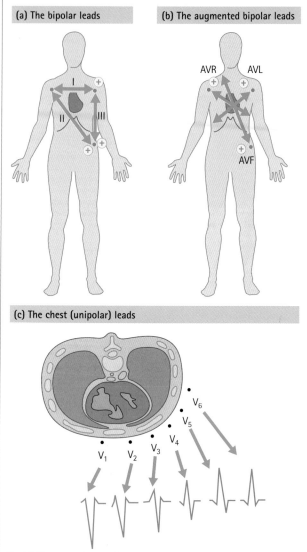

(a) The bipolar leads

(b) The augmented bipolar leads

(c) The chest (unipolar) leads

Fig. 9.3 The connections or directions that comprise the 12-lead ECG.

BOX 9.4. Performing an ECG

- Connect the ECG machine to a power point and switch on
- Connect the leads
- Limb leads
- Red to right arm
- Yellow to left arm
- Green to left leg
- Black (neutral) to right leg
- Chest leads
- V_1 Fourth intercostal space just to right of sternum
- V_2 Fourth intercostal space just to left of sternum
- V_3 Halfway between V_2 and V_4
- V_4 Fifth intercostal space left of mid-clavicular line
- V_5 On same horizontal as V_4 in anterior axillary line
- V_6 On same horizontal as V_4 in mid-axillary line
- Check that there is paper and that the paper speed is correct (25 mm/s)
- Ask the patient to keep still
- Press record/acquire ECG
- Label the ECG with the patient's name, and the date and time

Limb leads
- Six of the leads are obtained by recording from the limbs

Chest leads
- The other six leads record potentials between points on the chest wall and an average of the three limbs

Aspects of the heart (Fig. 9.4)
- V_1 and V_2 – right ventricle
- V_3 and V_4 – interventricular septum
- V_5 and V_6 – left ventricle
- Leads II, III and AVF – inferior aspect
- Leads I and AVL – lateral left ventricle

ECG paper
- Paper speed is 25 mm/s
- Therefore each small square = 0.04 s
- Each large square = 0.2 s

Normal ECG waveform and intervals
See Figures 9.5, 9.7.

Axis (Fig. 9.6)
- The normal axis of the heart is −30° and +90°
- Axis deviation can be identified by looking at the positive and negative deflections in leads I, II and III

Exercise ECG (Box 9.5)
- Assesses cardiac response to exercise
  - Treadmill or cycle ergometer

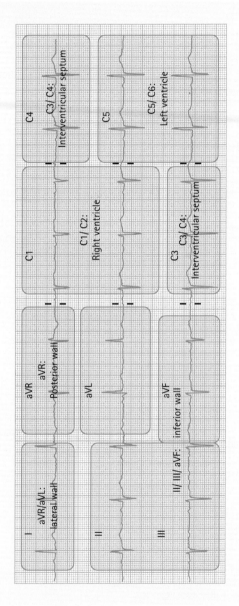

Fig. 9.4 Aspects of the ECG.

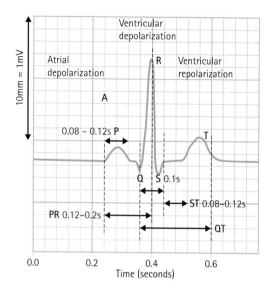

Fig. 9.5 Waves and intervals of the normal ECG.

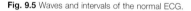

BOX 9.5. Procedure for exercise ECG

- Continuous recording of pulse rate and 12-lead ECG and intermittent BP recordings (every 60 seconds)
- The patient walks on a treadmill or cycles an exercise bike, slowly on the flat at first then graduating to high-speed walking (or running or cycling) on a gradient until a predesignated target heart rate (according to age) is reached or until symptoms or ECG abnormalities prevent further exertion
- The ECG is analysed for ischaemic changes

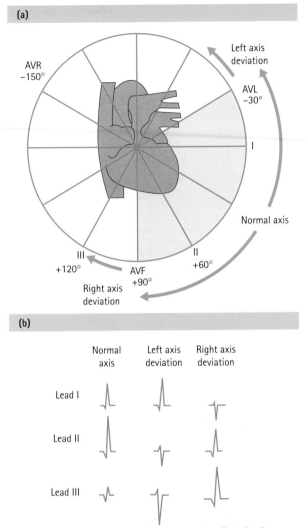

Fig. 9.6 The cardiac axis. (a) The hexaxial reference system, illustrating the six leads in the frontal plane, e.g. lead I is 0°, lead II is +60°, lead III is +120°. (b) Calculating the direction of the cardiac vector. In the first column, the QRS complex with zero net amplitude (i.e. when the positive and negative deflections are equal) is seen in lead III. The mean QRS vector is therefore perpendicular to lead III and is either −150° or +30°. Lead I is positive, so the axis must be +30°, which is normal. In left axis deviation (second column), the main deflection is positive (R wave) in lead I and negative (S wave) in lead III. In right axis deviation (third column), the main deflection is negative (S wave) in lead I and positive (R wave) in lead III. The frontal plane QRS axis is normal only if the QRS complexes in leads I and II are predominantly positive. *(Reproduced from Kumar P, Clark M. Kumar and Clark's Clinical Medicine, 8th edn. Edinburgh: Elsevier; 2012, with permission from Elsevier.)*

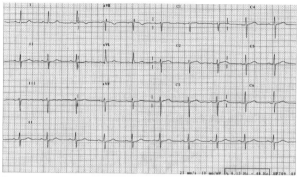

Fig. 9.7 The normal 12-lead ECG.

- Detects myocardial ischaemia (ST depression and T wave changes) during exertion
- May be coupled with stress echocardiography

Indications
- Investigation of chest pain
  - Sensitivity and specificity 70%
- Risk assessment after MI

Contraindications
- Recent MI or troponin positive ACS (within 1 week)
- Dynamic ECG changes suggestive of severe ischaemia
- Aortic stenosis
- Hypertrophic obstructive cardiomyopathy

24-hour ambulatory taped ECG

- 24-hour recording of ECG via a portable recorder
- Records transient changes, e.g. paroxysmal tachycardias or rhythm pauses
- Event recording can link symptoms to changes in the ECG

Echocardiography

- Non-invasive ultrasound examination of the heart
- Records dynamic anatomy of the four chambers and the valves
  - Wall movement abnormalities (hypokinesia when ischaemic)
  - Valvular stenosis or regurgitation
  - Heart valve vegetations (endocarditis)
- Doppler echo gives information about
  - Blood flow
  - Ejection fraction
  - Pressure gradients
  - Trans-oesophageal echo – higher resolution assessment of heart valves
  - Stress echocardiography – uses inotropes to induce ischaemia

Table 9.7 Functions of cardiac catheter

	Chambers and vessels examined
Direct pressure measurements	Right atrium
	Aorta
	Right ventricle
	Left ventricle
	Pulmonary artery
Indirect pressure measurements	Left atrium using pulmonary capillary wedge pressure
Blood sampling for P_aO_2	From all chambers to detect right to left shunts

Nuclear imaging (e.g. thallium scan, muga scan)

- Used to measure myocardial function and perfusion defects and position
- Detects reversible ischaemia, e.g. resting or stress-induced, and irreversible ischaemia, e.g. MI
- Useful in those with impaired mobility

Cardiac catheterization (Table 9.7)

- Uses intraluminal catheter inserted via peripheral blood vessel to perform pressure measurements and contrast imaging from within the heart chambers, great vessels and coronary arteries

Coronary angiography

- X-ray contrast medium is injected directly into the main coronary arteries via an intracardiac catheter

Indications

- Primary percutaneous intervention for ACS, e.g. coronary artery stenting/angioplasty
- Troponin positive acute coronary syndrome (ACS)
- Angina refractory to medical therapy
- Strongly positive exercise test
- Angina after MI
- Chest pain where cause is unclear
- Cardiac MRI
- Non-invasive imaging of heart structure

VALVULAR HEART DISEASE (TABLE 9.8)

Lesions of the heart valves that lead to dysfunction (either regurgitation or stenosis)

Mitral stenosis

Aetiology
- Rheumatic fever

Table 9.8 Typical ECG changes in acute MI	
STEMI	NSTEMI
Q waves	No Q waves
>1 mm broad and 2 mm deep	Deep ST depression
Negative deflection at start of QRS complex	T wave inversion
Normal in AVR and V_1	
ST elevation	
T wave inversion	

Clinical features

Symptoms Only occur in moderate or severe stenosis.
- Progressive breathlessness
- Paroxysmal nocturnal dyspnoea
- Orthopnoea } Secondary to pulmonary venous hypertension
- Haemoptysis
- Recurrent chest infections

Signs
- Mitral facies (malar flush – a cyanotic purple discoloration over the upper cheeks)
- Small-volume pulse
- Atrial fibrillation
- Tapping apex beat
- Loud first heart sound unless calcific mitral stenosis
- Opening snap (OS)
- 'Rumbling' mid-diastolic murmur at apex with the patient on their left, with presystolic accentuation (if in sinus rhythm)
- Signs of right ventricular failure (raised JVP, peripheral oedema)

Investigations
- Chest X-ray
  - Small heart with large left atrium (widened carina)
  - Convex left heart border
- ECG
  - Bifid P wave (P mitrale) or atrial fibrillation
  - Right ventricular hypertrophy (right axis deviation and tall R waves in V1)
- Echocardiogram
  - Reduced lumen area (normal =5 cm^2, severe = 1 cm^2)

Management

Medical
- Diuretics
- Digoxin for control of heart rate if in atrial fibrillation
- Anticoagulation if in atrial fibrillation

Surgical
- Non-responsive or severe disease
- Balloon valvotomy via femoral vein
- Closed valvotomy via the apex of the left ventricle
- Open surgical valvotomy

- Mitral valve replacement if:
  - Mitral regurgitation also present
  - Badly damaged valve leaflets
  - Left atrial thrombus resistant to anticoagulation

Mitral regurgitation

Aetiology
- Mitral valve prolapse
- Rheumatic heart disease (50% of all cases)
- Pre-existing aortic valve disease
- Acute rheumatic fever
- Infective endocarditis
- Ischaemic heart disease
  - Rupture of the cordae tendineae
  - Ischaemic cardiomyopathy
- Myocarditis/cardiomyopathy
  - HOCM
  - Dilated cardiomyopathy
- Autoimmune rheumatic disease
  - SLE
- Collagen synthesis disorders
  - Marfan syndrome
  - Ehlers–Danlos syndrome

Clinical features
Symptoms
- Palpitations secondary to increased stroke volume
- Pulmonary hypertension → dyspnoea and orthopnoea
- Reduced cardiac output → Fatigue and lethargy
- Right-sided heart failure

Signs
- Cardiac failure
- Apex: laterally displaced, hyperdynamic, systolic thrill

Heart sounds
- Soft first heart sound
- Loud pansystolic murmur at apex radiating to axilla
- Third heart sound

Investigations
- Chest X-ray
  - Left atrial and ventricular enlargement
  - Valve calcification
- Echocardiography
- Cardiac catheterization

Management
- Echocardiographic monitoring
- Endocarditis prophylaxis
- Surgery (valve replacement) if cardiac enlargement detected
- Symptomatic
  - ACE inhibitors, diuretics

Aortic stenosis

Aetiology
- Congenital (e.g. bicuspid valve)
- Rheumatic fever
- Calcific
- Non-valvular left ventricular outflow obstruction:
  - Hypertrophic obstructive cardiomyopathy (HOCM)
  - Congenital fibrous band above valve

Clinical features
Symptoms
- Often no symptoms until severe disease
- Exercise-induced angina, syncope, breathlessness
- Sudden death (usually within 3 years of symptom onset if not treated)
Signs
- Small-volume slow-rising pulse
- Sustained apex beat
- Systolic thrill in aortic area

Heart sounds
- Ejection systolic murmur in aortic area radiating to carotids
- Ejection click
- Soft second heart sound ± reversed split S_2
- Fourth heart sound

Investigations
- ECG – left ventricular hypertrophy/strain
  - Depressed ST segments and inverted T waves
  - Usually in I, AVL, V_5 and V_6
- Echocardiograph
  - Measures pressure gradient across valve
  - Gradient >50 mmHg suggests severe disease

Management
- Surgery – aortic valve replacement
- Avoid exercise
- Avoid vasodilators
- β-blockers for angina and palpitations

Aortic regurgitation

Aetiology
Acute
- Acute rheumatic fever
- Infective endocarditis
- Aortic dissection
Chronic
- Rheumatic heart disease
- Marfan syndrome
- Syphilitic aortitis
- Autoimmune rheumatic disease
  - Reiter syndrome
  - Ankylosing spondylitis
  - Rheumatoid arthritis
- Bicuspid aortic valve
- Severe hypertension

Clinical features
Symptoms
- No symptoms until left ventricular failure has occurred
- Palpitations
- Angina and dyspnoea

Signs
- Left ventricular failure
- Hyperdynamic circulation:
  - Pulsating nail beds (Quincke's sign)
  - Head nodding (De Musset's sign)
  - Collapsing/waterhammer pulse
  - Vigorous neck pulsation (Corrigan's sign)
  - 'Pistol shot' sound on auscultation of the femorals
  - Murmur over femorals (Duroziez's sign)

Heart sounds
- Apex (displaced laterally, diffuse, hyperdynamic)
- Soft high-pitched early diastolic murmur at left sternal edge
- Ejection systolic aortic flow murmur
- Austin Flint (mid diastolic) murmur – from mitral valve leaflets in severe AR

Management
- Surgery – valve replacement – best done prior to onset of heart failure
- Medical – treat heart failure

Tricuspid regurgitation

Aetiology
- Functional TR secondary to right ventricular dilatation (e.g. cor pulmonale)
- Infective endocarditis in intravenous drug users
- Pulmonary hypertension
- Carcinoid syndrome

Clinical features
- Exertional breathlessness
- Gastrointestinal upset secondary to congestion
- Elevated JVP with giant v wave
- Enlarged pulsatile liver
- Peripheral oedema
- Ascites
- Pleural effusions
- Right ventricular impulse at left sternal edge

Heart sounds
- Pansystolic murmur at lower left sternal edge, louder in inspiration

Management
- Medical – treat right ventricular failure
- Surgical valve resection – for infective endocarditis
- Valve surgery
- Valve repair
  - Maintains anatomy of heart muscle
  - Avoids anticoagulation

Tricuspid stenosis

Aetiology
- Rheumatic heart disease
- Women » men
- Carcinoid syndrome

Clinical features
- Almost always associated with another valve lesion
- Only when severe:
  - Hepatomegaly → abdominal pain
  - Ascites
  - Peripheral oedema

Heart sounds
- Low pitched mid-diastolic murmur

Management
- Diuretics
- Surgical valvotomy/replacement

Pulmonary stenosis

Aetiology
- Usually congenital
- Rheumatic fever
- Carcinoid syndrome

Clinical features
- Right heart failure → peripheral oedema

Heart sounds
- Harsh mid-systolic murmur

Management
- Diuretics
- Balloon valvotomy

ISCHAEMIC HEART DISEASE

Myocardial demand for oxygen/nutrients greater than delivery via coronary arteries.

Aetiology
- Occlusive coronary artery disease
  - Atherosclerosis
  - Thrombosis
  - Spasm
  - Embolus
  - Coronary arteritis, e.g. SLE
- Reduced oxygen delivery:
  - Anaemia
  - Hypotension
- Increased oxygen requirements
  - Thyrotoxicosis
  - Aortic stenosis

Risk factors for coronary artery disease
- Age
- Male sex (equalizes after the menopause)
- Family history

- Hyperlipidaemia
- Diet and obesity (30% of deaths are related to poor diet)
- Smoking (risk returns to normal 10 years after stopping)
- Hypertension (12–14% of deaths are HT related)
- Diabetes mellitus
- Hyperlipidaemia
- Newer risk factors
  - Sedentary lifestyle
  - Stress/depression/lack of social support
  - Binge alcohol consumption
  - High lipoprotein (a)
  - ACE gene deletion polymorphism
  - COX-2 inhibitors (e.g. rofecoxib)

Risk stratification and prevention

- Cardiovascular risk prediction
  - Established cardiovascular or peripheral vascular disease
  - Cholesterol >8 mmol/L
  - LDL cholesterol >6 mmol/L
  - BP >180/110 mmHg
  - Diabetes
  - Close relatives with early onset atherosclerosis

Angina

Clinical features
- Chest pain – heavy, tight, gripping
- Central, radiates to arms and jaw
- Breathlessness   } Exertional – relieved by rest
- Usually no clinical signs

Investigations
- Resting ECG (Table 9.9)
  - Normal
  - Evidence of previous acute myocardial infarction
  - Transient ST segment depression, T inversion
- Exercise ECG (ST depression >1 mm during exercise which reverts to normal – Fig. 9.8)
- Stress echo or nuclear imaging
- Coronary angiography and intervention

Pathology
- Myocardial ischaemia with reversible myocardial injury

Management
- Eliminate risk factors
  - Stop smoking
  - Treat hypertension
  - Optimize diabetes treatment
  - Treat hyperlipidaemia
- Aspirin to prevent progression
- Nitrates to reduce peripheral resistance
- β-blockers to reduce myocardial oxygen requirements
- Calcium channel blockers, e.g. amlodipine
- Potassium channel blockers, e.g. nicorandil

Table 9.9 The TIMI risk score in acute coronary syndrome (NSTEMI/UA)

Risk factor	Score
Age >65	1
More than three coronary artery disease risk factors – hypertension, hyperlipidaemia, family history, diabetes, smoking	1
Known coronary artery disease (coronary angiography stenosis >50%)	1
Aspirin use in the last 7 days	1
Severe angina (more than two episodes of rest pain in 24 hours)	1
ST deviation on ECG (horizontal ST depression or transient ST elevation >1 mm)	1
Elevated cardiac markers (CK-MB or troponin)	1

Total score	Rate of death/MI in 14 days (%)	Rate of death/MI/urgent revascularization (%)
0–1	3	4.75
2	3	8.3
3	5	13.2
4	7	19.9
5	12	26.2
6–7	19	40.9

(Reproduced from Kumar P, Clark M. Kumar and Clark's Clinical Medicine, 8th edn. Edinburgh: Elsevier; 2012, with permission from Elsevier.)

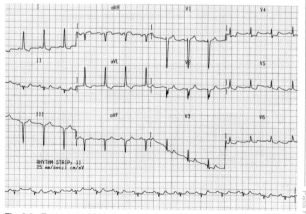

Fig. 9.8 Twelve-lead ECG in angina showing ST depression and T wave inversion.

- Revascularization
  - Percutaneous transluminal coronary angioplasty (PTCA)
  - Intracoronary stents
  - Coronary artery bypass grafting (CABG)

Acute coronary syndrome (Box 9.6)

- NSTEMI – non-ST elevation myocardial infarction
- STEMI – ST elevation myocardial infarction
- Unstable angina

Aetiology

- Coronary atheroma with overlying thrombus

Clinical features

- Chest pain
  - Severe
  - Sudden onset at rest
  - Persists several hours
- 'Silent' in 20%
- Sweating
- Breathlessness
- Nausea and vomiting
- Patient is pale, sweaty and grey
- Tachycardia

BOX 9.6. ACS – NSTEMI and unstable angina

Clinical features
- Pain at rest
- 'Crescendo' angina

Management
- Admission for bed rest with cardiac monitoring
- High-flow oxygen
- Aspirin 300 mg chewed stat then 75–150 mg daily

Pain relief
- Diamorphine 2.5–5 mg i.v. (plus antiemetic)

Anticoagulation
- Fondaparinux (Factor Xa inhibitor) or low molecular weight heparin subcutaneously to full anticoagulant dose, e.g. enoxaparin 1 mg/kg per day
- Continue aspirin 75 mg once a day and consider adding clopidogrel

Standard medical anti-anginal therapy
- β-blockers unless contraindicated
- Atenolol 50 mg orally
- Nitrates
- GTN i.v. infusion titrated to pain
- Isosorbide mononitrate 60 mg orally daily
- Consider – glycoprotein IIb/IIIa receptor inhibitors
- Prompt angiography and revascularization

- Heart failure
- Hypotension

Investigations

ECG See Figures 9.9–9.11 and Table 9.8.

Cardiac enzymes

- Troponin I or T peaks at 24–48 hours
- Creatine kinase (CK) peaks 24 hours after ACS
- Aspartate aminotransferase (AST) and lactate dehydrogenase (LDH) rise 2–5 days after MI

(a)

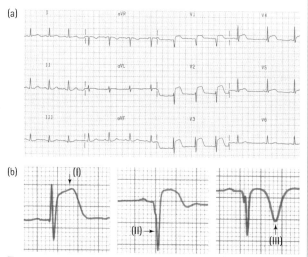

(b)

Fig. 9.9 Myocardial infarction. (a) Twelve-lead ECG showing full-thickness anterior MI with S–T elevation (STEMI). (b) Progressive ECG changes with time during an acute STEMI. ST elevation (I); Q waves (II); T inversion (III).

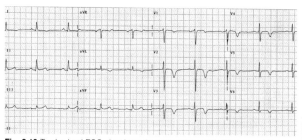

Fig. 9.10 Twelve-lead ECG showing subendocardial infarct. Widespread T wave inversion, no Q waves (NSTEMI).

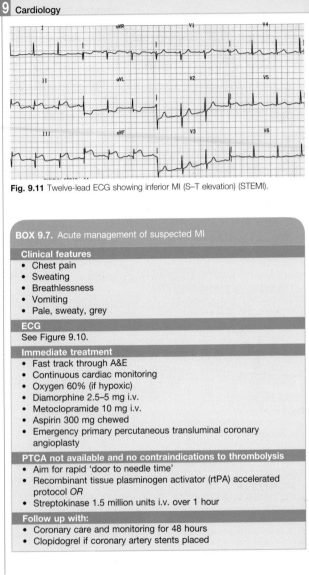

Fig. 9.11 Twelve-lead ECG showing inferior MI (S–T elevation) (STEMI).

BOX 9.7. Acute management of suspected MI

Clinical features
- Chest pain
- Sweating
- Breathlessness
- Vomiting
- Pale, sweaty, grey

ECG
See Figure 9.10.

Immediate treatment
- Fast track through A&E
- Continuous cardiac monitoring
- Oxygen 60% (if hypoxic)
- Diamorphine 2.5–5 mg i.v.
- Metoclopramide 10 mg i.v.
- Aspirin 300 mg chewed
- Emergency primary percutaneous transluminal coronary angioplasty

PTCA not available and no contraindications to thrombolysis
- Aim for rapid 'door to needle time'
- Recombinant tissue plasminogen activator (rtPA) accelerated protocol *OR*
- Streptokinase 1.5 million units i.v. over 1 hour

Follow up with:
- Coronary care and monitoring for 48 hours
- Clopidogrel if coronary artery stents placed

Assessment of infarct site
See Figure 9.4.

Assessment of prognosis
● TIMI score (Table 9.9)

Acute management
See Box 9.7.

Aftercare
Ongoing pain after thrombolysis
● i.v. β-blocker or nitrate
● Emergency angiography and revascularization
Pain-free with signs of heart failure
● Nitrate ± diuretic
● ACE inhibitor long term
Pain-free with no complications
● β-blocker long-term
● Return to work in 2–3 months
All patients
● Aspirin 75–150 mg/day
● β-blocker if no contraindications (maintain heart rate <60 b.p.m.)
● Statin
● ACE inhibitor (improves myocardial remodelling)
● Risk factor stratification
● Exercise ECG ± angiography
● Structured rehabilitation
● No driving for 1 month

Complications
Early
● Arrhythmias (ventricular tachycardia/AF/heart block)
● Sudden death
● Pericarditis
● Heart failure
● Cardiogenic shock
● Ruptured papillary muscle or chordae tendineae → mitral regurgitation
● Ventricular septal defect (VSD)
● Cardiac dilatation/rupture
Late
● Deep venous thrombosis (DVT), pulmonary embolism (PE)
● Mural thrombus
● Cardiac aneurysm
● Dressler syndrome (fever, chest pain, pericarditis secondary to autoimmune carditis)

Sudden cardiac death and acute life support
See Figures 9.12 and 9.13.

Prognosis
● 50% die acutely
● 6–7% die in hospital
● 20% die within 2 years
● 30-day mortality depending on other risk factors 1–35%

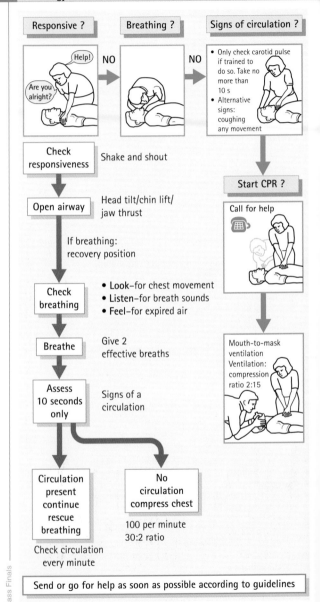

Fig. 9.12 Basic life support.

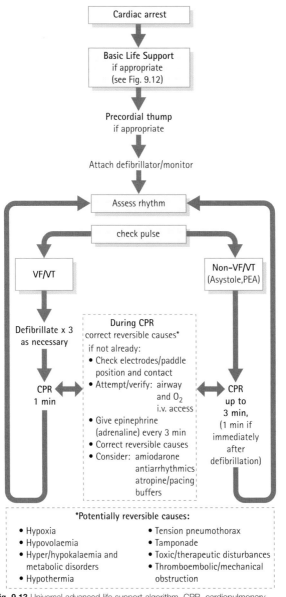

Fig. 9.13 Universal advanced life support algorithm. CPR, cardiopulmonary resuscitation; PEA, pulseless electrical activity; VF/VT, ventricular fibrillation/ventricular tachycardia. (Copyright European Resuscitation Council www.erc.edu – 2012/042, with permission.)

HEART FAILURE

- Occurs when the heart is unable to maintain sufficient cardiac output to provide a physiologically normal circulation

Pathophysiology
See Figure 9.14.

Aetiology
See Table 9.10.

Left heart failure

Aetiology
- Ischaemic heart disease (40%)
- Cardiomyopathy (35%)
- Hypertension (20%)
- Aortic/mitral valve disease
- Arrhythmias
- Congenital heart disease
- Pericardial disease

Clinical features
- Fatigue
- Exertional breathlessness
- Orthopnoea
- Paroxysmal nocturnal dyspnoea (PND)
- Pulmonary oedema → pink frothy sputum
- Distress
- Tachycardia
- Enlarged heart
- Gallop rhythm (triple fast rhythm due to third or fourth heart sound)
- Fine crackles at lung bases

Right heart failure

Aetiology
- Chronic lung disease = cor pulmonale
- Pulmonary emboli
- Pulmonary hypertension
- Left to right shunts
- Tricuspid regurgitation

Table 9.10 Causes of cardiac failure	
Myocardial dysfunction	High cardiac output
Ischaemic heart disease	Thyrotoxicosis
Cardiomyopathy	Anaemia
Hypertension	Paget's disease
Volume overload	Left to right shunts
Valve disease	Compromised ventricular filling
Fluid overload	Constrictive pericarditis
Obstruction to flow	Pericardial tamponade
Aortic stenosis	Altered rhythm
Chronic lung disease	Atrial fibrillation

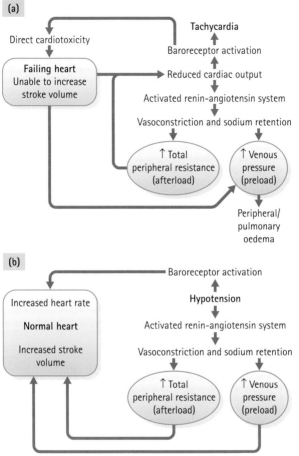

Fig. 9.14 Pathophysiology of heart failure.

Clinical features
- Tiredness
- Anorexia, nausea
- Gastrointestinal upset
- Raised JVP
- Dependent pitting oedema
- Pleural effusions
- Hepatic enlargement
- Ascites
- Functional tricuspid regurgitation

BOX 9.8. Acute pulmonary oedema

Clinical features
- Extreme breathlessness (often in middle of night)
- Wheeze
- Anxiety
- Cold sweat
- Cough with frothy pink sputum
- Grey and/or cyanosed
- Tachypnoea
- Peripherally shut down and cold
- Raised JVP
- Gallop rhythm
- Crackles and wheeze throughout chest
- Hypotension

Immediate investigations
- Chest X-ray – exclude pneumothorax
- Arterial blood gases – low PO_2, ± high PCO_2 ECG – arrhythmia

Immediate management
- Sit up
- High-flow oxygen
- i.v. furosemide (frusemide) 40–80 mg
- i.v. diamorphine 2.5–5 mg (not if BP <80 systolic)
- i.v. metoclopramide 10 mg
- i.v. GTN (if not hypotensive)
- Nebulized salbutamol 2.5 mg if bronchospasm

Investigation and treatment of cardiac failure

Investigations
- Chest X-ray
- ECG
- Serum BNP (if normal excludes heart failure)
- Echocardiogram
  - Left ventricular ejection fraction <45%
- Cardiac catheter and coronary angiography
  For management of acute pulmonary oedema, see Box 9.8.

Management
- Identify and treat lifestyle causes or aggravating factors
- Drugs
  - Diuretics (spironolactone, furosemide)
  - ACE inhibitors (reduce mortality)
  - β-blockers (reduce mortality)
  - Digoxin
  - Nitrates
  - Anticoagulation
- Surgery
  - CABG
  - Valve replacement
  - Pacemaker
  - Heart transplant

HYPERTENSION

Primary 'essential' hypertension

Aetiology
- Genetic
- Fetal (low birth weight)
- Obesity ± sleep apnoea
- Alcohol
- Sodium intake
- Stress

Secondary hypertension

Aetiology

Renal
- Diabetic nephropathy
- Renovascular disease
- Adult polycystic disease
- Chronic glomerulonephritis

Endocrine
- Conn syndrome
- Adrenal hyperplasia
- Phaeochromocytoma
- Cushing syndrome
- Acromegaly

Cardiovascular drugs
- Coarctation of the aorta
- Oral contraceptive pill
- Steroids
- NSAIDs/COX-II inhibitors

Pregnancy
- Second half of pregnancy
- Pre-eclampsia
- Hypertension and proteinuria

Clinical features
- Usually no symptoms
- Features of underlying cause
- Headaches
- Nose bleeds
- Nocturia
- Complications (see below)
- Elevated blood pressure
- Renal artery bruit
- Radiofemoral delay (coarctation of the aorta)
- Left ventricular hypertrophy

Retinal changes
- Grade 1 – tortuosity of retinal arteries and 'silver wiring'
- Grade 2 – grade 1 plus arteriovenous nipping
- Grade 3 – grade 2 plus flame haemorrhages and soft 'cotton wool' exudates
- Grade 4 – grade 3 plus papilloedema

Investigations
- Chest X-ray
- ECG (left ventricular hypertrophy and strain)
- Echocardiogram (left ventricular hypertrophy)
- Urinalysis for casts, protein and red cells
- Fasting blood glucose and lipids
- Serum urea, creatinine and electrolytes

Complications
- Cerebrovascular disease
- Coronary artery disease
- Retinopathy
- Renal disease

Management

General measures
- Weight loss
- Alcohol reduction

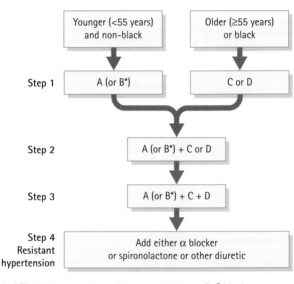

A: ACE inhibitor or angiotensin receptor blocker   B: β blocker
C: Calcium channel blocker   D: Diuretic (thiazide
                                                    and thiazide-like)

* Combination therapy involving B and D may induce more new onset
  diabetes compared with other combination therapies

Fig. 9.15 The British Hypertension Society Guidelines for combining blood
pressure lowering drugs. (Adapted from Williams B, Poulter NR, Brown MJ et al.
British Hypertension Society guidelines for hypertension management 2004
(BHS-IV): summary. BMJ 2004; 328:634–640.)

- Salt restriction
- Exercise
- Low fat diet
- Reassess after 6 months

Drug therapy See Figure 9.15 and Table 9.11.

Malignant hypertension

Clinical features
- Diastolic BP >140 mmHg
- Progressive renal failure, proteinuria and haematuria
- Cerebral oedema or haemorrhage
- Grade 4 retinopathy
- Hypertensive encephalopathy

Management
- Aim to reduce diastolic BP to 100–110 mmHg over 24–48 hours
- Oral treatment is usual
- In urgent situations, e.g. aortic dissection
- i.v. sodium nitroprusside or β-blockers

Table 9.11 Drug treatment of hypertension		
Class	Example	Side-effects
Thiazide diuretics	Bendroflumethiazide (bendrofluazide)	Hypokalaemia
Cardioselective β-blockers	Atenolol Bisoprolol	Bronchospasm Symptoms of hypoglycaemia Nightmares Cold peripheries Erectile dysfunction
ACE inhibitors	Enalapril Ramipril Lisinopril	Dry cough First-dose hypotension Renal function deterioration Hyperkalaemia
ACE II receptor antagonists	Losartan	
Calcium channel blockers α-blockers	Amlodipine	Erectile dysfunction
		Hypotension
	Doxazosin	Hypotension
Aldosterone antagonists	Spironolactone	Hyperkalaemia

CONGENITAL HEART DISEASE (TABLE 9.12)

- Affects 1% of live births ♂ >♀

Disease associations

- Maternal rubella infection
  - Patent ductus arteriosus
  - Pulmonary valve/artery stenosis
- Maternal drug/alcohol abuse
  - Septal defects
- Maternal radiation exposure
- Genetically inherited
  - Atrial septal defect
  - Congenital heart block
- Chromosomal abnormalities
  - Down syndrome → septal defects
  - Turner syndrome → coarctation of the aorta

Acyanotic – Left to right shunt

Ventricular septal defect (VSD)
- 1:500 live births

Clinical features
- Often no symptoms
- Fatigue
- Dyspnoea
- Loud pansystolic murmur at lower left sternal edge
- Thrill at lower left sternal edge
- Pulmonary hypertension

Table 9.12 Classification of congenital heart disease		
	Acyanotic	**Cyanotic**
	Normal or increased blood flow through lungs	Reduced blood flow through lungs
With shunts		
Presence of a bypass between heart chambers or great vessels	Atrial septal defect Ventricular septal defect Patent ductus arteriosus Partial anomalous venous drainage	Fallot's tetralogy Great vessel transposition Epstein's anomaly
Without shunts		
No bypass circuit	Coarctation of the aorta Congenital aortic stenosis	Severe pulmonary stenosis Tricuspid atresia Pulmonary atresia Hypoplastic left heart

Management
- Antibiotic prophylaxis for procedures
- Surgical closure

Complications
- Pulmonary hypertension
- Right ventricular hypertrophy
- Increased right sided pressures
- → right to left shunt: Eisenmenger's

Atrial septal defect (ASD)
Clinical features
- Usually none until adulthood
- Breathlessness
- Fatigue
- Right ventricular heave
- Loud pulmonary second sound
- Fixed splitting of second heart sound (A_2–P_2)
- Mid-diastolic murmur at left sternal edge

Management
- Angiographic transcatheter closure
- Surgical closure

Complications
- Pulmonary hypertension

Persistent ductus arteriosus
- Failure of closure of the ductus arteriosus
- → Shunt from aorta to pulmonary artery

Aetiology
- Idiopathic
- Prematurity
- Maternal rubella

Clinical features
- Left heart failure
- Congestive heart failure
- Infective endocarditis
- Continuous 'machinery' murmur
- May develop pulmonary hypertension (Eisenmenger's)

Management
- Surgical closure before pulmonary hypertension develops
- Angiographic ligation
- Aspirin
- Indomethacin in premature infants

Cyanotic – right to left shunt

Fallot's tetralogy
- VSD
- Overriding aorta
- Right ventricular outflow obstruction
- Right ventricular hypertrophy

Clinical features
- Breathlessness
- Fatigue
- Hypoxia on exertion – cyanosis ± syncope
- Squatting – to improve venous return and reduce shunt

- Right parasternal heave
- Systolic ejection murmur
- Central cyanosis
- Finger clubbing
- Polycythaemia

Management
- Surgical correction
- Antibiotic prophylaxis

Eisenmenger syndrome

- Reversal of shunt in large VSD due to secondary pulmonary hypertension giving right to left shunt and cyanosis

No shunt

Coarctation of the aorta

- ♂ > ♀
- Turner syndrome
- Associated with bicuspid aortic valve and aortic stenosis

Clinical features
- Hypertension in upper limbs
- Radiofemoral delay
- Mid to late systolic murmur over the back

Investigations
- CXR
  - Dilated aorta
  - Rib notching (due to large collateral arteries eroding ribs)

Management
- Surgical excision

INFLAMMATORY AND INFECTIVE DISEASES OF THE HEART

Acute pericarditis

- Acute inflammation of the pericardium
- Associated with a pericardial effusion

Aetiology
- Infective
  - Viral: Coxsackie/mumps/HIV
  - Bacterial: *Staphylococcus*/*Strep. pneumoniae*
  - Tuberculous
- Post-MI (acute in 20% of full-thickness anterior MI)
- Dressler syndrome (type 3 hypersensitivity 3 weeks after MI)
- Uraemic
- Malignant: metastatic > primary

Clinical features
- Chest pain
  - Substernal
  - Sharp
  - Worse on breathing
  - Relieved by sitting forward
  - Worse on lying flat

- Fever
- Malaise
- Pericardial friction rub (sounds like 'walking on snow')

Investigations
- ECG (widespread 'saddle-shaped' ST elevation)

Management
- Anti-inflammatory drugs
- Rest
- Treat underlying cause
- 20% recur

Pericardial effusion

Aetiology
Acute
- MI with ventricular rupture
- Aortic dissection
- Post-cardiac surgery
- Post-transseptal puncture at cardiac catheterization
Subacute and chronic
- Metastatic malignant disease
- Tuberculous pericarditis
- Dressler syndrome

Clinical features
- Raised JVP
- Kussmaul's sign (JVP elevates during inspiration)
- Pulsus paradoxus
- Failure to locate apex beat
- Quiet heart sounds

Investigations
- ECG (low-voltage complexes)
- Chest X-ray (large globular heart)
- Echocardiogram
- Pericardiocentesis for diagnosis and to treat incipient tamponade

Constrictive pericarditis

- Pericardial calcification or fibrosis

Aetiology
- Tuberculosis
- Haemopericardium
- Bacterial infection
- Rheumatic fever

Clinical signs
- Increased JVP during inspiration (Kussmaul's)
- Fall in JVP during diastole (Freidreich's)
- Fall is systolic BP during inspiration (pulsus paradoxus)
- Venous congestion → oedema/ascites/hepatomegaly

Investigation
- CXR: cardiac calcification in 50%/small heart
- ECG: low voltage QRS
- Echo

Myocarditis

Aetiology
- Viral
  - Coxsackie
  - Influenza
  - Rubella
  - Polio
- Protozoal
  - *Trypanosoma cruzi* (Chagas disease)
  - *Toxoplasma gondii*
- Toxins
  - Lead poisoning
  - Radiation injury
  - Drugs: methyl dopa, penicillins
- Bacterial infection
  - Diphtheria
  - Q fever
  - *Coxiella burnetti*
- Autoimmune disease

Clinical features
- Fatigue
- Palpitations
- Chest pain
- Acute cardiac failure
- Fever

Investigations
- Chest X-ray
- ECG
  - ST and T wave abnormalities
  - Arrhythmias
- Cardiac enzymes elevated
- Viral antibody titres
- Echocardiography
- Endomyocardial biopsy

Management
- Treat heart failure
- Treat underlying cause

Cardiomyopathy

Aetiology
- Dilated
  - Alcohol
  - Post-pregnancy
  - Hypertension
  - Valvular heart disease
- Hypertrophic
  - Familial/autosomal dominant
- Restrictive
  - Amyloid
  - Sarcoidosis
  - Endomyocardial fibrosis
  - Loeffler's endocarditis

Rheumatic fever

Aetiology
- Group A streptococcal infection

Clinical features (Table 9.13)
- General
  - Fever
  - Malaise
- Carditis
  - New or changing murmurs
  - Cardiac failure
  - Pericardial effusion
- Arthritis
  - Fleeting polyarthritis of large joints
- Sydenham's chorea (St Vitus' dance)
  - Choreoathetoid movements
- Skin
  - Erythema marginatum
  - Subcutaneous nodules (painless)

Investigations
- Throat swab
- Antistreptolysin-O titre
- ESR
- CRP

Management
- Penicillin to eradicate streptococci
- Bed rest
- High-dose aspirin
- Corticosteroids (prednisolone 60–120 mg/day)

Infective endocarditis (Box 9.9)

- Sometimes acute. Usually insidious (subacute)
- Most commonly affects rheumatic or congenitally abnormal valves, VSD or patent ductus
- Prosthetic valves may also be affected

Table 9.13 Duckett Jones diagnostic criteria in rheumatic fever

Two or more major *or* one major *plus* two or more minor *plus* evidence of recent streptococcal infection

Major	Minor
Carditis	Fever
Polyarthritis	Arthralgia
Chorea	Previous rheumatic fever
Erythema marginatum	Raised erythrocyte sedimentation rate (ESR)/C-reactive protein (CRP)
Subcutaneous nodules	Raised white cell count
	Prolonged PR interval

BOX 9.9. Duke's criteria for the diagnosis of infective endocarditis

- Diagnosis can be made in the presence of:
- 2 major criteria
- 1 major and 3 minor
- 5 minor criteria

Major	Minor
Positive blood culture:	Fever ≥38°C
Expected organism	Predisposing condition
Persistent positivity (3 of 3 or 4 cultures, separated by 12 hours)	Consistent but not diagnostic echo
	Immunological phenomena present (Roth Spots/ Osler's nodes/ glomerulonephritis/ rheumatoid)
Evidence of endocardial involvement:	
Echo: vegetation or abscess	Positive blood cultures
New valvular regurgitation	Vascular phenomena (arterial emboli/mycotic aneurysm/ conjunctival haemorrhage/ Janeway lesions)

Aetiology
- *Streptococcus viridans* (50% of cases)
- *Enterococcus faecalis*
- *Staphylococcus aureus*
  - Often acute
  - Associated with central venous catheters, temporary pacing wires and in i.v. drug users
  - Poor prognosis
- *Staphylococcus epidermidis*
  - i.v. drug users
  - Alcoholics
- *Coxiella burnetti* (Q fever)

Clinical features (Table 9.13)
[a]Seen in >50% of cases.
- General
  - Malaise[a]
  - Clubbing
- Cardiac
  - Murmurs[a]
  - Cardiac failure[a]
- Arthralgia
- Pyrexia[a]
- Skin lesions
  - Osler's nodes
  - Splinter haemorrhages
  - Janeway lesions
  - Petechiae[a]

- Eyes
  - Roth spots
  - Conjunctival haemorrhage
- Splenomegaly
- Neurological (cerebral emboli)
  - Mycotic aneurysm
  - Renal (haematuria[a])

Investigations

Blood

- Anaemia
- Raised serum CRP and ESR
- Mildly abnormal liver biochemistry
- Raised total serum immunoglobulins
- Raised total complement and C3

Urinalysis

- Proteinuria with casts
- Microscopic haematuria

Blood cultures

- At least six sets from different veins at different times (positive in 75% of cases)

Echocardiography

- Trans-oesophageal echocardiography (TOE) is best for visualizing vegetations and is mandatory in non-native valves

Management

Antibiotics

- Bactericidal antibiotics chosen on the basis of blood culture results and sensitivities
- i.v. antibiotics for 2–6 weeks with back-titrations to confirm bactericidal serum levels

Indications for surgery

- Significant extensive valve damage
- Early infection of prosthetic valve
- Persistent infection with negative blood cultures
- Embolization
- Progressive cardiac failure
- Tricuspid valve infection in i.v. drug users

Prophylaxis

CARDIAC ARRHYTHMIAS

- Bradycardia – heart rate <60 b.p.m.
- Tachycardia – heart rate >100 b.p.m.

Sinus arrhythmia

- Due to normal changes in autonomic tone
- Heart rate increases in inspiration and falls in expiration

Sinus bradycardia

Aetiology

- Hypothermia
- Hypothyroidism
- Raised intracranial pressure

(a)

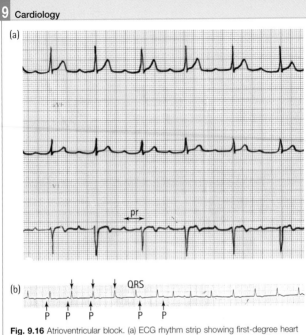

(b)

Fig. 9.16 Atrioventricular block. (a) ECG rhythm strip showing first-degree heart block with prolongation of the PR interval. (b) Complete heart block with dissociation of the P waves and QRS complexes.

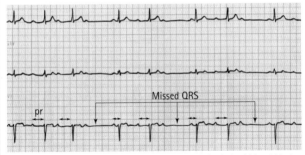

Fig. 9.17 ECG rhythm strip showing second-degree 'Wenckebach' heart block, with prolongation of the PR interval and missed QRS.

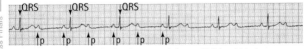

Fig. 9.18 ECG rhythm strip showing second-degree '2:1' heart block.

- Drugs (β-blockers, digoxin)
- Ischaemia

Sinus tachycardia

Aetiology
- Fever
- Exertion
- Emotion
- Pregnancy
- Anaemia
- Cardiac failure
- Thyrotoxicosis
- Drugs (sympathomimetics)

Sinus node disease (sick sinus syndrome)

Aetiology
- Ischaemia
- Infarction
- Degenerative disease

Clinical features
- Combinations of fast and slow supraventricular rhythms

Investigations
- ECG – long interval between P waves >2 seconds

Management
- Permanent pacemaker
- Antiarrhythmic drugs to combat tachycardia
- Anticoagulation

Atrioventricular block

First-degree
- Prolonged PR interval (Fig. 9.16)

Second-degree
- Some P waves conduct to ventricles
- Mobitz type 1 ('Wenckebach' – Fig. 9.17)
  - Progressive elongation of PR interval until failure to conduct
- Mobitz type 2
  - Dropped QRS conduction without progressive PR elongation
- 2:1 or 3:1 block
  - Every second or third P wave conducts to ventricles (Fig. 9.18)

Third-degree (complete heart block)
- No P waves conduct
- Ventricular rhythm is maintained by spontaneous escape rhythm from ventricular myocardium with broad complexes

Aetiology
- Ischaemic heart disease
- Cardiac surgery
- Dilated cardiomyopathy
- Drugs

Clinical features
- May be no symptoms (first- and second-degree)
- Dizziness

- Syncope
- Blackouts (Stokes–Adams attacks) (third-degree)
- Cannon 'a' waves in JVP in third-degree

Management
- Permanent pacemaker for symptomatic bradycardias

Bundle branch block

Aetiology

Right bundle branch block (RBBB – Fig. 9.19)
- Congenital heart disease
- Cor pulmonale
- Pulmonary embolus
- Myocardial infarction
- Cardiomyopathy
- Hyperkalaemia
- Can be normal

Left bundle branch block (LBBB – Fig. 9.20)
- Aortic stenosis
- Hypertension
- Acute MI
- Severe coronary artery disease
- Cardiomyopathy

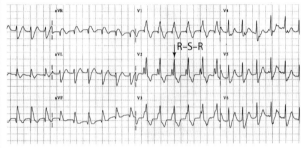

Fig. 9.19 Twelve-lead ECG showing right bundle branch block and right axis deviation.

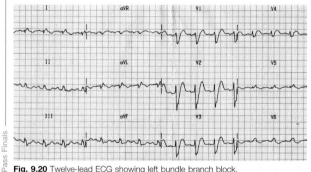

Fig. 9.20 Twelve-lead ECG showing left bundle branch block.

Management
- Permanent pacemaker for symptomatic cases

Atrial tachyarrhythmias

Aetiology
- Ischaemic heart disease
- Rheumatic heart disease
- Thyrotoxicosis
- Cardiomyopathy
- Wolff–Parkinson–White syndrome
- Pneumonia
- Atrial septal defect
- Pericarditis
- Pulmonary embolus

Atrial flutter

- Atrial rate about 300/min with 2:1 or 3:1 AV conduction

Investigations
- ECG (Fig. 9.21) – sawtooth atrial flutter waves between QRS complexes

Management
- Electrical cardioversion
- Class III antiarrhythmic drugs
- Radiofrequency catheter ablation

Atrial fibrillation

- Uncoordinated rapid continuous activation of atria from multiple foci

Aetiology
See above.

Clinical features
- No symptoms
- Reduced exercise tolerance
- Palpitations
- Heart failure
- Embolic events
- Completely irregular pulse

Investigations
- ECG (Fig. 9.22)
  - No P waves
  - Irregular rapid QRS rhythm

Management
- Treat the cause
- Control ventricular rate
  - β-blockers
  - Digoxin
  - Verapamil

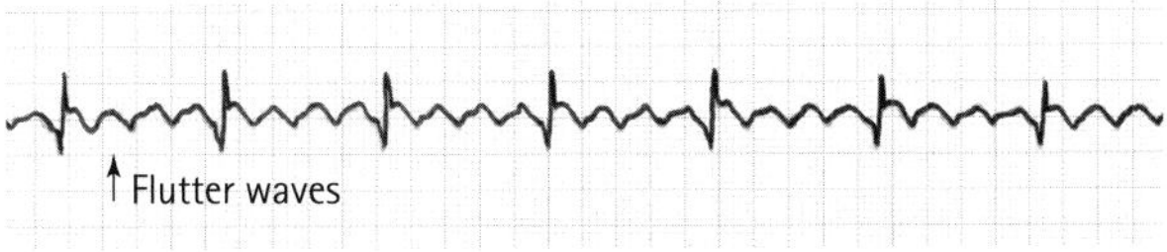

↑ Flutter waves

Fig. 9.21 ECG rhythm strip showing atrial flutter.

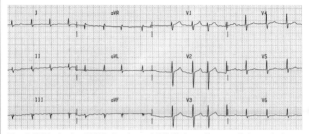

Fig. 9.22 Twelve-lead ECG showing atrial fibrillation with controlled ventricular rate (no P waves).

- Cardioversion
  - Electrical DC cardioversion
  - Drugs (amiodarone, flecainide)
- Prophylaxis against thrombotic events
  - Warfarin
- AV node ablation and permanent pacemaker insertion

Supraventricular tachycardia

- AV junctional tachycardias

Aetiology
- Provoked by
  - Exertion
  - Caffeine
  - Alcohol
  - β_2-agonists
- Congenital (re-entry tachycardias)
  - Abnormal conduction from ventricle to atria:
    1. Wolff–Parkinson–White syndrome
    2. Lown–Ganong–Levine syndrome

Clinical features
- Palpitations
- Chest pain
- Breathlessness
- Syncope
- Polyuria
- Rapid regular pulse 140–280/min

Investigations (Fig. 9.23)
- ECG
  - Narrow complex QRS tachycardia
  - Occasionally broad complex when associated with interventricular conductance disturbances

Management (Fig. 9.24)
- Vagotonic manoeuvres
- Carotid sinus massage
- Ocular pressure
- Valsalva manoeuvre

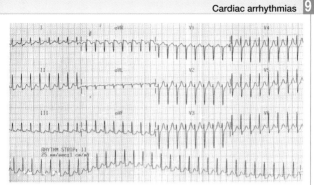

Fig. 9.23 Supraventricular tachycardia.

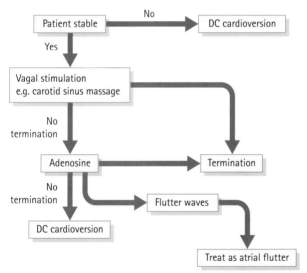

Fig. 9.24 Management of supraventricular tachycardia.

- Drugs
  - Adenosine in increasing i.v. doses with continuous rhythm monitoring (avoid in asthma)
- Prophylaxis
- Accessory pathway ablation

Ventricular tachyarrhythmias

Sustained ventricular tachycardia
- Rapid ventricular rhythm at 120/minute for more than 30 seconds

Clinical features
- Palpitations
- Dizziness
- Syncope
- Angina

Investigations (Fig. 9.25)
- ECG – broad complex tachycardia

Acute management
See Figure 9.26

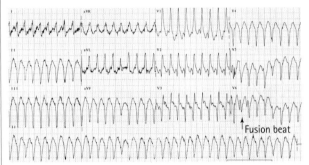

Fig. 9.25 Twelve-lead ECG showing ventricular tachycardia.

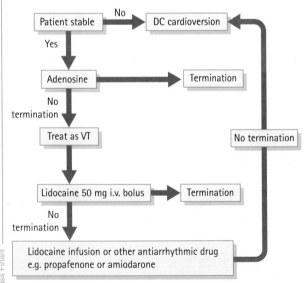

Fig. 9.26 Management of broad complex tachycardia.

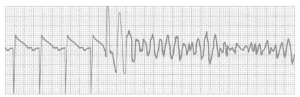

Fig. 9.27 Four beats of sinus rhythm followed by a ventricular ectopic beat that initiates ventricular fibrillation. The ST segment during sinus rhythm is elevated owing to acute MI in this case.

Long-term management
● Drugs – class III antiarrhythmics
● Accessory pathway ablation
● Implantable cardioverter defibrillator (ICD)

Torsades de pointes

Causes
● Congenital long QT
● Electrolyte disturbances
● Drugs

Investigations
● ECG VT with alternating polarity
● Prolonged QT

Management
● ICD

Ventricular fibrillation

● See Figure 9.27
● Pulseless rapid irregular ventricular activity with no mechanical effect

MULTIPLE CHOICE QUESTIONS

Multiple choice questions (single best answer)

1. Which one of the following is a feature of aortic stenosis:
    A. Collapsing pulse
    B. Pan-systolic murmur
    C. Syncope on exertion
    D. Austin flint murmur
    E. Opening snap
2. Which one of the following is a feature of mitral stenosis:
    A. Atrial fibrillation
    B. Thrusting apex beat
    C. Early diastolic murmur
    D. Loud second heart sound
    E. Sudden death
3. In mitral regurgitation:
    A. The pulse is characteristically collapsing
    B. There is an apical pansystolic murmur radiating to the axilla
    C. The ECG shows left ventricular hypertrophy

D. The commonest cause is hypertension

E. Atrial fibrillation is uncommon

4. In tricuspid regurgitation:
   A. There is a pansystolic murmur radiating to the axilla
   B. Pulmonary hypertension is a cause
   C. There may be pulsatile splenomegaly
   D. Cannon waves are seen in the jugular venous pulse
   E. Complete heart block is common

5. In acute myocardial infarction:
   A. The ECG always shows raised ST segments
   B. The pain is characteristically left-sided and worse on inspiration
   C. Diamorphine is contraindicated
   D. Creatine kinase levels are maximally elevated 2–4 hours after the onset of pain
   E. Treatment with streptokinase reduces mortality

6. The following are signs of congestive cardiac failure:
   A. Raised jugular venous pressure
   B. Splinter haemorrhages
   C. Splenomegaly
   D. Papilloedema
   E. Lymphoedema

7. In unstable angina:
   A. The most common heart rhythm is atrial fibrillation
   B. The ECG shows ST depression and T wave inversion
   C. Creatine kinase is elevated
   D. Treatment of choice is anticoagulation with warfarin
   E. 30-day mortality is 50%

8. In systemic hypertension:
   A. The commonest cause is renal artery stenosis
   B. Complications include diabetes mellitus
   C. Effective treatment reduces the incidence of stroke
   D. Presents most commonly with headache
   E. The first-line treatment is methyldopa

9. The following are usual features of tetralogy of Fallot:
   A. Episodes of cyanosis
   B. Atrial septal defect
   C. Ebstein's anomaly
   D. Normal life expectancy
   E. Right ventricular dilatation

10. The following are features of acute rheumatic fever:
    A. Recent staphylococcal throat infection
    B. Clubbing
    C. Roth spots
    D. Sydenham's chorea
    E. Osler's nodes

11. In acute pericarditis:
    A. The chest pain is characteristically crushing and radiates down the right arm
    B. The ECG shows widespread concave ST elevation
    C. There is usually pulsus paradoxus
    D. Viral infections are an uncommon cause
    E. High-dose prednisolone is the treatment of choice

12. The following are features of infective endocarditis:
    A. Spider naevi
    B. Osler's nodes
    C. Huntingdon's chorea
    D. Jaundice
    E. Past history of pulmonary TB
13. In patients with atrial fibrillation:
    A. The cardiac rhythm becomes more regular with exertion
    B. Common causes include rheumatoid arthritis and obstructive jaundice
    C. A fourth heart sound is always absent
    D. Digoxin should always be given
    E. Complications include stroke and mesenteric infarction
14. In supraventricular tachycardia:
    A. The onset is characteristically sudden
    B. The QT interval is prolonged
    C. Carotid sinus massage causes the heart rate to accelerate
    D. First-line treatment is atropine
    E. There is often underlying heart disease
15. The following are features of complete heart block:
    A. Syncopal attacks
    B. Giant V waves in the jugular venous pulse
    C. A delta wave on ECG
    D. It responds to an atrial pacemaker
    E. Shortened P–R interval on the ECG
16. Which one of the following criteria strongly supports the diagnosis of infective endocarditis?
    A. Positive Coxsackie virus serology
    B. Aortic sclerosis
    C. Temperature 37.5°C
    D. Positive blood cultures 12 hours apart
    E. Positional chest pain
17. A 56-year-old man was admitted with central chest pain. Which of the following is most effective in discounting ischaemic heart disease as a cause?
    A. Normal chest X-ray
    B. Normal ECG
    C. Normal creatine kinase
    D. Normal blood pressure
    E. Normal troponin I
18. A 66-year-old woman was seen with sudden onset central chest pain and widespread ST elevation on her ECG with a pulse rate of 50 b.p.m. What is the most appropriate management?
    A. Percutaneous coronary intervention
    B. Thrombolysis with alteplase
    C. Intravenous unfractionated heparin
    D. Oral indomethacin
    E. Oral atenolol
19. A 69-year-old man presents with an acute coronary syndrome. He is prescribed Fondaparinux. Which one of the following does fondaparinux?
    A. Glycoprotein IIb/IIIa
    B. Factor Xa

C. Vitamin K dependent clotting factors
D. Thromboxane A2
E. Endothelin

20. A 61-year-old man was found to have a blood pressure of 160/90 mmHg while being assessed for a colonoscopy. What is the most appropriate management?
   A. Delay the procedure until the blood pressure is controlled
   B. Carry out the procedure and advise him to consult his GP
   C. Give a single dose of bisoprolol to cover the procedure
   D. Start amlodipine orally
   E. Commence i.v. fluids during the colonoscopy

Extended matching questions

Question 1 Theme: Central chest pain

A. Reflux oesophagitis
B. Angina
C. Acute coronary syndrome
D. Dissecting thoracic aortic aneurysm
E. Mitral valve prolapse
F. Costochondritis
G. Gallstones
H. Duodenal ulcer
I. Pneumothorax
J. Mesothelioma
K. Pulmonary embolus

For each of the following questions, select the best answer from the list above:

I. A 20-year-old male with Marfan syndrome presents with severe chest pain at rest associated with nausea and shortness of breath. Blood pressure is decreased in the right arm compared with the left arm. What is the most likely diagnosis?

II. A 55-year-old male smoker with diabetes presents with a history of self-limiting central chest pain lasting 2 minutes, associated with nausea and shortness of breath which starts every time he plays football with his grandson. What is the most likely diagnosis?

III. A 45-year-old obese female smoker presents with episodic burning chest pain, worse at night and after spicy foods. What is the most likely diagnosis?

Question 2 Theme: Ankle swelling

A. Left ventricular failure
B. Cardiomyopathy
C. Deep venous thrombosis
D. Nephrotic syndrome
E. Cellulitis
F. Ruptured Baker's cyst
G. Liver failure
H. Gout
I. Charcot's joints

For each of the following questions, select the best answer from the list above:

I. A 60-year-old male alcoholic present with a 3-month history of swelling of the abdomen and ankles, and shortness of breath on exertion. On examination there are no signs of chronic liver disease. His pulse is 120/minute with atrial fibrillation and the apex beat is displaced laterally and inferiorly; he has ascites and ankle oedema. What is the most likely diagnosis?

II. A 70-year-old female with a history of myocardial infarction 10 years ago, and who returned from Australia 1 week ago, presents with swollen ankles, worse on the right, and shortness of breath on exertion. What is the most likely diagnosis?

III. A 50-year-old diabetic female on enalapril presents with a painful swollen right ankle which started 10 days ago. Examination reveals erythema and oedema, with a small painless ulcer on the right heel. What is the most likely diagnosis?

Question 3 Theme: Palpitations

A. Supraventricular tachycardia
B. Atrial fibrillation
C. Wolff–Parkinson–White syndrome
D. Anxiety
E. Thyrotoxicosis
F. Hypertension
G. Stokes–Adams attacks
H. Digoxin toxicity
 I. β₂-agonists
 J. Cocaine abuse

For each of the following questions, select the best answer from the list above:

 I. A 69-year-old female smoker being investigated for chest pains presents with sudden onset of rapid palpitations associated with dizziness and shortness of breath. Her pulse is irregular, rate 160/minute and BP is 90/60. The ECG shows no P waves. What is the most likely diagnosis?

II. A 68-year-old female recently saw her GP for wheeze and shortness of breath, and was prescribed some treatment. She now presents with episodes of dizziness, palpitations and tremor. On examination her pulse is regular, 130/min. The ECG shows a sinus tachycardia. What is the most likely diagnosis?

III. A 22-year-old law student presents with intermittent episodes of palpitations, shortness of breath and tingling in his fingers and round his lips. Examination is normal. Thyroid function tests a year ago (for similar symptoms) were normal. What is the most likely diagnosis?

EXAMINING THE ABDOMEN

Examination should include all of the following and be done in the following order:

Expose the abdomen

- Lie the patient flat for abdominal examination
- Pay attention to the dignity of the patient and cover/uncover as needed

General examination: hands/face/neck/thorax

Look for:
- Jaundice (Table 10.1)
- Weight loss/malnutrition
- Anaemia
- Stigmata of chronic liver disease (Table 10.2)
- Spider naevi – demonstrate filling from the central arteriole by pressing in the centre
  - >5 in men or 7 in women pathological
- Koilonychia – iron deficiency anaemia – concave nails
- Leuconychia – hypoalbuminaemia – white nails
- Lymphadenopathy – supraclavicular fossae (a node in the left fossa may indicate oesophageal or gastric cancer)

Table 10.1 Causes of jaundice

Pre-hepatic	Haemolysis	Autoimmune haemolytic anaemia Malaria
Hepatic	Abnormal bilirubin metabolism	Gilbert syndrome Benign recurrent idiopathic cholestasis (BRIC) Crigler–Najjar syndrome
	Hepatocellular dysfunction	Viral hepatitis Drugs Alcohol Autoimmune Pregnancy Infiltrations
Post-hepatic	Cholestasis	Primary biliary cirrhosis
	Biliary obstruction	Sclerosing cholangitis Gallstones Pancreatic carcinoma Cholangiocarcinoma

Table 10.2 Stigmata of chronic liver disease

Skin	Abdomen
Jaundice	Ascites
Spider naevi	Hepatomegaly
Caput medusae	Splenomegaly
Distended abdominal	**Eyes**
veins	Anaemia
Bruising	Jaundice
Striae	Xanthelasma
Hands	**Mouth**
Liver flap	Fetor hepaticus
Leuconychia	Bleeding gums
Dupuytren's contractures	**Genitals/breasts**
Palmar erythema	Gynaecomastia
Clubbing	Testicular atrophy/loss of body
Muscle wasting	hair

Abdomen

Look for:
- Shape of the abdomen and signs of distension
- Obvious masses
- Visible peristalsis
- Scratch marks due to obstructive jaundice
- Stretch marks
- Hernias (periumbilical, inguinal and femoral)
- Stomas
  - Bowel: ileostomy or colostomy
  - Urinary: ileal conduit
- Operation scars

Palpation

- Ask if the abdomen is tender and, if so, where
- Start palpating away from this point; always look at the patient's face during palpation
- Start gently, with the flat of the fingers, eliciting tenderness and obvious masses
- Palpate more deeply in an ordered way around the abdomen looking for deep masses
- Describe the location of findings as per the regions shown in Figure 10.1

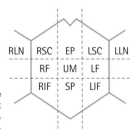

Fig. 10.1 Anatomical regions of the abdomen. EP, epigastrium; SC, subcostal; LN, loin; UM, umbilical; F, flank; SP, suprapubic; IF, iliac fossa.

Liver (Tables 10.3 and 10.4)

- The normal liver is only just palpable in slim people on inspiration
- Start from the right iliac fossa
- Use the pulps of the finger or the side of the index finger (with the hand flat)
- Ask the patient to take deep breaths in and out
- On inspiration the diaphragm flattens, pushing the liver down towards your fingers. Note the position of the lowest palpable point, e.g. 'three finger breaths below the costal margin'
- The upper limit is defined by percussing in the mid-clavicular line from the nipple and noting the boundary between resonance and dullness (normally the sixth intercostal space)
- Note any tenderness or palpable texture

Spleen (Tables 10.4 and 10.5)

- Start from the right iliac fossa
- Palpate towards the left hypochondrium
- The normal spleen is not palpable
- Ask the patient to roll onto his or her right side to bring the spleen forward, making it easier to feel
- You will not be able to feel the upper margin
- An enlarged spleen moves down and medially on inspiration and is dull to percussion

Table 10.3 Causes of hepatolmegaly

Infective	Metabolic
Acute viral hepatitis	Haemochromatosis
Epstein–Barr virus	Malignant
Malaria	Hepatocellular cancer
Kala-azar	Chronic leukaemia
Inflammatory	Secondary malignancy
Alcoholic liver disease	Cardiovascular
Primary biliary cirrhosis	Right ventricular failure
Infiltration	Tricuspid regurgitation
Amyloid fat	

Table 10.4 Causes of hepatosplenomegaly

Hepatic	Infection
Chronic liver disease with portal hypertension	Viral hepatitis
	Epstein–Barr infection
	Schistosomiasis
Malignancy	Infiltration
Leukaemia	Amyloid
Lymphoma	Sarcoid

Table 10.5 Causes of splenomegaly

Malignancy	Infective
Myelofibrosis	Malaria
Lymphoma	Kala-azar
Chronic myeloid leukaemia	EBV
Infiltration	Chronic liver disease
Gaucher's disease	Portal hypertension
Amyloid	

Table 10.6 Causes of enlarged kidneys

Bilateral	Unilateral
Polycystic kidney disease	Renal carcinoma
Hydronephrosis	Hydronephrosis
Amyloid	Large renal cyst

Table 10.7 Causes of ascites

Hepatic	Hypoalbuminaemia
Chronic liver disease (portal	Nephrotic syndrome
hypertension)	Protein-losing enteropathy
Peritoneal	Protein malnutrition
Peritoneal malignancy	Vascular
Infection	Hepatic vein thrombosis
Tuberculosis	Budd–Chiari syndrome

Kidneys (Table 10.6)

- Place your hand under the loin just below the level of the costal margin
- Use this hand to push the kidney up towards your other hand (balloting)
- If you are able to feel the kidney, just below the hypochondrium, it is enlarged
- You should be able to feel the upper pole of an enlarged kidney
- Always check for a transplanted kidney, usually in the right iliac fossa
- Check for an arteriovenous fistula (for haemodialysis) on the forearm

Ascites (Table 10.7)

- Eliciting shifting dullness is the easiest and most appropriate test

Shifting dullness
- Percuss the abdomen from the umbilicus laterally until the boundary between resonance and dullness is apparent
- Position your hand so that this boundary is between the middle and ring fingers of your splayed hand

- Ask the patient to roll towards you keeping your hand on the abdomen
- Allow the fluid to settle (at least 15–20 seconds), then percuss again to demonstrate that the boundary has moved

Fluid thrill

Do not do this in an exam unless asked to by the examiner.

- Ask the examiner or the patient to place the lateral aspect of his or her hand firmly on the abdomen in the midline, then flick or tap the lateral aspect of the abdomen with one hand
- The other hand is placed on the opposite side to detect the vibration

Hernial orifices

- Palpate the hernial orifices
- Ask the patient to cough and feel for an impulse
- Repeat with the patient standing

Tell the examiner

- That you would like to examine the genitalia, test the urine and carry out a rectal exam

GASTROINTESTINAL INVESTIGATIONS

Radiology

See Chapter 5.

Endoscopy

Video endoscopes are used to examine the macroscopic appearances of the GI mucosa; samples can be taken for histopathology, cytology and microbiology. Therapeutic procedures can also be performed:
- Dilatation and stenting (inserting tubes used to bypass obstructions) of strictures
- Injection of bleeding lesions
- Polypectomy/excision of tissues
- Insertion of feeding tubes, e.g. percutaneous gastrostomy feeding tubes

Gastroscopy

- Examines the oesophagus, stomach and parts one and two of the duodenum

Colonoscopy

- Examines the rectum, colon and terminal ileum
- Used for patients with positive faecal occult blood tests during colorectal cancer screening

Sigmoidoscopy

- Examines the rectum and sigmoid colon

Endoscopic retrograde cholangiopancreatography (ERCP)

- Outlines the pancreatic duct and biliary tree
- Useful to examine dilated pancreatic and bile ducts
- Can be used to remove gallstones from the bile duct

Enteroscopy

- Examines the stomach and proximal small bowel

Video (wireless) capsule endoscopy

- Swallowed capsule incorporating camera, light source and transmitter
- Allows for examination of entire small bowel mucosa
  - Anaemia/obscure GI bleeding – if gastroscopy and colonoscopy normal
  - Detect small bowel Crohn's disease
- Cannot be used to biopsy mucosa

Radioisotope studies

- ^{13}C urea breath test for *Helicobacter pylori* infection
- SeHCAT scan for bile salt malabsorption
- Gastric emptying
- White cell scan to look for inflammation/collections
- Meckel's scan
- Octreotide/MIBG scans to evaluate neuroendocrine tumours and metastases
- Red cell scan in obscure GI bleeding
- Hydrogen breath test for bacterial overgrowth

Stool tests

Microscopy and culture
- Infections

Faecal occult blood
- Used in population screening for colorectal malignancy

Faecal elastase
- Used to detect pancreatic insufficiency

OESOPHAGEAL DISEASE

Gastro-oesophageal reflux disease (GORD)

- Prolonged contact of gastric contents with the oesophageal mucosa
- Acid or bile causes mucosal irritation

Aetiology
See Figure 10.2.

Clinical features
- Retrosternal burning pain (heartburn)
- Can be worse during the night or when bending over
- Associated bitter taste in the mouth
- Sore throat/dysphonia
- Excessive salivation (water-brash)
- Nocturnal cough or bronchospasm (aspiration)
- Dysphagia (difficulty in swallowing)

Investigations
- Trial of antacid/proton pump inhibitor
- Upper GI endoscopy to look for oesophagitis
- Oesophageal pH studies and manometry (particularly if surgery to be considered)

Management
- Lifestyle changes: lose weight, reduce precipitants, e.g. smoking, alcohol

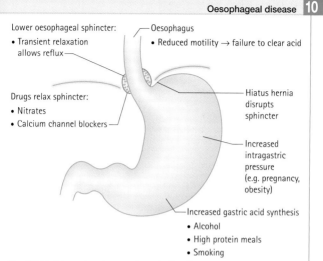

Lower oesophageal sphincter:
- Transient relaxation allows reflux

Oesophagus
- Reduced motility → failure to clear acid

Drugs relax sphincter:
- Nitrates
- Calcium channel blockers

Hiatus hernia disrupts sphincter

Increased intragastric pressure (e.g. pregnancy, obesity)

Increased gastric acid synthesis
- Alcohol
- High protein meals
- Smoking

Fig. 10.2 Aetiology of gastro-oesophageal reflux disease.

- Over the counter meds (OTC)
  - Antacids
  - Histamine$_2$-receptor blockers, e.g. ranitidine
- Proton pump inhibitors, e.g. omeprazole
- Prokinetics, e.g. domperidone
- (Laparoscopic) Nissen fundoplication

Complications
- Peptic oesophageal strictures
- Barrett's oesophagus

Hiatus hernia

See Box 10.1 and Figure 10.2.

Barrett's oesophagus

- Normal squamous mucosa is replaced with columnar epithelium with intestinal metaplasia as a consequence of severe GORD
- ♂ >> ♀
- 0.12–0.5% develop oesophageal adenocarcinoma per year
- Endoscopic screening/surveillance to detect dysplasia is controversial

Oesophageal carcinoma

- 40% squamous cell carcinomas
- 60% adenocarcinomas
- Prevalence: 10–15/100 000 and increasing

Clinical features
- Dysphagia: progressive: solids then liquids
- Weight loss
- Anorexia
- Lymphadenopathy

Investigations
- Upper GI endoscopy and biopsy
- CT scanning for staging
- Endoscopic ultrasound and PET scanning to stage, if CT shows lesion is not advanced

Management
- 10% 5-year survival
- Surgery gives best chance of cure but patients often present with advanced disease or poor performance status
- Neoadjuvant (preoperative) chemotherapy
- Chemoradiation (radiotherapy + chemotherapy)
- Radiotherapy for palliation
- Endoscopic palliation: oesophageal stents reduce dysphagia
- Palliative thermal ablation, e.g. laser

Achalasia

- Rare: 1 : 100 000 incidence
- Oesophageal aperistalsis and failure of relaxation of lower oesophageal sphincter
- → Dysphagia (intermittent to solids and liquids)

Investigations
- Barium swallow – shows the poor peristalsis and dilatation, swan neck deformity
- Endoscopy – to exclude malignancy
- Oesophageal manometry
  - Measurement of sphincter pressure (raised, non-relaxing)
  - Aperistalsis or non-propulsive contractions

Management
- Nifedipine or sidenafil can be tried but rarely give durable relief
- Endoscopic balloon dilatation of sphincter
- Injection of *Botulinum* toxin into sphincter
- Surgery (Heller's procedure: division of muscle)

THE STOMACH

Dyspepsia

- Symptoms referable to the upper gastrointestinal tract
- Heartburn
- Epigastric pain
- Discomfort or 'fullness' after eating/bloating
- Nausea

Alarm signals

- Dysphagia
- Weight loss
- Vomiting
- Haematemesis, melaena or anaemia
- Anorexia
- Previous gastric ulcer or gastric surgery

Epidemiology

- 80% of population get symptoms at some time

Aetiology

- Non-ulcer (functional) dyspepsia
- GORD
- Gastritis (NSAIDs, *H. pylori,* bile)
- Peptic ulcer disease
- Gastric malignancy

Investigations

- ^{13}C urea breath/serology/stool antigen test for *H. pylori*
- Upper GI endoscopy if alarm symptoms or if new symptoms over 45 years old

Management

- Treatment of cause, e.g. GORD, peptic ulcer
- Consider a trial of proton pump inhibitors if no alarm signals and age over 45

Peptic ulceration

- Breaches in the mucosa in the stomach or duodenum

Aetiology

- Gastric ulcers
  - *H. pylori* (60%)
  - NSAIDs and selective COX II inhibitors
  - Adenocarcinoma, lymphoma
  - Associated/worsened with steroids, bisphosphonates, chronic kidney disease, hypercalcaemia
- Duodenal ulcers
  - *H. pylori* (80%)
  - NSAIDs
  - Zollinger–Ellison syndrome

Clinical features

- Upper abdominal pain
- Pain at night or related to food
- Nausea
- GI haemorrhage (haematemesis or melaena)

- Anaemia
- Tender abdomen

Investigations
- Gastroscopy
- Testing for *H. pylori*
- Biopsy for histology (imperative for gastric ulcers to exclude malignancy)

Management
- *H. pylori* eradication therapy (proton pump inhibitor and two antibiotics for 7 days)
- Stop NSAIDs or other injurious agents
- Proton pump inhibitors for 8 weeks
- Follow-up gastroscopy at 6 weeks for gastric ulcer to ensure healing
- Non-healing ulcers should be treated surgically

Complications
- Haemorrhage → haematemesis/melaena
- Perforation → peritonism and air under diaphragm on chest X-ray
- Gastric outlet obstruction

Gastritis

- Inflammation of the gastric mucosa diagnosed histologically

Aetiology
- *H. pylori*
- NSAIDs
- Autoimmune (pernicious anaemia)
- Chemical, e.g. bile, alcohol

Management
- of cause e.g. *H. pylori* eradication, avoid NSAIDs

Upper GI bleeding

Aetiology
- Oesophageal or gastric varices
- Ulceration
- Mallory–Weiss tear (associated with vomiting)
- Malignancy

Clinical features

- Nausea
- Haematemesis
- Melaena
- Dizziness due to hypovolaemia
- Hypotension
- Tachycardia
- Stigmata of chronic liver disease
  - Splenomegaly
  - Ascites
  - Spider naevi
  - Caput medusae

  } Portal hypertension

Investigations
- Full blood count – low haemoglobin, high platelets
- Urea and electrolytes – high urea

- Liver biochemistry – abnormal in liver disease
- Coagulation – elevated prothrombin time
- Group and cross-match blood
- Gastroscopy to identify and treat cause

Management
- See Box 10.2
- 80% will stop spontaneously
- Gastroscopy
- Therapy depends on cause (see below)

Varices
- Endoscopic therapy
  - Elasticated bands around varices
  - Fibrin glue for gastric varices
- Non-endoscopic therapy
  - Vasopressin analogues, e.g. terlipressin
  - Sengstaken tube
  - Transjugular intrahepatic portosystemic shunt (TIPS)

Ulcers
- Endoscopic:
  - Adrenaline (epinephrine) injection
  - Clipping of bleeding vessel
  - Thermal coagulation
- Intravenous PPI infusions reduce re-bleeding following endoscopy
- Angiography and embolization of feeding vessel if endoscopy fails to find a source
- Surgery for uncontrollable bleeding

Gastric tumours: Adenocarcinoma

Epidemiology
- Incidence in men is twice that of women
- 15/100 000 men/year in UK
- Wide geographical variation, e.g. more common in Japan

Aetiology/associations
- H. pylori
- Smoking

- Alcohol
- High dietary salt
- Mediterranean diet may be protective
- Family history
- Pernicious anaemia
- Previous gastric surgery

Clinical features
- May be asymptomatic
- Abdominal pain
- Early satiety
- Weight loss
- Nausea and vomiting
- Upper GI bleeding
- Palpable epigastric mass
- Left supraclavicular lymph node (Virchow's)
- Enlarged liver due to metastases

Investigations
- Gastroscopy
- CT
- Laparoscopy } To stage tumour
- Endoscopic ultrasound
- PET scanning

Management
- Surgery for low-stage tumours
- Palliation for high-stage tumours
- Palliative chemotherapy/radiotherapy
- 10% 5-year survival

Stromal tumours

- GI stromal tumours (GIST) can occur anywhere in gut but most common in stomach
- May ulcerate → bleeding
- Treated with surgery or imatinib (blocks the activated receptor tyrosine kinase activity of c-kit)

Malt lymphoma

- Mucosa-associated lymphoid tissue lymphoma of stomach
- Associated with *H. pylori*
- 80% are cured by eradication of *H. pylori*
- 90% 5-year survival

SMALL BOWEL DISEASE

Coeliac disease

- Hypersensitivity to gluten in wheat, barley, rye → small intestinal inflammation

Epidemiology
- England 1:300; Ireland 1:100, can occur at any age, peak diagnosis is in 5th decade
- Caucasians mainly
- Family history 10–15% of first-degree relatives affected

Pathology
- → Subtotal villous atrophy (Table 10.8)
  - Loss of villi
  - Crypt hyperplasia
- → Malabsorption (Table 10.9)

Clinical features
- Abdominal pain
- Diarrhoea
- Steatorrhoea/malabsorption
- Weight loss
- Symptoms of anaemia
- Mouth ulceration
- Anaemia → pale conjunctivae (50% iron deficiency)
- Dermatitis herpetiformis (blistering rash on extensor surfaces)

Investigations
- Anti-endomysial antibodies ⎫
- Tissue transglutaminase ⎬ Negative after gluten-free diet
- Endoscopy and duodenal biopsy is the diagnostic test
- Full blood count
  - Anaemia (macrocytic or microcytic)
  - Hyposplenism, Howell–Jolly bodies
- Dexa scan

Disease associations
- Thyroid disease
- Diabetes
- Inflammatory bowel disease
- Primary biliary cirrhosis
- Autoimmune hepatitis
- Sjögren syndrome

Complications
- Ulcerative jejunitis
- Unresponsive coeliac disease – associated with enteropathy-associated T cell lymphoma (EATCL)

Table 10.8 Causes of villous atrophy

Coeliac disease	Infection enteritis in children
Whipple's disease	Kwashiorkor
Small bowel lymphoma	Cow's milk protein intolerance
Primary hypogammaglobulinaemia	Zollinger–Ellison syndrome

Table 10.9 Causes of small bowel malabsorption

Coeliac disease	Crohn's disease
Dermatitis herpetiformis	Whipple's disease
Tropical sprue	Radiation enteritis
Bacterial overgrowth	Giardia intestinalis
Intestinal resection	Lymphoma

- Oesophageal and small bowel carcinoma
- Osteomalacia and osteoporosis

Management
- Gluten-free diet
- Iron/folate supplementation
- Treatment/prevention of osteoporosis

Bacterial overgrowth

- Bacterial colonization of the small bowel
- Commonly *Escherichia* or *Bacteroides*
- → Bacterial consumption of vitamin B_{12}
- → Breakdown of bile salts
- → Bacterial synthesis of folate

Aetiology
- Small bowel structural abnormalities, e.g. diverticulum
- Strictures

Clinical features
- Diarrhoea
- Steatorrhoea

Investigations
- Lactulose hydrogen breath tests
- Low vitamin B_{12}
- High folate

Management
- Correct structural cause if possible
- Rotating antibiotics, e.g. tetracycline, ciprofloxacin or metronidazole

Whipple's disease

- Due to *Tropheryma whippleii*
- → Villous atrophy
- Diarrhoea and steatorrhoea
- Rare

Management
- Antibiotics

Small bowel tumours

- Lymphomas
- Adenocarcinomas (rare)
- Carcinoids

Carcinoid syndrome

- Occurs in only 5% of carcinoid tumours
- Due to serotonin (5-hydroxytryptamine, 5-HT), bradykinin and histamine secretion by liver metastases

Clinical features
- Flushing
- Diarrhoea
- Right heart failure
- Hepatomegaly
- Pulmonary valve stenosis
- Tricuspid regurgitation

Investigations
- 24-hour urinary 5-hydroxyindoleacetic acid (5-HIAA)
- CT or ultrasound of liver
- Octreotide-labelled scan

Management
- Octreotide to reduce symptoms
- Embolization of hepatic secondaries

INFLAMMATORY BOWEL DISEASE

Inflammatory diseases of the GI tract are of unknown aetiology. Both Crohn's disease and ulcerative colitis demonstrate a defective mucosal immune system producing an inappropriate response to luminal antigens which results in uncontrolled inflammation.

Crohn's disease

Epidemiology
- Prevalence = 50–60/100 000
- More common in Caucasian races
- Familial association
- Genetic predisposition

Pathology
- Any part of gut from mouth to anus
- Skip lesions – patchy disease with normal mucosa in between
- Commonly terminal ileum and ascending colon
- → Inflammation, ulceration, abscesses and fistulae
- Full bowel wall thickness involved
- Inflammatory infiltrates
- Non-caseating granulomata

Clinical features
- Depend on the area of bowel involved
- Mouth ulcers
- Diarrhoea
- Abdominal pain – colicky
- Nausea/vomiting
- Low-grade pyrexia
- Generally unwell, lethargy, weight loss
- Cutaneous fistulae (often perianal)

Disease associations (Fig. 10.3)
- Small joint arthritis
- Sacroiliitis
- Ankylosing spondylitis
- Iritis/uveitis/conjunctivitis
- Erythema nodosum – tender lower leg lesions
- Pyoderma gangrenosum – skin ulceration
- Sclerosing cholangitis

Investigations
- Blood tests: FBC, ESR, CRP, LFTs, Vitamin B_{12} and Red Cell folate,
- Colonoscopy and terminal ileal biopsy
- Small bowel imaging – MRI, wireless capsule endoscopy or Barium follow through (involves radiation)
- Faecal calprotectin can be used to detect disease activity

Management

- Induction of remission:
  - i.v. or oral glucocorticoids
  - Enteral nutrition
  - Azathioprine or 6MP (usually with oral glucocorticoids for first few weeks)
- Maintenance of remission:
  - 5-aminosalicylic acid (5-ASA), e.g. mesalazine for colonic disease
  - Azathioprine/6MP
- Treatment of therapy resistant disease:
  - Anti-TNF-a antibodies (infliximab and adalimumab)
  - Other biologicals in clinical trials
- Antibiotics for perianal disease
- Surgery for resistant disease but recurrence is inevitable

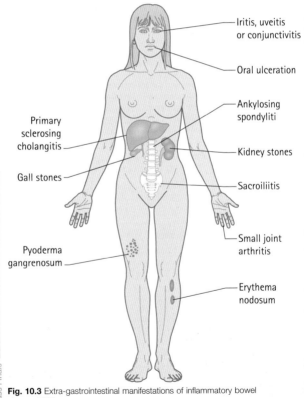

Fig. 10.3 Extra-gastrointestinal manifestations of inflammatory bowel disease (IBD).

Complications
- Vitamin B_{12} deficiency
- Short bowel syndrome after surgery
- Toxic megacolon in colitis
- Kidney stones
- Gallstones
- Malnutrition
- Osteoporosis
- Colonic cancer
- Venous and arterial thromboembolism

Ulcerative colitis

Epidemiology
- Prevalence = 80–120/100 000
- Uncommon in smokers

Pathology
- Limited to colon, inflammation spreads proximally from the rectum
- Mucosal inflammation → erythema, oedema and ulceration
- Microscopically → chronic inflammatory infiltrate, crypt abscesses, goblet cell depletion

Clinical features
- Diarrhoea
- Blood or mucus per rectum
- Mouth ulcers

Disease associations
- Uveitis/iritis/conjunctivitis
- Erythema nodosum/pyoderma gangrenosum
- Arthritis/sacroiliitis/ankylosing spondylitis
- Sclerosing cholangitis

Investigations
- Blood for inflammatory markers particularly CRP
- Stool cultures to exclude infection
- Plain abdominal X-ray for acute severe colitis to look for toxic megacolon
- Colonoscopy and biopsy

Indicators of acute severe colitis urgent treatment
- >Six stools per day with blood
- Fever >37.5°C
- Tachycardia >90 b.p.m.
- ESR >30 mm/h
- Haemoglobin <100 g/L
- Albumin <30 g/L

Management
- 5-ASA, e.g. mesalazine oral and topical, e.g. enemas or suppositories
- Steroids, e.g. prednisolone
- Azathioprine
- i.v. cyclosporin or infliximab for acute severe colitis
- Surgery for toxic megacolon, perforation, failure of medical therapy or malignancy
- Probiotics for pouchitis

> **BOX 10.3.** Toxic megacolon
>
> - Dilatation of the (transverse) colon with a high risk of perforation
> - Signs: fever, abdominal pain, bloody diarrhoea, tachycardia, hypotension
> - i.v. access and fluid resuscitation
> - Plain abdominal film to monitor colon diameter
> - Erect chest X-ray to rule out perforation
> - i.v. steroids and s.c. heparin
> - Early surgical involvement
> - Daily plain abdominal film
> - Intravenous antibiotics
> - If poor response to treatment → consider colectomy

Complications
- Toxic megacolon (Box 10.3)
- Iron deficiency anaemia
- Increased risk of colorectal cancer
- Thromboembolism

COLONIC DISEASE

Colorectal cancer

Epidemiology
- 1 in 27 of the population
- 10% are familial
- See Table 10.10 for other risk factors

Aetiology
- Genetic predisposition to promote accumulation of defects in growth regulating genes
  - *apc* gene mutation and loss
  - K-*ras* mutation
  - Smad2/4 loss
  - *p53* gene mutation and loss
- Microsatellite instability (failure of DNA repair)

Pathology
Adenomatous polyps → adenocarcinoma
- Most commonly in sigmoid colon or rectum
Microsatellite instability tumours
- Not associated with polyp formation
- More common in ascending colon and caecum

Familial cancers
Familial adenomatous polyposis (FAP)
- *apc* gene mutation
- → Multiple adenomatous polyps
- → Very high risk of malignant change
Hereditary non-polyposis colorectal cancer (HNPCC)
- Associated with microsatellite instability
- Associated increased risk of upper GI and gynaecological cancers

Table 10.10 Risk factors in colorectal cancer

Increased risk
  Increasing age
  Animal fat (saturated) and red meat consumption
  Sugar consumption
  Colorectal polyps
  Family history of colon cancer or colonic polyps
  Chronic inflammatory bowel disease
  Obesity (body and abdominal)
  Smoking
  Acromegaly
  Abdominal radiotherapy
  Ureterosigmoidostomy
Decreased risk
  Vegetable, garlic, milk, calcium consumption
  Exercise (colon only)
  Aspirin (including low dose) and other NSAIDs

(Reproduced from Kumar P, Clark M. Kumar & Clark's Clinical Medicine, 8th edn. Edinburgh: Elsevier; 2012, with permission from Elsevier.)

Clinical features
- Change in bowel habit to diarrhoea
- Rectal blood/mucus
- Asymptomatic with iron deficiency anaemia
- Population FOB screening

Investigations
- Full blood count – iron deficiency anaemia
- Colonoscopy
- CT colonography for failed colonoscopy
- CT to stage the cancer (Table 10.11)
- MRI to stage and plan treatment for rectal cancers
- Pet scanning with CT staging finds suspicious lesions

Management
- MDT approach
- Surgical resection
- Adjuvant chemotherapy
- Preop radiotherapy for rectal cancer

Complications
- Bowel obstruction
- Iron deficiency anaemia
- Hepatic metastases

Screening
- High-risk individuals (e.g. family history, previous polyps or cancer and ulcerative colitis)
- Population FOB screening

Diverticular disease

- Presence of mucosal pouches protruding outside the bowel
- Very common: 50% of those >50 years old

Table 10.11 Staging and survival of colorectal cancers

TNM classification			Modified Dukes' classification	5-year survival (%)
Stage I (N0, M0)	Tumours invade submucosa	T1	A	90
	Tumours invade muscularis propria	T2		
Stage IIA (N0, M0)	Tumours invade into subserosa	T3	B	70
IIB	Tumours invade directly into other organs	T4		65
Stage III (M0)	T1, T2 + 1–3 regional lymph nodes involved	N1	C	60
IIIB	T3, T4 + 1–3 regional lymph nodes involved	N1		35
IIIC	Any T + 4 or more regional lymph nodes	N2		25
Stage IV	Any T, any N + distant metastases	M1	D	7

(Reproduced from Kumar P, Clark M. Kumar & Clark's Clinical Medicine, 8th edn. Edinburgh: Elsevier; 2012, with permission from Elsevier.)

Clinical features
- 95% asymptomatic, incidental finding
- Erratic in bowel habit
- Left iliac fossa pain
- Acute diverticulitis
  - Severe left iliac fossa pain
  - Fever and tachycardia
  - Abdominal tenderness, guarding ± mass

Investigations
- CT

Management
- High-fibre diet
- Antibiotics for diverticulitis
- Surgery for complications

Complications
- Diverticulitis – inflammation/infection
- Diverticular abscess
- Lower GI bleeding
- Perforation

Functional bowel disease

- GI symptoms without an identified pathology
- Irritable bowel syndrome

Clinical features

- Left iliac fossa pain
- Alternating diarrhoea and constipation

BOX 10.4 Approaches to management of the irritable bowel syndrome (IBS)	
	Action
End organ treatment	
Explore dietary triggers	Refer to dietician
High-fibre diet ± fibre supplements for constipation FODMAP diet for bloating	Refer to dietician
Anti-diarrhoeal drugs for bowel frequency	Loperamide Codeine phosphate Co-phenotrope
Constipation	$5HT_4$ receptor agonist, e.g. prucalopride
Smooth muscle relaxants for pain	Mebeverine hydrochloride Dicycloverine hydrochloride Peppermint oil
Central treatment	
Explain physiology and symptoms	At consultation (leaflets with diagrams help)
Psychotherapy	Refer to clinical psychologist (see p. 1163)
Hypnotherapy	
Cognitive behavioural therapy	Refer to psychiatrist
Antidepressants	Functional diarrhoea – clomipramine Diarrhoea-predominant IBS – tricyclic group, e.g. amitriptyline Constipation-predominant IBS – SSRI, e.g. paroxetine
Alter the microbiota	Rifaximin has shown short-term benefit in IBS patients without Pro- and pre-biotics constipation (Target I and II trials)

(Reproduced from Kumar P, Clark M. Kumar & Clark's Clinical Medicine, 8th edn. Edinburgh: Elsevier; 2012, with permission from Elsevier.)

- Bloating
- Rabbit pellet stools
- Sensation of incomplete evacuation

Investigations
- Normal physical examination
- Rule out gynaecological problems
- Full blood count, CRP, TFTs and coeliac serology
- Gastroscopy and colonoscopy if atypical or alarm symptoms

Management
See Box 10.4.

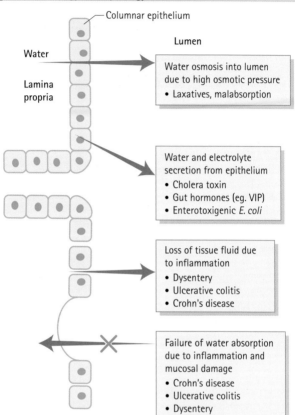

Fig. 10.4 Mechanisms of diarrhoea.

CHANGE IN BOWEL HABIT

Diarrhoea (Fig. 10.4)

An increase in stool weight to >250 g/day, usually associated with an increase in stool frequency.

Osmotic diarrhoea

Non-absorbable hypertonic substances in the bowel lumen
- → Osmotic pressure draws water into the bowel

Aetiology
- Purgatives, e.g. magnesium sulphate
- Malabsorption → solutes in the bowel, e.g. glucose
- Absorptive defects, e.g. lactase deficiency
- Diarrhoea stops when the patient stops eating or taking the purgative

Secretory diarrhoea

- Increased secretion and decreased absorption of fluid and electrolytes

Aetiology
- Cholera toxin
- *E. coli* heat-labile and stable toxins
- Hormones, e.g. vasoactive intestinal peptides
- Bile salts and fatty acids following terminal ileal resection
- Some laxatives

Inflammatory diarrhoea

- Mucosal inflammation → loss of fluid and blood
- May also → absorptive failure
- e.g. Ulcerative colitis, Crohn's disease, dysentery due to *Shigella*

Increased stool frequency: Abnormal GI tract motility

- Post-vagotomy
- Diabetic autonomic neuropathy
- Hyperthyroidism

Structural abnormalities

- Diverticular disease
- Colorectal carcinoma

Other

- Faecal impaction and overflow

Constipation

Aetiology
- Old age and immobility
- Low-volume/fibre diets
- Intestinal obstruction
- Colonic disease, e.g. colorectal carcinoma
- Hypothyroidism
- Hypercalcaemia
- Depression
- Parkinson's disease
- Spinal cord lesions
- Drugs
  - Opiates
  - Iron
  - Antidepressants
  - Aluminium antacids

Management
- High fibre diet and adequate fluid intake
- Bulking laxatives – fibre/bran
- Stimulants – anthraquinones (senna), bisacodyl
- Osmotics – magnesium sulphate/macrogols
- Suppositories – bisacodyl
- Enemas – phosphate

GASTROINTESTINAL INFECTIONS

A very common cause of morbidity and mortality, notably in the developing world.

Viral infections

Aetiology
- More common in children than adults
- Rotavirus → epidemic diarrhoea in children
- Noroviruses → epidemic diarrhoea and vomiting in children (also involve adults)

Management
- Supportive

Bacterial infections

Cholera
- *Vibrio cholerae*
- Faecal–oral transmission
- 'Ricewater' high-volume stools
- Secretory diarrhoea due to cAMP activation
- Treat with oral rehydration therapy
- Ciprofloxacin or azithromycin if severe

Salmonella
- *Salmonella enteritidis* and *typhimurium*
- Eggs and poultry products
- 2–3 days of diarrhoea and malaise
- Rarely bloody diarrhoea
- Treat with oral rehydration
- Complications – cholecystitis and chronic carriage with re-infection

Staphylococcus
- *Staphylococcus aureus*
- Toxin-related gastroenteritis
- Short-lived diarrhoea and vomiting

Escherichia coli
- ETEC (enterotoxigenic) → watery diarrhoea
- EIEC (enteroinvasive) → dysentery
- EHEC (enterohaemorrhagic) → haemorrhagic colitis ± haemolytic uraemic syndrome, associated with serotype O157:H7

Yersinia
- *Yersinia enterocolitica* and *paratuberculosis*
- Enterocolitis, terminal ileitis
- → Fever, diarrhoea and abdominal pain
- → arthritis and Reiter syndrome

Campylobacter
- *Campylobacter jejuni*
- Mucosal ulcer and inflammation, colitis
- → Diarrhoea ± blood, fever
- Cramping abdominal pains
- Self-limiting, use azithromycin if severe
- Complications – Guillain–Barré syndrome

Shigellosis

- *Shigella dysenteriae, flexneri, sonnei*
- Usually affects children
- → Fever, abdominal pain, watery diarrhoea

- → Bloody diarrhoea and abdominal cramps
- Treat symptoms; ciprofloxacin for severe cases

Bacillus cereus
- Toxin-mediated
- Short-lived vomiting
- 'Fried rice poisoning'

Clostridial infections

Clostridium perfringens
- Spores in food
- Watery diarrhoea and pain

Clostridium difficile
- A and B toxins
- Antibiotic associated diarrhoea, e.g. cephalosporins
- Pseudo-membranous colitis → Bloody diarrhoea
- Treat by stopping antibiotics; oral metronidazole or vancomycin

Protozoal infections

Amoeba
- *Entamoeba histolytica*
- → Dysentery and colitis, liver abscess
- Treat with metronidazole

Giardia
- *Giardia intestinalis*
- Diarrhoea and malabsorption (partial villous atrophy)
- Treat with metronidazole

Cryptosporidium
- *Cryptosporidium parvum*
- Water-borne
- Fever and diarrhoea
- Self-limiting, in HIV can be severe and protracted

Helminths

Nematodes
- *Strongyloides stercoralis*
- Hookworm (*Ancylostoma duodenale*)
- Roundworm (*Ascaris lumbricoides*)
- Threadworm (*Enterobius vermicularis*)

Trematodes
- Schistosomiasis

Cestodes
- Tapeworms (*Taenia saginata/solium*)

PANCREATIC DISEASE

Acute pancreatitis

- Acute inflammation of the pancreas

Aetiology
- Alcohol
- Gallstones

Table 10.12 Causes of a raised serum amylase

Pancreatic	Hepatic
Acute/chronic pancreatitis	Gallstones
	Acute hepatitis
Pseudocysts	Salivary
Carcinoma	Adenitis, tumours, mumps
Abdominal	Others
Perforation, duodenal ulcer	Diabetic ketoacidosis
	Alcohol
Ectopic pregnancy	Anorexia
Ovarian tumours	Burns

- Infections, e.g. mumps, coxsackie B
- Pancreatic tumours
- Drugs, e.g. azathioprine, steroids, oral contraceptive
- Iatrogenic, e.g. post-ERCP
- Hyperlipidaemia
- Other
  - Trauma
  - Cardiac surgery
  - Scorpion bites
- Idiopathic

Clinical features
- Abdominal pain radiating to back
- Nausea and vomiting
- Abdominal tenderness and guarding
- Flank bruising (Cullen and Grey–Turner signs) if severe necrotizing

Investigations
- Amylase – elevated greater than 3 times (Table 10.12)
- Plain abdominal X-ray – pancreatic calcification suggests previous chronic disease
- CRP, full blood count, urea and electrolytes, liver function tests, calcium, glucose and blood gases for baseline and at 24 and 48 hours monitoring of severity
- Ultrasound – to diagnose gallstones
- CT at 72 hours to assess pancreatic necrosis for prognosis and look for complications
- MRI useful to see if a mass is solid or liquid

Management
- Oxygen requirements determined by ABGs
- i.v. fluids
- NG tube for suction if abdominal distension
- i.v. antibiotics
- Analgesia
- Feeding – usually enterally NG or NJ
- Early ERCP for obstructing gallstones

Complications
- Sepsis
- Multi-organ failure

Table 10.13 Poor prognostic indicators in acute pancreatitis in the first 48 hours

Age	>55 years
WCC	$>15 \times 10^9$/mL
Glucose	>10 mmol/L
Urea	>16 mmol/L
Albumin	<30 g/L
ALT	>200 U/L
Calcium	<2 mmol/L
LDH	>600 IU
P_aO_2	<8 kPa

- Hypocalcaemia (fat saponification)
- Pseudocyst formation

Prognosis
See Table 10.13.

Chronic pancreatitis

- Long-standing or repeated attacks of pancreatitis resulting in fibrosis

Aetiology
- Alcohol
- Autoimmune pancreatitis
- Hereditary, e.g. cystic fibrosis
- Tropical
- Hypercalcaemia

Clinical features
- Chronic abdominal pain
- Weight loss
- Exocrine or endocrine deficiency
- Steatorrhoea

Investigations
- Amylase is usually normal
- Plain abdominal X-ray or ultrasound shows pancreatic calcification
- Faecal elastase
- Blood sugar – elevated due to diabetes
- CT scan and MRCP

Management
- Analgesia
- Treatment of steatorrhoea with pancreatic enzymes
- Treatment of diabetes

Pancreatic malignancy

- Majority are adenocarcinomas
- Often present late and so have poor prognosis

Clinical features

- Painless jaundice – bile duct compression
- Anorexia
- Weight loss

Investigations

- Ultrasound to assess biliary obstruction
- CT to stage for operability
- ERCP for cytology
- MRI/endoscopic ultrasound
- Percutaneous biopsy if not operable and chemotherapy possible

Management

- ERCP stenting to relieve jaundice
- Surgical resection of primary (only 20% cases operable)
- Chemotherapy 5FU and gemcitabine
- Palliative care

Pancreatic neuroendocrine tumours

- Gastrinomas and rarely other hormone-secreting tumours (e.g. insulinomas)
- Symptoms depend on hormone secreted

Zollinger–Ellison syndrome

- Gastrin-secreting tumour
- → High gastric acid secretion
- → Multiple gastroduodenal ulcers
- Diarrhoea

JAUNDICE

See Table 10.1 and Figure 10.5.

HEPATITIS (TABLE 10.14)

Acute hepatocyte breakdown leading to release of aminotransferases (ALT, AST) and jaundice. Prolonged or severe damage results in synthetic failure, leading to a reduction in the synthesis of albumin and clotting factors (causing an elevated prothrombin time).

Causes

- Viral hepatitis
- Drugs (Table 10.14)
- Autoimmune hepatitis

Table 10.14 Causes of chronic hepatitis	
Viruses	Hereditary
Hepatitis B ± D	Haemochromatosis
Hepatitis C	α_1-antitrypsin disease
Autoimmune hepatitis	Wilson's disease
Drugs	Others
Methyldopa	Alcohol
Isoniazid	

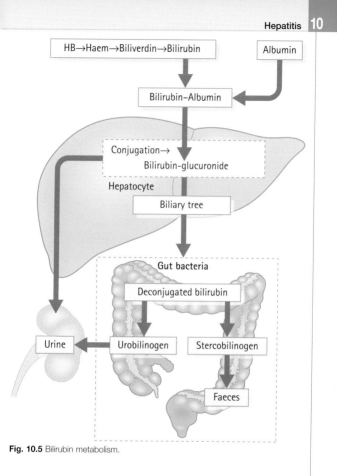

Fig. 10.5 Bilirubin metabolism.

- Alcohol
- Haemochromatosis
- Wilson's disease

Viral hepatitis

Hepatitis A (HAV) RNA virus
- Faecal–oral spread (e.g. shellfish)
- Incubation 2–3 weeks
- No progression → chronic liver disease

Clinical features
- Nausea
- Anorexia
- Jaundice ± hepatomegaly/rash

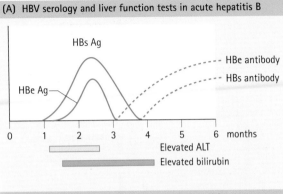

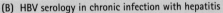

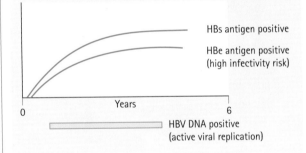

Fig. 10.6 Hepatitis B. (a) HBV serology and liver biochemistry in acute hepatitis B. (b) HBV serology in chronic infection with hepatitis.

Investigations
- Anti-HAV IgM
- Elevated ALT/aspartate aminotransferase (AST)
- Elevated bilirubin (may be subclinical)

Management
- Supportive

Hepatitis B (HBV) DNA virus (Figs 10.6, 10.7)
- Blood/saliva/sexual/vertical spread
- Incubation 1–5 months
- 10–15% carriage in Africa and Far East

Clinical features
- Jaundice/malaise ± rash
- May be asymptomatic

Investigations (Fig. 10.6)
- Liver biochemistry – ALT elevated first then bilirubin

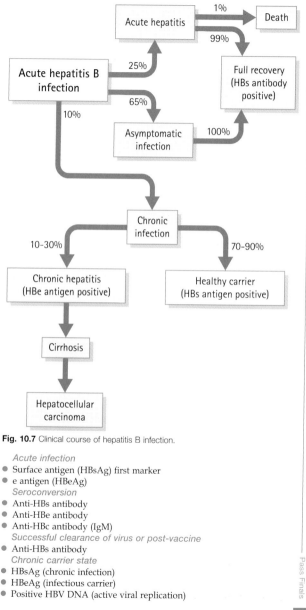

Fig. 10.7 Clinical course of hepatitis B infection.

Acute infection
- Surface antigen (HBsAg) first marker
- e antigen (HBeAg)
Seroconversion
- Anti-HBs antibody
- Anti-HBe antibody
- Anti-HBc antibody (IgM)
Successful clearance of virus or post-vaccine
- Anti-HBs antibody
Chronic carrier state
- HBsAg (chronic infection)
- HBeAg (infectious carrier)
- Positive HBV DNA (active viral replication)

Management
- Treat symptoms in acute infection and monitor viral markers
- Antivirals for chronic infection: interferon, lamivudine, adefovir, entecavir and tenofovir

Complications
- Chronic infection → chronic liver disease
- Hepatocellular carcinoma
- 1% → fulminant acute hepatitis → death

Hepatitis D
- Only causes hepatitis when it co-infects with hepatitis B
- Commonest in i.v. drug abusers
- Diagnosis by detection of specific antibodies

Hepatitis C (HCV; Fig. 10.8)
- RNA virus
- Blood spread (rarely sex/saliva)
- Acute infection often asymptomatic
- 80% → chronic liver disease
- 30% of these → cirrhosis
- 5% of these → hepatocellular carcinoma

Investigations
- Anti-HCV antibodies
- HCV RNA in blood

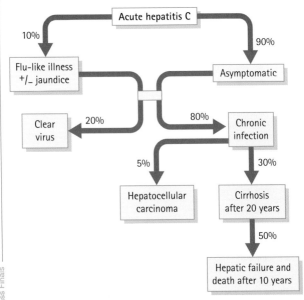

Fig. 10.8 Clinical course of hepatitis C infection.

- Abnormal liver function in chronic infection
- Ultrasound and α-fetoprotein to detect hepatocellular carcinoma

Management
- Antivirals, e.g. interferon and ribavirin to clear the virus
- Newer antiviral agents have better efficacy, e.g. telapravir, bocepravir
- Efficacy depends on genotype
- Liver transplantation is considered for those with decompensated cirrhosis

Others
- Hepatitis E (1–2% mortality in pregnancy)
- Epstein–Barr virus (EBV)
- Cytomegalovirus (CMV)
- Yellow fever

Autoimmune hepatitis

Epidemiology
- ♀ > ♂
- Associated with other autoimmune disease, e.g. thyroid, diabetes

Clinical features
- May be asymptomatic
- Jaundice
- Bruising
- Signs of acute or chronic liver disease

Investigations
- Antinuclear antibodies
  - Anti-smooth muscle antibodies Type I
- Anti-soluble liver antigen antibodies
  - Anti-liver/kidney microsomal antibodies Type II

Management
- Steroids/azathioprine

Fulminant hepatic failure

Aetiology
- Hepatitis A B (D) and E
- Drugs, e.g.
  - Paracetamol
  - Volatile liquid anaesthetics
  - Isoniazid
  - Ecstasy
- Wilson's disease
- Pregnancy
- Reye syndrome
- Budd–Chiari
- Autoimmune hepatitis

Clinical features
- Jaundice
- Encephalopathy
- Drowsiness → coma
- Hypoglycaemia
- Low potassium or calcium
- Coagulopathy and haemorrhage

Management

- Treat on a specialist unit
- Supportive therapy
- Liver transplant

CIRRHOSIS

Liver cell necrosis followed by nodular regeneration and fibrosis, resulting in increased resistance to blood flow and deranged liver function.

Aetiology

- Alcohol
- Hepatitis B or C
- Biliary cirrhosis
- Autoimmune hepatitis
- Haemochromatosis
- Wilson's disease
- α_1-antitrypsin disease
- Cystic fibrosis
- Non-alcoholic steatohepatitis (NASH)
- Hepatic venous congestion
- Budd–Chiari
- Drugs, e.g. methotrexate

Clinical features

Chronic liver dysfunction

- Jaundice
- Anaemia
- Bruising
- Palmar erythema
- Dupuytren's contracture

Portal hypertension

- Splenomegaly
- Ascites
- Spider naevi
- Caput medusae
- Oesophageal/rectal varices

Investigations (Table 10.15)

- ALT/AST may be high or normal
- Alkaline phosphatase is usually high
- Bilirubin is usually high
- Albumin falls as cirrhosis worsens

Table 10.15 Liver function tests

Hepatocellular damage (hepatitis)	Synthetic function
Aminotransferases (ALT/AST)	Albumin
γ-Glutamyl transpeptidase (γ-GT)	Prothrombin time
Cholestasis (bile ducts)	
Bilirubin	
Alkaline phosphatase	

- Prothrombin time often prolonged
- Sodium low in severe disease
- α-fetoprotein – hepatocellular carcinoma
- Ultrasound – liver may be large, normal or small; splenomegaly
- Endoscopy for oesophageal varices

Management
- Stop drinking
- Treat complications
- Transplantation

Complications (Table 10.16)
- Ascites
- Transudate (protein <30 g/L in fluid) (Table 10.17)
  Treatment:
  - Spironolactone + loop diuretics
  - Ascitic drainage
  - Venous shunt, e.g. TIPS
- Serum-ascites albumin gradient
  - >11 g suggests transudate
  - More sensitive than absolute protein
- Spontaneous bacterial peritonitis
  - → Worsening of clinical state
  - Diagnosis: ascitic tap
  - Treatment: parenteral antibiotics
- Variceal bleeding
- Encephalopathy
- Hepatorenal syndrome
- Hepatocellular carcinoma

Table 10.16 Indicators of poor prognosis in cirrhosis

Albumin <25 g/L	Persistent jaundice
Sodium <120 mmol/L	Ascites
Prolonged prothrombin time	Variceal bleeding

Table 10.17 Causes of ascites

Transudate (protein <30 g/L)	Exudate (protein >30 g/L)
Portal hypertension	Infections
Cirrhosis of the liver	Peritoneal tuberculosis
Portal vein thrombosis	Malignancy
Low serum protein	Ovarian carcinoma
Liver disease	Peritoneal metastases
Nephrotic syndrome	Inflammatory
Malnutrition	Pancreatitis
Others	
Right ventricular failure	
Myxoedema	

Primary biliary cirrhosis

- Chronic destruction of bile ducts
- ♀ > ♂

Clinical features

- Jaundice
- Itching
- Xanthelasma
- Hepatosplenomegaly

Investigations

- Antimitochondrial (M2) antibodies
- High alkaline phosphatase
- Relatively normal ALT
- Ultrasound
- Liver biopsy

Management

- Ursodeoxycholic acid may normalize liver biochemistry
- Supplement fat-soluble vitamins (A, D, E, K)
- Cholestyramine for itching
- Consider liver transplant when bilirubin >100 mmol/L

Hereditary haemochromatosis

- Autosomal recessive
- 1:400 homozygous
- → Abnormalities of iron transportation
- → Accumulation of iron in epithelial cells
- ♂ = ♀ but women less severely affected due to menstruation

Clinical features

- Heart: cardiomyopathy
- Pancreas: diabetes
- Pituitary hypogonadism
- Liver: hepatitis and cirrhosis, hepatocellular carcinoma
- Skin: pigmentation
- Calcium pyrophosphate deposition in joints – arthritis
- Testes: infertility

Investigations

- Ferritin >500 µg/L
- Serum iron >30 µmol/L
- Transferrin saturation >60%
- Liver biopsy
- HFE gene; also screen family

Management

- Venesection to normalize ferritin

Wilson's disease

- Autosomal recessive
- Defect of copper transport
- → Failure of biliary copper excretion

Clinical features

- Liver: chronic hepatitis → cirrhosis
- Basal ganglia: tremor, dysarthria, dementia

- Kidneys: tubular degeneration
- Eyes: Kayser–Fleischer rings

Investigations
- Reduced serum copper and caeruloplasmin
- Elevated urinary copper
- Liver biopsy

Management
- Penicillamine – chelates copper

α_1-antitrypsin deficiency

- Inherited deficiency of α_1-antitrypsin
- Autosomal dominant
- Liver cirrhosis
- Early emphysema in smokers

Alcohol-related liver disease and alcoholism

Pathology
- Fatty change
- Alcoholic hepatitis
- Cirrhosis

Clinical features
- Those of the stage of liver disease (see above)

Investigations
- Abnormal liver function
- γ-GT elevation.
- AST:ALT >1
- Liver biopsy
- Ultrasound
- α-fetoprotein for hepatocellular carcinoma

Management
- Cessation of alcohol consumption
- Support during physical withdrawal (Table 10.18)
- Psychological support

Complications
- Hepatocellular carcinoma (10–15%)
- End-stage liver disease
- Wernicke–Korsakoff syndrome (see below)
- Encephalopathy
- Dementia
- Epilepsy (5–10%)

Table 10.18 Withdrawal syndrome with benzodiazepines	
Insomnia	Perceptual distortions
Anxiety	Hallucinations (which may be visual)
Tremulousness	Hypersensitivities (light, sound, touch)
Muscle twitchings	Convulsions

(Reproduced from Kumar P, Clark M. Kumar & Clark's Clinical Medicine, 8th edn. Edinburgh: Elsevier; 2012, with permission from Elsevier)

Wernicke–Korsakoff syndrome
- Thiamine deficiency
- → Acute Wernicke syndrome
  - Nystagmus, ataxia, confusion
- → Chronic Korsakoff syndrome
  - Dementia, chronic amnesia, confabulation
- Investigations: red cell transketolase
- Management: parenteral thiamine

Hepatic encephalopathy

- Reversible neuropsychiatric deficit

Clinical features (Box 10.5)
- Flapping tremor of hands
- Decreased level of consciousness
- Personality changes
- Intellectual deterioration
- Slow, slurred speech
- Constructional apraxia – unable to copy a drawn five-pointed star
  Worsened by:
- Sepsis
- Constipation, diarrhoea or vomiting
- Diuretics
- GI bleeding
- Alcohol withdrawal

Investigations
- Urea and electrolytes
- Full blood count
- Liver function tests
- EEG
- Blood cultures to detect sepsis
- Ascitic tap for spontaneous bacterial peritonitis

Management
- Laxatives e.g. lactulose
- Treat sepsis

BOX 10.5. Assessing hepatic encephalopathy

Presence of 'liver flap'
- Straight arms and hyperextended wrist with fingers splayed
- Slow wrist flexion

Assessment of conscious level
- Glasgow coma score

Assessment of cognition
- Mini-mental test

Assessment of apraxia
- Ask patient to copy a five-pointed star
- Repeat on a daily basis to demonstrate changes in encephalopathy

- Careful fluid balance
- Supportive treatment

OTHER DISEASES OF THE LIVER

Liver abscess

- Single or multiple abscesses
- *E. coli*
- *Enterococcus faecalis*
- *Staphylococcus aureus*
- *Entamoeba histolytica* (amoeba)
- → Fever, rigors, vomiting, weight loss, shock

Investigations
- Blood count – anaemia and leucocytosis
- Blood cultures
- Amoeba serology
- Ultrasound and aspiration for culture and sensitivities

Management
- Broad-spectrum antibiotics
- Ultrasound-guided drainage
- Consider underlying bowel disease, e.g. colorectal cancer

Budd–Chiari syndrome

- Hepatic vein thrombosis
- → Hepatic failure
- Clinical ascites, abdominal pain and vomiting
- Hepatomegaly

Pregnancy related liver disease

- Fatty liver
- Hepatitis
- Cholestasis
- Eclampsia → hepatic necrosis
- HELLP syndrome (haemolysis, elevated liver enzymes, low platelets)

Hepatocellular carcinoma

- Common worldwide
- Alcohol, hepatitis B or C-related
- Investigations: ultrasound and α-fetoprotein
- Local treatment with surgery or radiofrequency ablation
- Transplantation if poor synthetic function

Hepatic metastases

- Commonest hepatic tumours
- GI tract, breast and lung carcinomas

Hepatic steatosis

- 'Fatty liver'
- ALT usually elevated
- Commonly asymptomatic
- Commonly associated with alcohol
- Hyperlipidaemia
- Obesity
- Diabetes mellitus

Table 10.19 Risk factors for gallstones

Increasing age	Weight loss
♀ > ♂	Contraceptive pill
Multiparity	Ileal resection/disease
Obesity	Diabetes
Diet high in animal fat	

Nash: Non-alcoholic steatohepatitis
- Fat deposition and inflammation in the liver
- Can progress to cirrhosis

Nafld: Non-alcoholic fatty liver disease
- Fat deposition
- Does not require inflammation for the diagnosis
- Excludes alcohol as a cause

Table 10.20 Drugs and the liver

Drugs causing hepatitis	Hypersensitivity-mediated damage
Isoniazid	Sulphonamides
Methyldopa	Penicillins
Enalapril	Amoxicillin
Nifedipine	Flucloxacillin
Ketoconazole	NSAIDs
Volatile anaesthetics	Salicylates
Rifampicin	Diclofenac
Atenolol	Allopurinol
Verapamil	Phenytoin
Amiodarone	Diltiazem
Cytotoxics	Antithyroid
Drugs causing cholestasis	Carbimazole
Oestrogens	Propylthiouracil
Ciclosporin	Miscellaneous
Chlorpromazine	Necrosis
Cimetidine	Carbon tetrachloride
Erythromycin	Paracetamol
Imipramine	Salicylates
Azathioprine	Cocaine
Haloperidol	Fibrosis
Ranitidine	Methotrexate
Nitrofurantoin	Retinoids
Hypoglycaemics	Tumours
	High-oestrogen OCP
	Chronic hepatitis
	Methyldopa
	Isoniazid
	Nitrofurantoin

DISEASES OF THE BILIARY TREE

Gallstones (Table 10.19)

- 10–20% of the population
- Often an incidental finding at ultrasound

Types
- Cholesterol stones
- Bile pigment stones

Clinical features
- 80% asymptomatic
- Acute cholecystitis – impacted stone leading to inflammation → right hypochondrial and shoulder tip pain, fever, vomiting ± jaundice
- Biliary obstruction by a gallstone → pain and jaundice; ERCP may be required to remove stone

Complications
- Pancreatitis
- Biliary – enteric fistula
- Gallstone ileus

Cholangiocarcinoma

- Primary tumour of bile ducts
- → Obstructive jaundice

Primary sclerosing cholangitis

- Multiple bile duct strictures
- Associated with ulcerative colitis
- Increased risk of cholangiocarcinoma
- Investigations: MRCP, liver biopsy and ERCP

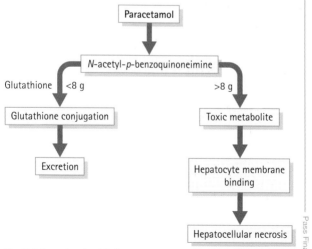

Fig. 10.9 Paracetamol metabolism.

DRUGS AND THE LIVER

The liver is responsible for the initial metabolism of oral drugs (first-pass metabolism) prior to the drug reaching the systemic circulation. Many drugs are also metabolized or excreted by the liver after reaching the systemic circulation. As a result, drugs can be responsible for hepatic disease (see Table 10.20, Fig. 10.9).

SELF-ASSESSMENT QUESTIONS

Multiple choice questions (single best answer)

1. Which of the following is the likeliest cause of jaundice in a 24-year-old man in the UK?
   A. Cancer of the head of the pancreas
   B. Sulphonamide antibiotics
   C. Malaria
   D. Iron deficiency anaemia
   E. Epstein–Barr virus

2. Exudative ascites occurs secondary to:
   A. Ovarian cancer
   B. Alcohol misuse
   C. Anaemia
   D. Coeliac disease
   E. Hypoalbuminaemia

3. Which of the following is the most sensitive method of diagnosing *Helicobacter pylori* infection?
   A. Blood urease test
   B. Endoscopy and biopsy
   C. *H. pylori* antigen in stool
   D. ^{13}C urea breath test
   E. Serum *H. pylori* antibodies

4. Which one of the following is most likely to cause hepatomegaly?
   A. Portal vein thrombosis
   B. Carcinoma of the head of the pancreas
   C. Burkitt's lymphoma
   D. Primary biliary cirrhosis
   E. Right heart failure

5. Which one of the following is a common complication of chronic gastro-oesophageal reflux disease?
   A. Bronchospasm
   B. Headache
   C. Gastric ulcer
   D. Achalasia
   E. Squamous metaplasia

6. Which one of the following increases the risk of oesophageal carcinoma:
   A. Omeprazole
   B. Aspirin
   C. Acid reflux
   D. Ascorbic acid
   E. *H. pylori*

7. Which one of the following is a characteristic finding in Barrett's oesophagus?
   A. The presence of goblet cells
   B. Transitional cell metaplasia of the oesophageal mucosa
   C. Increased risk of oesophageal squamous cell carcinoma
   D. Villous formation
   E. Mucosal dysplasia

8. Which one of the following is associated with oesophageal varices?
   A. Hyposplenism
   B. Acute viral hepatitis
   C. Nodular regeneration and fibrosis of the liver
   D. Portal hypotension
   E. Increased risk of bleeding with propranolol

9. Which one of the following increases oesophageal sphincter tone?
   A. Alcohol
   B. Nifedipine
   C. Achalasia
   D. Isosorbide mononitrate
   E. Botulinum toxin

10. Which of the following is the commonest cause of gastric ulcer?
    A. Ibuprofen
    B. Proton pump inhibitors
    C. Gastric lymphoma
    D. *H. pylori*
    E. Alendronate

11. Which of the following is associated with gastritis?
    A. Salmonella enteritidis
    B. Chlorpromazine
    C. Pantoprazole
    D. Renal failure
    E. Thyrotoxicosis

12. Which one of the following is true of gastric MALT lymphoma?
    A. Is a tumour arising from basophils in the gastric mucosa
    B. May be effectively treated by omeprazole, clarithromycin and amoxicillin
    C. Frequently metastasizes
    D. Can arise anywhere in the gastrointestinal tract
    E. Is a Hodgkin's lymphoma

13. Which one of the following is associated with a decreased risk of gastric adenocarcinoma?
    A. High dietary ascorbic acid
    B. Active *H. pylori* infection
    C. Gastric intestinal metaplasia
    D. Smoking
    E. Coeliac disease

14. Which one of the following is useful in the management of peptic duodenal ulcers?
    A. Omeprazole
    B. Aspirin
    C. Gluten free diet
    D. Iron sulphate
    E. Mesalazine

15. Which one of the following is associated with coeliac disease?
    A. Steatohepatitis
    B. Colon cancer
    C. Hypersplenism
    D. Dermatitis herpetiformis
    E. Thiamine deficiency

16. Which one of the following is characteristic of coeliac disease?
    A. Crypt shortening
    B. Decreased lamina propria lymphocytes
    C. Villus shortening
    D. Crypt abscesses
    E. Jejunal ulceration

17. Which one of the following is true of carcinoid syndrome?
    A. Lung metastases result in right-sided cardiac valve lesions
    B. Flushing and diarrhoea usually occurs
    C. Octreotide is of little therapeutic use
    D. The primary tumour is commonly in the liver
    E. Elevated Serum 5-HIAA is diagnostic

18. Which one of the following would favour the diagnosis of ulcerative colitis rather than Crohn's disease?
    A. Non-caseating granulomata
    B. Crypt abscesses
    C. Enterovesical fistula formation
    D. Oral ulceration
    E. Failure to respond to oral methotrexate

19. Which one of the following is a recognized manifestation of Crohn's disease?
    A. Retinitis pigmentosa
    B. Erythema multiforme
    C. Discoid lupus erythematosus
    D. Dermatitis herpetiformis
    E. Uveitis

20. Which one of the following is a risk factor for the development of colorectal cancer?
    A. NSAID consumption
    B. Chronic idiopathic constipation
    C. Alcohol consumption
    D. Ulcerative colitis
    E. Diverticulosis

21. A 28-year-old man presents with increased stool frequency and rectal mucus. What is the most likely diagnosis?
    A. Diverticular disease
    B. Irritable bowel syndrome
    C. Tubulovillous adenoma of the rectum
    D. Colorectal cancer
    E. Thyrotoxicosis

22. Which one of the following symptoms is more suggestive of colonic carcinoma than irritable bowel syndrome?
    A. Rectal bleeding
    B. Weight loss
    C. Alternating diarrhoea and constipation
    D. Sensation of incomplete evacuation of stool
    E. Bloating

23. Which one of the following is most useful in the management of irritable bowel?
    A. Mebeverine
    B. Ibuprofen
    C. Phenelzine
    D. Prednisolone
    E. Mesalazine

24. Which one of the following causes diarrhoea?
    A. Iron sulphate
    B. Octreotide
    C. Vasoactive intestinal peptide (VIP)
    D. Loperamide
    E. Hypothyroidism

25. Which one of the following may cause increased stool frequency?
    A. Vagotomy
    B. Diabetes insipidus
    C. Smoking
    D. Hypercalcaemia
    E. Hyperparathyroidism

26. The following are clinical features of cirrhosis of the liver except:
    A. Palmar erythema
    B. Caput medusae
    C. Macrocytosis
    D. Portal hypotension
    E. Bruising

27. Which one of the following drugs causes abnormalities of liver function?
    A. Ursodeoxycholic acid
    B. Flucloxacillin
    C. Folic acid
    D. Verapamil
    E. Thyroxine

Multiple choice questions (true or false)

28. The following organisms cause diarrhoea mainly via the mechanism given:
    A. Cholera – mucosal inflammation
    B. *E. coli* – enterotoxin production
    C. *Campylobacter* – mucosal inflammation
    D. *Bacillus cereus* – colonic ulceration
    E. *Giardia* – malabsorption of water

29. The following are true of pseudomembranous colitis:
    A. Diagnosis is based on the presence of *Clostridium difficile* in stool
    B. It is best treated with intravenous vancomycin
    C. Risk of the disease is increased by intravenous cephalosporins
    D. It may result in bloody diarrhoea
    E. The causal bacterium is a normal commensal gut organism

30. The following are recognized causes of acute pancreatitis:
    A. Gallstones
    B. Prednisolone
    C. Thyroxine

D. Coxsackie virus infection

E. Hyperlipidaemia

31. The following are indicators of poor prognosis in acute pancreatitis:

    A. Glucose <6 mmol/L

    B. Hypocalcaemia

    C. Hypoxia

    D. Albumin >30 g/L

    E. P_aCO_2 <5 kPa

32. The following favour a diagnosis of pancreatic carcinoma over acute viral hepatitis in painless jaundice:

    A. Weight loss

    B. Dilated bile ducts on ultrasound scanning

    C. Elevated alkaline phosphatase

    D. Unconjugated hyperbilirubinaemia

    E. Bilirubin >300 μmol/L

33. The following are associated with an elevated serum gastrin:

    A. Omeprazole therapy

    B. Zollinger–Ellison syndrome

    C. Hyperchlorhydria

    D. Vagotomy

    E. Hypoglycaemia

34. The following are causes of a conjugated hyperbilirubinaemia:

    A. Gilbert syndrome

    B. Carcinoma of the head of the pancreas

    C. Cholangiocarcinoma

    D. Viral hepatitis

    E. Haemolytic anaemia

35. The following are associated with acute hepatitis A infection:

    A. Elevated alanine transaminase

    B. Nausea and vomiting

    C. Bilirubin level always greater than 100 μmol/L

    D. Progression to chronic hepatitis

    E. Food-related outbreaks

36. The following statements are correct in the interpretation of hepatitis B serology:

    A. HBs (surface) antibody positive – previous exposure to infection

    B. HBe antigen positive – high infectivity risk

    C. HBc (core) antibody positive – seroconversion

    D. HBs antigen positive – successful immunization

    E. HBe antibody positive – seroconversion after acute infection

37. The following are associated with hepatitis C infection:

    A. Cryoglobulinaemia

    B. Hepatocellular carcinoma

    C. Primary sclerosing cholangitis

    D. Hepatic cirrhosis

    E. Ascites

38. The following are causes of viral hepatitis:

    A. Epstein–Barr virus

    B. Isolated hepatitis D virus

    C. Cytomegalovirus in immunosuppressed patients

    D. Coxsackie virus

    E. Adenovirus

39. The following are causes of fulminant hepatic failure:
    A. Paracetamol
    B. Hepatitis A
    C. Aspirin in childhood
    D. Halothane
    E. Haemochromatosis
40. The following are causes of transudative ascites:
    A. Right heart failure
    B. Peritoneal tuberculosis
    C. Ovarian malignancy
    D. Nephrotic syndrome
    E. Liver cirrhosis

Extended matching questions

Question 1 Theme: Diarrhoea

A. *E. coli*
B. Thyrotoxicosis
C. Hypercalcaemia
D. Autonomic neuropathy
E. Laxative abuse
F. Osmotic diarrhoea
G. Ulcerative colitis
H. Tubulovillous adenoma
 I. Diverticular disease
 J. Coeliac disease
K. Giardiasis
L. Pseudomembranous colitis

For each of the following questions, select the best answer from the list above:

 I. A 65-year-old man with known diabetes mellitus is reviewed as he has worsening diarrhoea. Upper gastrointestinal endoscopy, duodenal biopsy and colonoscopy were all normal. Stool culture carried out on three occasions did not reveal any abnormality. Blood testing revealed normal urea and electrolytes, calcium and liver function. What is the most likely cause for his diarrhoea?

 II. A 38-year-old man is admitted with profuse mucus per rectum and generalized weakness. His potassium is noted to be 2.9 mmol/L. What is the most likely diagnosis?

III. A 27-year-old woman is admitted with abdominal discomfort, profuse bloody diarrhoea and a low-grade fever. Investigations reveal an iron deficiency anaemia. What is the most likely reason for her diarrhoea?

Question 2 Theme: Abdominal pain

A. Sigmoid volvulus
 B. Acute appendicitis
 C. Cholecystitis
 D. Duodenal ulceration
 E. Bowel ischaemia
 F. Diverticulosis
 G. Crohn's disease
 H. Irritable bowel syndrome
 I. Acute pancreatitis
 J. Colorectal carcinoma

K. Carcinoid syndrome

L. Ovarian cysts

M. Ectopic pregnancy

For each of the following questions, select the best answer from the list above:

I. A 76-year-old man complains of pain in the abdomen after eating. This is associated with mild diarrhoea. In the past he has had a myocardial infarction and several episodes of angina. He has type II diabetes mellitus. He smokes 20 cigarettes a day and drinks 10 units of alcohol a week. Suggest a likely cause for his pain.

II. A 32-year-old woman is referred by her GP with abdominal pain, nausea, weight loss and diarrhoea. She is also complaining of a bruise-like rash on her lower legs and mild joint pains. On examination she has multiple oral aphthous ulcers and tender bruise-like lesions over her shins. What is the cause of her abdominal pain?

III. A 47-year-old woman is referred with left iliac fossa pain, bloating and alternating diarrhoea and constipation. Her weight is gradually increasing. The discomfort comes and goes but is relieved by defaecation. What is the most likely diagnosis?

Question 3 Theme: Malabsorption

A. Pernicious anaemia

B. Coeliac disease

C. Whipple's disease

D. Primary biliary cirrhosis

E. Chronic pancreatitis

F. Cystic fibrosis

G. Bacterial overgrowth

H. Surgery for ileal Crohn's disease

I. Partial gastrectomy

J. Chronic alcohol-related liver disease

K. Carcinoma of the head of the pancreas

For each of the following questions, select the best answer from the list above:

I. A 15-year-old man is referred with a 6-year history of abdominal pain, bloating and weight loss. He is 1.78 m (5 feet 2 inches) tall and weighs 47 kg (7 stones 6 pounds). He has diarrhoea 2–3 times a day. What is the most likely diagnosis?

II. A 56-year-old woman is noted to be vitamin B_{12}-deficient and anaemic. She has known autoimmune hypothyroidism but is otherwise well. What is causing her B_{12} deficiency?

III. A 49-year-old man with a long history of alcohol abuse is reviewed due to worsening diarrhoea and abdominal pain. The stools are reported as foul-smelling and difficult to flush. His liver function tests are mildly deranged. What is the cause of his symptoms?

Question 4 Theme: Intestinal bleeding

A. Oesophageal varices

B. Gastric ulcer

C. Duodenal ulcer

D. Coeliac disease

E. Small bowel angiodysplasia

F. Meckel's diverticulum

G. Terminal ileal Crohn's disease

H. Caecal carcinoma

I. Diverticular bleeding

J. Haemorrhoids

For each of the following questions, select the best answer from the list above:

I. A 56-year-old man was admitted with haematemesis, melaena, hypotension and a tachycardia. He had recently been taking indomethacin for joint pains. What is the likeliest cause for his symptoms?

II. A 76-year-old woman was seen with 3 months of diarrhoea and weight loss. What is the most likely diagnosis?

III. A 32-year-old woman was seen with bright red bleeding. What is the likeliest diagnosis?

STRUCTURE AND FUNCTION

The muscular skeletal system comprises bones, joints and connective tissues.

Connective tissues

- Cartilage
- Tendons
- Ligaments

Extracellular matrix

- Macromolecule matrix contained in all connective tissues
- Components:
  - Collagens
  - Elastin
  - Glycoproteins
  - Proteoglycans

Joints

- Synovial
- Fibrocartilaginous
- Fibrous

Synovial joints (see Fig. 11.1 for the components)

- Ball and socket joints, e.g. hip joint
- Hinge joints, e.g. interphalangeal

Fibrocartilaginous joints

- Intervertebral discs
- Sacroiliac joints
- Pubic symphysis
- Costochondral joints

EXAMINING THE MUSCULOSKELETAL SYSTEM

Examination should include all of the following and be done in roughly this order:

Examination of individual joints

- Ask the patient if the joint is painful; proceed with care if it is
  Look for:
- Swelling

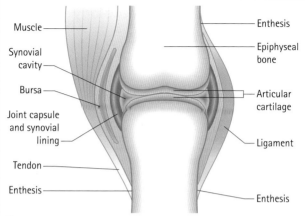

Fig. 11.1 The synovial joint.

- Erythema/rash
- Deformity
- Muscle-wasting
  Feel for:
- Tenderness
- Warmth
- Swelling
  - Hard swelling = bony
  - Fluctuant swelling = fluid/effusion
  - Boggy swelling = synovial swelling
    Move the joint:
- Passively first
- Assess for crepitus

Examination of the hands

- Expose both arms to the shoulders
- Ask if they are painful
- Describe particular features of osteoarthritis or rheumatoid arthritis if present (Table 11.1 and Fig. 11.2)
- Then proceed as for individual joints above
- Also examine the nails and feel for nodules on the forearms

Examination of the gait

- Ask the patient to walk a short distance away from you, turn, walk towards you and stand still

ARTHRITIS

Osteoarthritis

See Tables 11.1 and 11.2 and Figures 11.2 and 11.3.

Table 11.1 Some common particular features of osteoarthritis and rheumatoid arthritis in the hands

	Hand joints usually affected	Particular features
Osteoarthritis	DIP joints (Heberden's nodes) PIP joints (Bouchard's nodes) Carpometacarpal joint	Square hand
Rheumatoid arthritis	PIP joints MCP joints	Ulnar deviation Palmar subluxation of MCP joints Fixed flexion of PIP joints (Boutonnière deformity) Fixed hyperextension of PIP joints (swan neck deformity)

(a)

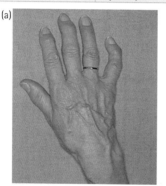

(b)

Fig. 11.2 The hands in arthritis. (a) Nodal osteoarthritis. Heberden's and Bouchard's nodes and squaring of the thumb bases. The synovial joints are seen. (b) Rheumatoid arthritis.

Table 11.2 Comparison of osteoarthritis and rheumatoid arthritis

	Osteoarthritis (OA)	Rheumatoid arthritis (RA)
Description	Pain and disability associated with joint space narrowing; altered cartilage osteophyte formation	Systemic disease with chronic, symmetrical polyarthritis synovitis; non-articular features
Epidemiology	Most common type of arthritis	0.5–1% of the population (falling)
	Prevalence increases with age	Presents at all ages
	X-ray OA very common >60 years	Commonly presents 30–50 years
		♀ > ♂ before menopause
		Familial or sporadic
		HLA-DR4 in 50–70%
Aetiology	Primary idiopathic	Unexplained
	Secondary:	T cell activation
	Trauma, e.g. previous fracture	Presence of rheumatoid factors
	Chondrocalcinosis	
	Haemochromatosis	
	Acromegaly	
	Haemophilia	
	Avascular necrosis, e.g. steroids	
	Sickle cell disease	
Clinical features	Joint pain/swelling/instability	Slow onset but progressive
	Morning stiffness	Symmetrical peripheral polyarthritis
	Joint effusion and crepitus	Joint pain and morning stiffness
	Bony swelling	Eased by gentle activity
	Muscle wasting	Joints warm and tender
	Limitation of movement and loss of function	Limitation of movement and deformity
		Joint effusion
		Muscle-wasting
		Lethargy, malaise
		Non-articular features (Fig. 11.3)

Clinical subtypes

Nodal OA

- Develops in late middle age
- Polyarticular involvement of the hand
- Particularly distal interphalangeal joints (Heberden's nodes)
- Generally good long-term functional outcome
- Predisposes to OA of the knee, hip and spine
- X-ray – marginal osteophyte and joint space loss

Erosive OA

- Rare
- DIP and PIP joints
- Poor functional outcome
- X-ray – marked subchondral cysts
- May develop into rheumatoid arthritis

Generalized OA

- May occur in combination with nodal OA
- Hands, knees, first MTP joints and hips

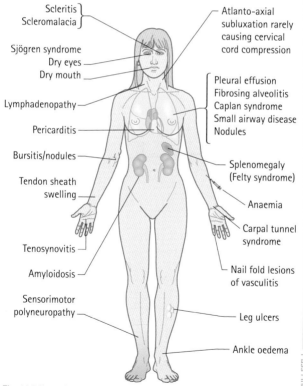

Fig. 11.3 Non-articular manifestations of rheumatoid arthritis.

- Familial
- ♀ >> ♂
- May be autoimmune
- Large joint OA
- Knees and hips

Crystal-associated OA (chondrocalcinosis)
- Calcium pyrophosphate crystal deposition
- Knees and wrists commonly affected
- X-ray – may show calcification in the cartilage

Investigations
- Inflammatory markers not elevated
- No autoantibodies
- X-rays abnormal if damage severe
- MRI can show early cartilage changes
- Arthroscopy – early fissuring and cartilage surface erosion

Management
- Treat symptoms and disability, not X-rays
- Explain diagnosis and reassure
- Weight loss and exercise
- Hydrotherapy (particularly lower limb joints)
- Heat/massage
- Analgesia
- Patients often use complementary medicine
- Joint replacements/other surgery

Rheumatoid arthritis

See Table 11.1 and 11.2 and Figures 11.2 and 11.3.

Clinical subtypes
Palindromic
- Monoarticular
- Progresses to other types

Transient
- Self-limiting
- Usually Rh factor-negative

Remitting
- Active for years then remits

Chronic persistent
- Most typical form
- Relapsing and remitting

Rapidly progressive
- Remorseless
- Progressive
- Rh factor-positive
- ACPA (anti-citrullinated peptide antibodies)-positive, are a better predictor for prognosis
- Associated with non-articular fractures

Investigations
- Anaemia
- ↑ inflammatory markets
- Rheumatoid factors (in 70%)
- X-rays – erosions

Table 11.3 Side-effects of steroids	
General	Cardiovascular
Weight gain	Hypertension
Fluid retention	Eyes
Skin	Cataracts
Acne	Bones
Thin skin with easy bruising	Osteoporosis
Endocrine	
Diabetes	
Cushing syndrome	

Management

- Explain diagnosis and reassure
- Multidisciplinary team approach
- NSAIDs and analgesics
- Disease-modifying antirheumatic drugs (DMARDs):
- Sulphasalazine
- Methotrexate
- Leflunomide
- Anti-TNF drugs:
  - Etanercept
  - Infliximab
  - Adalimumab
- Corticosteroids (see Table 11.3 for side-effects)
- Less commonly used:
  - Gold
  - Penicillamine
  - Hydroxychloroquine
  - Azathioprine
  - Ciclosporin
  - Anakinra
  - Joint replacements/other surgery

Septic arthritis

Aetiology

- Direct injury
- Blood–borne infection
- → Susceptibility in
  - Chronically inflamed joints
  - Immunosuppressed patients
  - Artificial joints

Organisms

- *Staphylococcus aureus*
- *Streptococcus* and other *staphylococci*
- *Neisseria gonorrhoeae*
- *Haemophilus influenzae*
- Gram-negative organisms

Clinical features

- Joint pain
- Muscle spasm

- Joint hot, red and swollen
- Signs of the source of infection

Investigations
- Urgent joint aspiration
  - Microscopy and culture/gram stain
- Elevated white cell count
- Blood cultures

Management
- Two i.v. antibiotics for 2 weeks (start antibiotics immediately diagnosis suspected)
- Followed by 6 weeks of oral antibiotics
- Initial immobilization of the joint
- Early physiotherapy
- Consider surgical drainage and washout

Seronegative spondyloarthropathies

- Conditions affecting the spine and peripheral joints which cluster in families and are associated with HLA-B27

Ankylosing spondylitis

- Episodic inflammation of spine and sacroiliac joints
- Asymmetrical large joint arthritis
- HLA-B27 in >90%
- Associated with uveitis and costochondritis
- Inflammatory markers elevated
- X-rays
  - Erosions and sclerosis of affected joints
  - Syndesmophytes
  - Bamboo spine
- Treated with preventative exercises and NSAIDs, TNF-α blocking drugs if severe

Psoriatic arthritis

Clinical features
- Arthritis in association with psoriasis
- May predate skin lesions
- DIP most common joints affected
- Dactylitis
- Erosions on X-rays (centre of joint unlike juxta-articular erosions in RA)
- 5% have arthritis mutilans
- Nail dystrophy in 85% of cases
- HLA-B27 in 50%

Management
- Treated with:
  - NSAIDs
  - Steroid injections to joints
  - Sulfasalazine
  - Methotrexate/ciclosporin
  - TNF-α blocking drugs, e.g. infliximab

Reactive arthritis

- Sterile synovitis following dysentery or a sexually acquired infection

Aetiology
- Trigger organism
  - *Salmonella*
  - *Shigella*
  - *Yersinia*
  - *Chlamydia*
  - *Ureaplasma*

Clinical features
- Acute asymmetrical lower limb arthritis
- ♂ > ♀
- Often also an enthesitis, e.g. plantar fasciitis
- Non-articular features
  - Acute anterior uveitis (see above)
  - Circinate balanitis
  - Keratoderma blenorrhagica
  - Nail dystrophy
  - Conjunctivitis
- Reiter's disease = urethritis, arthritis and conjunctivitis

Management
- Treatment usually symptomatic with NSAIDs or steroid injections
- Treat underlying infection with antibiotics

Inflammatory bowel disease (IBD)-associated arthritis

- 10–15% of patients with IBD
- Lower limb joints
- In ulcerative colitis treatment of bowel disease may improve arthritis
- In Crohn's disease, arthritis persists even when bowel is disease inactive
- 5% have sacroiliitis (independent of activity of IBD)
- Treatment with intra-articular steroids and sulfasalazine

Gout

- Inflammatory arthritis associated with hyperuricaemia and urate crystal deposition

Epidemiology
- 5% of population have hyperuricaemia
- 0.2% of population have gout
- ♂ > ♀
- Commonly presents between 30 and 50 years
- Rare in women before the menopause
- Familial or sporadic
- HLA-DR4 positive in 50–70%

Aetiology
- Causes of hyperuricaemia (Table 11.4)

Clinical features
- Acute onset
- Acute painful, red, swollen joint
- Often affects first MTP joint
- Precipitated by
  - Alcohol
  - Excess food

Table 11.4 Causes of hyperuricaemia

Impaired excretion of uric acid
  Chronic kidney disease (clinical gout unusual)
  Drug therapy, e.g. thiazide diuretics, low-dose aspirin
  Hypertension
  Lead toxicity
  Primary hyperparathyroidism
  Hypothyroidism
  Increased lactic acid production from alcohol, exercise, starvation
  Glucose-6-phosphatase deficiency (interferes with renal excretion)
Increased production of uric acid
  Increased purine synthesis *de novo* due to
    Hypoxanthine-guanine-phosphoribosyl transferase (HGPRT)
      reduction (an X-linked inborn error causing the Lesch–Nyhan
      syndrome)
    Phosphoribosyl-pyrophosphate synthetase overactivity
    Glucose-6-phosphatase deficiency with glycogen storage
      disease type 1 (patients who survive develop hyperuricaemia
      due to increased production as well as decreased excretion)
  Increased turnover of purines due to:
    Myeloproliferative disorders, e.g. polycythaemia vera
    Lymphoproliferative disorders, e.g. leukaemia
    Others, e.g. carcinoma, severe psoriasis

- Dehydration
- Diuretics

Investigations
- Joint fluid microscopy – needle-shaped crystals
- Serum urate
- Urea and electrolytes

Management
- NSAIDs
- Colchicine (particularly if NSAIDs cannot be used)
- If attacks are frequent give allopurinol to reduce urate 4–6 weeks after acute attack
- Lifestyle advice, e.g. diet, reduce alcohol intake

Chronic tophaceous gout
- Very high serum urate
- White urate deposits (tophi) in skin particularly ear lobes and around joints
- Associated with renal failure or use of diuretics

AUTOIMMUNE RHEUMATIC DISEASE

Systemic lupus erythematosus (SLE)

- Inflammatory multisystem disorder with arthralgia and rashes as common symptoms, and cerebral and renal disease as serious problems

Epidemiology
- ♂ > ♀
- Black > Caucasian
- Peak age of onset 20–40 years

Aetiology
- Familial
- ↑ HLA-B8 and DR3 in Caucasians
- Inherited deficiency of complement (C2 and 4)
- ?Related to female sex hormones
- Loss of immunological tolerance
- Environmental triggers
  - Drugs – hydralazine, isoniazid, methyldopa, oral contraceptive pill/HRT
  - Ultraviolet light

Clinical features
- The result of vasculitis (Fig. 11.4)

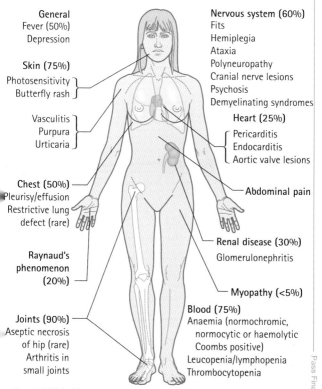

General
Fever (50%)
Depression

Skin (75%)
Photosensitivity ⎤
Butterfly rash ⎦

Vasculitis ⎤
Purpura
Urticaria ⎦

Chest (50%)
Pleurisy/effusion
Restrictive lung defect (rare)

Raynaud's phenomenon (20%)

Joints (90%)
Aseptic necrosis of hip (rare)
Arthritis in small joints

Nervous system (60%)
Fits
Hemiplegia
Ataxia
Polyneuropathy
Cranial nerve lesions
Psychosis
Demyelinating syndromes

Heart (25%)
⎡ Pericarditis
⎢ Endocarditis
⎣ Aortic valve lesions

Abdominal pain

Renal disease (30%)
Glomerulonephritis

Myopathy (<5%)

Blood (75%)
Anaemia (normochromic, normocytic or haemolytic Coombs positive)
Leucopenia/lymphopenia
Thrombocytopenia

Fig. 11.4 Clinical features of systemic lupus erythematosus.

Investigations

Blood tests

- Normochromic normocytic anaemia
- Leucopenia
- Thrombocytopenia
- ± Autoimmune haemolytic anaemia
- ↑ ESR
- Normal CRP
- Antinuclear antibody (ANA) positive
- Double-stranded DNA positive in 50%, SLE-specific
- Low complement during attacks
- Rh factor-positive in 30–50%
- False positive syphilis serology
- Raised IgG and M

Histology

- e.g. Renal biopsy
- Characteristic histology and immunofluorescence

CT/MRI

- e.g. Brain, may show infarcts/haemorrhage

Management

- Explain diagnosis
- Avoid UV light if photosensitive
- NSAIDs for arthralgia
- Antimalarials (e.g. chloroquine) for skin and joint disease
- Steroids for active disease
- Immunosuppressants
  - Azathioprine/cyclophosphamide/mycophenolate if severe

Course and prognosis

- Episodic
- Periods of complete remission
- 10-year survival 90%

Antiphospholipid syndrome

- A syndrome associated with the presence of antibodies to phospholipids

Clinical features

- Arterial and venous thromboses
- Recurrent miscarriage
- Thrombocytopenia
- Chorea, migraine and epilepsy
- Valvular heart disease
- Skin disease, e.g. livedo reticularis
- A few patients will have SLE

Investigation

- Anticardiolipin antibodies
- Lupus anticoagulant antibodies
- ESR and ANA usually normal
- Prolonged APTT

Management

- Aggressive anticoagulation
  - Aspirin
  - Heparin/warfarin

Systemic sclerosis

- A rare multisystem disease with widespread obliterative damage to small blood vessels associated with fibrosis of the skin and internal organs

Clinical features

Raynaud's phenomenon

- 97% of cases
- Arterial spasm of hands and feet
- Three phases
  - Pallor
  - Cyanosis
  - Erythema
- Numbness and pain

Skin

- Hands, face, feet, forearms
- Tight, waxy and tethered
- 'Beaking' of nose
- Microstomia
- Digital ulcers
- Telangiectasia
- Nail fold capillary loops

GI Tract

- Oesophagus
  - Reflux
  - Poor motility
  - Dilatation
- Small bowel
  - Bacterial overgrowth
  - Malabsorption

Renal

- Renal failure
- Malignant hypertension

Cardiorespiratory system

- Pulmonary fibrosis (common cause of death)
- Primary or secondary pulmonary hypertension
- Arrhythmias
- Conduction defects
- Pericarditis

Crest syndrome (Limited cutaneous scleroderma – LcSSc)

- **C**alcinosis (calcium deposits in skin and elsewhere)
- **R**aynaud's phenomenon
- **O**esophageal involvement
- **S**clerodactyly
- **T**elangiectasia

Investigations

- Normocytic normochromic anaemia
- Urea and electrolytes and urinalysis including creatinine clearance
- Autoantibodies
  - Speckled/nucleolar/anticentromere – 70–80%
  - Rheumatoid factor – 30%
- Chest X-ray – reticulonodular shadowing
- Other tests according to organ involved

Management

- Education, counselling and family support
- Hand-warmers and vasodilators for Raynaud's
- Proton pump inhibitors and motility agents
- Antibiotics and nutritional supplements
- Antihypertensives
- i.v. prostacyclin

VASCULITIS

- Inflammation of blood vessel walls (Table 11.5)

BONE DISEASE (TABLE 11.6)

Osteoporosis

- Low bone mass and micro-architectural deterioration of bone leading to bone fragility and increased fracture risk
- In osteoporosis the bone is mineralized normally but deficient in quantity and quality, including structural integrity

Epidemiology

- Common problem
- Lifetime risk of hip fracture in:
  - ♀ aged 50 years – 15%
  - ♂ aged 50 years – 5%

Risk factors

See Table 11.7.

Clinical features

Vertebral crush fractures

- Back pain
- Weight loss
- Kyphosis

Fractures associated with falls

- Colles' fracture
- Fractured neck of femur

Investigations

- Ca^{++}, PO_4 and alkaline phosphatase normal
- X-rays identify fractures
- DXA scanning
  - Measurement of bone density in lumbar spine and neck of femur
  - Osteoporosis is defined as bone density <2.5 SDs below the mean value of age-, sex- and race-matched controls
- Bone scan differentiates from bony metastases

Management

- Prevention
- Identification and monitoring of patients at risk

Non-drug therapies

- Diet rich in calcium and vitamin D
- Exercise
- Stopping smoking
- Reducing the risk of falls

Table 11.5 Vasculitides

Name	Type of vessel	Clinical features	Diagnosis	Treatment
Giant cell arteritis (GCA) and polymyalgia rheumatica (PMR)	Large vessel (e.g. temporal artery)	>50 years GCA Headache Scalp tenderness Jaw claudication Malaise, tiredness Fever Sudden painless vision loss PMR Pain and stiffness in shoulders, neck, hips and spine Malaise Tiredness Fever Weight loss Depression Worse in mornings	Raised ESR Temporal artery biopsy (shows a giant cell arteritis)	Steroids
Polyarteritis nodosa	Medium-sized vessels	Middle-aged men usually Fever Malaise Weight loss Myalgia Neurological (mononeuritis multiplex) Abdominal (GI bleeding, infarction of viscera) Renal (hypertension and acute kidney injury) Cardiac (myocardial infarction and heart failure) Skin (gangrene, livedo reticularis)	Raised ESR Renal/hepatic/gut microaneurysms ANCA–usually negative	Steroids Azathioprine

Table 11.5 (continued)

Name	Type of vessel	Clinical features	Diagnosis	Treatment
ANCA-positive vasculitis Wegener's granulomatosis Churg–Strauss syndrome Microscopic polyangiitis	Small vessels	Wegener's (Granulomatosis with polyangitis) and Churg–Strauss Microscopic polyarteritis Crescentic glomerulonephritis Associated with hepatitis B	ANCA	Steroids Immunosuppressants
Non-ANCA vasculitis Henoch-Schönlein purpura	Small vessels	Henoch-Schönlein purpura Children mostly, after upper respiratory tract infection Purpura Polyarthritis Abdominal pain Glomerulonephritis	Most self-limiting	Steroids if severe
Cryoglobulinaemic vasculitis		Purpura Glomerulonephritis Arthralgia, hepatitis C		
Behçet's disease	Small and large vessels	Japan, Turkey, Iran and countries bordering the Mediterranean Recurrent oral and genital ulceration Uveitis Erythema nodosum Papulopustular and pseudofolliculitis skin lesions Arthritis GI symptoms Neurological symptoms	Pathergy reaction	Steroids Ciclosporin Colchicine Thalidomide (not in pregnancy) Anti-TNF for severe cases

Table 11.6 Biochemical abnormalities in common bone disorders

Disease	Ca^{++}	PO$_4$	Alkaline phosphatase
Osteoporosis	→	→	→
Osteomalacia	↓	↓	↑
Paget's disease	→	→	↑
Bony secondary deposits	↑	↑ or →	↑

Table 11.7 Osteoporosis risk factors, associated disease and drug therapies

Risk factors
  Female sex
  Increasing age
  Early menopause (including surgical)
  White race/Asian
  Slender habitus
  Lack of exercise/immobility
  Smoking
  Family history
  Excess alcohol
  Nutrition (very low calcium diet, high protein intake for a long time)
Drug therapy
  Corticosteroids
  Heparin
  Ciclosporin
  Cytotoxic therapy

Disease
  Endocrine
    Cushing syndrome
    Hyperparathyroidism
    Hypogonadism (including orchidectomy)
    Acromegaly
    Type I diabetes mellitus
  Joints
    Rheumatoid arthritis
  Other
    Chronic kidney disease
    Chronic liver disease
    Mastocytosis
    Anorexia nervosa
  Inflammatory bowel disease

Drugs
- Calcium and vitamin D supplements
- Bisphosphonates
- Raloxifene
- Recombinant human parathyroid hormone peptide 1–34
- Strontium
- Androgens in hypogonadal men

Osteomalacia

- Defective bone mineralization associated with low levels of vitamin D
- In children, the effects on the growth plates lead to rickets

Aetiology
See Table 11.8.

Table 11.8 Causes of rickets and osteomalacia

Vitamin D deficiency
    Inadequate synthesis in skin
    Low dietary intake
    Malabsorption
        Coeliac disease
        Intestinal resection
        Chronic cholestasis, e.g. primary biliary cirrhosis
Renal disease
    Chronic kidney disease
    Renal osteodystrophy
    Bone disease due to dialysis
    Tubular disorders, e.g. renal tubular
    acidosis, Fanconi syndrome
Miscellaneous
    Multiple myeloma
    Vitamin D-dependent rickets types I and II
    X-linked hypophosphataemia (vitamin D-resistant rickets)
    Mesenchymal tumours

Clinical features

Adults
- Bone/muscle pain and tenderness
- Subclinical fractures
- Proximal myopathy
- Tetany (low calcium)

Children
- Bowed legs
- 'Rickety rosary' costochondritis
- Myopathy

Investigations
- $\downarrow Ca^{++}$, $\downarrow PO_4$, $\uparrow$ alkaline phosphatase
- $\downarrow$ 25-hydroxy vitamin D
- X-ray – defective mineralization
- 'Looser's zones' on X-ray

Management
- Correction of cause
- Replacement of vitamin D

Paget's disease

- Disorder of bone remodelling associated with excessive bone resorption and excess structurally abnormal new bone formation

Epidemiology
- Europe (especially northern England) » USA/Africa
- Patients >40 years
- Asymptomatic X-ray evidence very common
- Patients less commonly have symptoms

Aetiology
- Genetic component
- Geographical/ethnic clusters
- Viral aetiology has been suggested

Clinical features
- Commonly none
- Bone pain (spine/pelvis)
- Joint pain (near to involved bone)
- Deformities (tibia and skull)

Complications
- Nerve compression
  - VIIIth cranial nerve leads to deafness
  - Also IInd, Vth and VIIth cranial nerves
- Increased bone blood flow
  - → High-output cardiac failure
- Pathological fractures
- Osteogenic sarcoma (<1%)

Investigations
- Normal Ca^{++} and PO_4, ↑ alkaline phosphatase
- X-rays – excess abnormal bone

Management
- Simple analgesics for pain
- Bisphosphonates
- Surgery, e.g. joint replacement/osteotomy

DISORDERS OF CALCIUM METABOLISM

Hypercalcaemia

Aetiology
See Table 11.9.

Clinical features
- Tiredness
- Malaise
- Depression
- Renal stones
- Polyuria
- Bone pains
- Abdominal pain
- Peptic ulcer disease
- Ectopic calcification, e.g. corneal

Investigations
- Ca^{++}, PO_4, alkaline phosphatase
- Urea and electrolytes
- Chest X-ray
- Parathormone (PTH)
- Thyroid-stimulating hormone (TSH)
- Serum electrophoresis

Management
- Rectify cause
- i.v. Saline rehydration
- Bisphosphonates

Table 11.9 Causes of hypercalcaemia

Excessive parathormone (PTH) secretion
    Primary hyperparathyroidism (commonest by far), adenoma,
       hyperplasia or carcinoma
    Tertiary hyperparathyroidism
    Ectopic PTH secretion (very rare indeed)
Excess action of vitamin D
    Iatrogenic or self-administered excess
    Granulomatous diseases, e.g. sarcoidosis, TB
    Lymphoma
Excessive calcium intake
    'Milk-alkali' syndrome
Malignant disease (second commonest cause)
    Secondary deposits in bone
    Production of osteoclastic factors by tumours
    PTH-related protein secretion
    Myeloma
Other endocrine disease (mild hypercalcaemia only)
    Thyrotoxicosis
    Addison's disease
Drugs
    Thiazide diuretics
    Vitamin D analogues
    Lithium administration (chronic)
    Vitamin A
Miscellaneous
    Long-term immobility
    Familial hypocalciuric hypercalcaemia

Hypocalcaemia

Aetiology
See Table 11.10.

Clinical features
- Paraesthesiae
- Circumoral numbness
- Cramps
- Anxiety
- Tetany
- Fits
- Dystonia
- Psychosis
- Chvostek's sign – tapping over the facial nerve produces twitching of facial muscles
- Trousseau's sign – compression of the upper arm (e.g. with blood pressure cuff) produces tetany spasms of the hands

Investigations
- Ca^{++}, PO_4, alkaline phosphatase
- Urea and electrolytes
- X-rays

Table 11.10 Causes of hypocalcaemia

Increased phosphate levels
  Chronic kidney disease (common)
  Phosphate therapy
Hypoparathyroidism
  Surgical – after neck exploration (thyroidectomy parathyroidectomy
    – common)
  Congenital deficiency (DiGeorge syndrome)
  Idiopathic hypoparathyroidism (rare)
  Severe hypomagnesaemia
Vitamin D deficiency
  Osteomalacia
  Vitamin D resistance
Resistance to PTH
  Pseudohypoparathyroidism
Drugs
  Calcitonin
  Bisphosphonates
Miscellaneous
  Acute pancreatitis (quite common)
  Citrated blood in massive transfusion (not uncommon)
  Malabsorption, e.g. coeliac disease

- Parathyroid hormone
- Vitamin D

Management
- Rectify cause
- Calcium/vitamin D

DISORDERS OF COLLAGEN

- Collagen is part of the extracellular matrix
- It consists of three polypeptide chains wound round one another in a triple helical conformation

Ehlers–Danlos syndrome

- Ten different types, mainly autosomal dominant
- Varying degrees of
  - Skin fragility
  - Skin hyperextensibility
  - Joint hypermobility

Clinical features
- Easy bruising
- Extensible velvety skin
- Hypermobile joints

Pseudoxanthoma elasticum

- Abnormal collagen and elastin

Clinical features

Skin
- Loose, lax, wrinkled ('plucked chicken skin')
- Particularly in the flexures

Other
- GI bleeding
- Angioid streaks in the eye
- Early myocardial infarction
- Claudication

Marfan syndrome

- Autosomal dominant
- Mutation of the collagen fibrillin
- Chromosome 15

Clinical features
- Tall stature
- Arachnodactyly (long thin digits)
- Long arm span
- High arched palate
- Recurrent joint dislocations
- Inguinal/femoral herniae
- Spontaneous pneumothorax
- Emphysema
- Aortic/mitral incompetence
- Aortic aneurysm
- Dislocation of the lens

SELF-ASSESSMENT QUESTIONS

Multiple choice questions (single best answer)

1. The following are features of osteoarthritis but not rheumatoid arthritis:
   A. Joint swelling
   B. Heberden's nodes
   C. More common in women
   D. Negative rheumatoid factor
   E. Treatment may include joint replacements

2. In rheumatoid arthritis:
   A. 90% of patients have positive rheumatoid factors
   B. Infliximab is used as treatment in all patients
   C. HLA DR4 is present in 25%
   D. T cells are activated
   E. X-rays demonstrate the presence of osteophytes

3. In septic arthritis:
   A. Artificial joints are not affected
   B. Gram-positive organisms are usually the cause
   C. The joint is not usually swollen
   D. Immunosuppressants are used as treatment
   E. Treatment should wait for results of antibiotic sensitivities

4. Regarding autoantibodies:
   A. ANA occurs in 90% of cases of antiphospholipid syndrome
   B. Rheumatoid factor occurs in 40% of cases of systemic lupus erythematosus (SLE)

   C. Rheumatoid factor occurs in 90% of cases of systemic sclerosis

   D. Double-stranded DNA is specific for SLE

   E. Anticentromere antibodies occur in 20% of cases of systemic sclerosis

5. Which of the following is seen in systemic sclerosis:
   A. Butterfly skin rash
   B. Pleural effusion
   C. Thrombocytopenia
   D. Hemiplegia
   E. 'Beaking' of the nose

6. In systemic sclerosis:
   A. Steroids are used
   B. Malabsorption is caused by villous atrophy
   C. Pulmonary fibrosis is a common cause of death
   D. Raynaud's phenomenon occurs in few cases
   E. Hands are rarely affected

7. In osteoporosis:
   A. Plasma calcium may be low
   B. Diagnosis is made when bone density rises 2.5 SDs above the mean for sex- and race-matched controls
   C. Fracture risk can be reduced by bisphosphonates
   D. Men and women are equally affected
   E. Calcaneal fractures are common

8. In polymyalgia rheumatica:
   A. The ESR is usually low
   B. There can be an association with giant cell arteritis
   C. Disease is unresponsive to steroids
   D. Weight loss makes the diagnosis unlikely
   E. Symptoms are worse at night

9. Osteomalacia:
   A. Is treated with steroids
   B. Is associated with normal bone biochemistry
   C. Does not cause myopathy
   D. Can be caused by inadequate exposure to sunlight
   E. Is rare in primary biliary cirrhosis

10. Causes of hypocalcaemia include:
    A. Secondary deposits in bone
    B. Addison's disease
    C. Hyperparathyroidism
    D. Thiazide diuretics
    E. Massive blood transfusion

11. In hypocalcaemia:
    A. Tapping on the facial nerve may induce twitching of the facial muscles
    B. Tetany does not occur
    C. Treatment with bisphosphonates can be useful
    D. Treatment with calcitonin can be useful
    E. i.v. Calcium is contraindicated

12. In relation to serum bone biochemistry which statement is incorrect?
    A. Calcium is normal and alkaline phosphatase elevated in Paget's disease
    B. Phosphate is high in hypocalcaemia associated with chronic kidney disease

   C. Calcium is low and alkaline phosphatase elevated in osteomalacia
   D. Calcium is low in hyperparathyroidism
   E. Calcium is high and phosphate low in hyperparathyroidism

Extended matching questions

Question 1 Theme: Back pain
A. Osteoporosis
B. Osteoarthritis
C. Rheumatoid arthritis
D. Ankylosing spondylitis
E. Gout
F. Reactive arthritis
G. Systemic lupus erythematosus
H. Osteomalacia
I. Paget's disease

For each of the following questions, select the best answer from the list above:

   I. A 28-year-old male who has intermittent episodes of back pain has a raised ESR and is HLA-B27-positive. X-rays show syndesmophytes. What is the most likely diagnosis?

   II. A 60-year-old male smoker presents with progressive increasing episodes of back pain. His symptoms are worse in the mornings when he has stiffness. X-rays show no erosions. The ESR and alkaline phosphatase are normal. What is the most likely diagnosis?

   III. A 72-year-old female presents with an episode of severe back pain. She fractured her wrist recently during a fall and has a long history of asthma. She has normal alkaline phosphatase and calcium. What is the most likely diagnosis?

Question 2 Theme: Painful hands
A. Systemic sclerosis
B. Osteoarthritis
C. Rheumatoid arthritis
D. Gout
E. Reactive arthritis
F. Systemic lupus erythematosus
G. Septic arthritis
H. Psoriatic arthritis

For each of the following questions, select the best answer from the list above:

   I. A 56-year-old businessman has acute episodes of pain in the joints of his hands and feet. The episodes occur particularly in the distal and interphalangeal joints of the hands and first metatarsophalangeal joint of the great toe. His body mass index is 30 and the serum urate is elevated. What is the most likely diagnosis?

   II. A 35-year-old female presents with episodes of pain in the metacarpophalangeal joints of the hands. She has a fever and a rash on the face and the following blood results: rheumatoid factor positive, antinuclear antibody positive, ESR 15, CRP 145. What is the most likely diagnosis?

   III. A 72-year-old female presents with pains in the joints of her hands and her neck. On examination she has bony expansion of the distal interphalangeal joints of both hands. ESR is 35. What is the most likely diagnosis?

Question 3 Theme: Autoantibodies

A. Systemic sclerosis
B. Osteoarthritis
C. Rheumatoid arthritis
D. Gout
E. Reactive arthritis
F. Systemic lupus erythematosus
G. Septic arthritis
H. Antiphospholipid syndrome

For each of the following questions, select the best answers from the list above:

I. A 32-year-old female with a previous history of epilepsy presents with a history of recurrent miscarriage. She has a prolonged APTT and a positive anti-cardiolipin antibody. What is the most likely diagnosis?

II. A 35-year-old female presents with episodes of pain in the metacarpophalangeal joints of the hands. She has a fever. There are erosions on hand X-rays. Blood results show: rheumatoid factor negative, antinuclear antibody negative. What is the most likely diagnosis?

III. A 66-year-old retired schoolteacher has numbness and pain in her hands and feet. She has a positive-anticentromere antibody. What is the most likely diagnosis?

Dermatology 12

FUNCTIONS OF THE SKIN

- Physical barrier
- Protection against infection, chemicals and UV
- Prevention of excessive water loss or absorption
- UV-induced synthesis of vitamin D
- Temperature regulation
- Sensation
- Antigen presentation/immunological reactions and wound healing

EXAMINATION OF THE SKIN

Look at the rash
For useful terms, see Table 12.1.

Note its distribution
Useful terminology:
- Flexural/extensor (remember psoriasis is usually extensor and eczema is usually flexural)
- Localized/widespread
- Symmetrical/unilateral
- Facial
- Centripetal (trunk > limbs)
- Acral (hands and feet)
- Linear/annular
- Reticulate (lacy network)

Feel the rash
- Use gloves if necessary

Examine
- Nails
- Hair
- Mouth

INFECTIONS

Bacterial infections

Impetigo
- Weeping exudative areas with honey-coloured crust
- Highly infectious
- 90% due to *Staphylococcus aureus*
Management
- Topical/oral antibiotics

Cellulitis
- Hot tender area of confluent erythema
- Often on lower legs

Table 12.1 Useful terms to describe skin lesions

Term	Meaning
Atrophy	Thinning of skin
Bulla	Large fluid-filled blister
Crusted	Dried exudate
Ecchymosis	Large 'bruise'
Erosion	Small denuded area of skin
Excoriation	Scratch mark
Fissure	Deep linear crack
Lichenified	Thickened skin with normal markings
Macule	Flat, circumscribed non-palpable lesion
Nodule	Large papule (>0.5 cm)
Papule	Small palpable circumscribed lesion
Petechia	Pinpoint-sized macule of blood in the skin
Plaque	Large flat-topped palpable lesion
Purpura	Larger macule of blood in the skin which does not blanch on pressure
Pustule	Pus-filled lesion (white/yellow)
Scaly	Visible flakes/shedding of skin surface
Telangiectasia	Abnormal visible dilatation of blood vessels
Ulcer	Larger denuded area of skin
Vesicle	Small fluid-filled blister
Wheal	Raised erythematous swelling (dermal swelling)

- Can affect face (erysipelas)
- Caused by *streptococci*

Management
- Oral/i.v. antibiotics

Viral infections

Herpes simplex

HSV Type 1 – direct contact, droplet infection
- Vesicular lesions
- May be recurrent, e.g. cold sores

Management
- Topical aciclovir/oral valciclovir

HSV Type 2 – sexually transmitted
- Affect genital area

Herpes zoster (shingles)

Varicella zoster virus (VZV)
- Reactivation of infection
- There may be a prodrome of tingling pain

- Unilateral blistering eruption
  - Single dermatomal distribution usually
  - Otoscopy demonstrates vesicles in the external auditory meatus

Management
- Analgesia
- Oral valciclovir/famciclovir or aciclovir

Complications
- Post-herpetic neuralgia (pain)
- Ocular involvement (ophthalmic nerve)

Fungal infections (mycoses)

Dermatophyte infections
Tinea corporis
- Body ringworm
- Slightly itchy asymmetrical scaly patch with central clearing and raised edge
Tinea cruris
- Groin ringworm
Tinea pedis
- Athlete's foot
Tinea capitis
- Scalp ringworm
Management
- Antifungal cream
- Oral agents for feet/severe infections

Candida albicans
- Flexural areas
- Red areas with ragged edges
- Satellite lesions
Risk factors
- Immunosuppression including steroids
- Diabetes mellitus
Management
- Topical/oral antifungal agents

INFESTATIONS

Scabies

- *Sarcoptes scabiei*
- Itchy red papules
- Skin burrows visible in web spaces
- Diagnosis by skin scrapings

Treatment
- Malathion or permethrin
- Treat all skin below neck
- Treat all close contacts

ECZEMA (DERMATITIS) (TABLE 12.2)

- Acute – inflamed weeping skin with vesicles
- Subacute – erythema, dry/flaky skin, crusted
- Chronic – lichenified skin

Table 12.2 Classification of eczema

Endogenous	Exogenous
Atopic eczema	Contact eczema – irritant
Discoid eczema	Contact eczema – allergic
Hand eczema	Photosensitive eczema
Seborrhoeic eczema	Lichen simplex/nodular prurigo
Venous ('gravitational') eczema	
Asteatotic eczema	

Epidemiology
- 40% of population have an episode associated with atopy
- Atopic individuals have a tendency to
  - Asthma
  - Eczema
  - Hay fever
  - Allergic rhinitis

Atopic eczema

Aetiology
- Genetic – polygenic
- Environmental triggers
  - Detergents/chemicals
  - Infection
  - Stress/anxiety
  - Animal fur
  - Foods (dairy products in the very young)

Clinical features
- Itchy erythematous scaly patches
- Often flexural
- May be associated with nail pitting

Investigations
- May have raised IgE or eosinophils
- Skin-patch testing

Management
- Education and explanation
- Avoid irritants
- Emollients
- Bath oil or soap substitutes
- Topical steroids or immunomodulators (tacrolimus)
- Antibiotics for secondary infection
- Antihistamines
- Second-line agents
  - Phototherapy – Ultraviolet (UV) light
  - Oral steroids
  - Ciclosporin/azathioprine

PSORIASIS

- Common disorder characterized by red scaly plaques

Epidemiology
- 2% of the population
- ♂ = ♀

Aetiology
- T lymphocyte-driven
- Genetic – polygenic
- Environmental triggers
  - Infection
  - Drugs, e.g. lithium
  - UV light
  - Alcohol
  - Stress/anxiety

Clinical features
Chronic plaque psoriasis
- Purplish/red scaly plaques, particularly on extensor surfaces
- Scalp frequently involved
- Can occur in areas of skin trauma (Köbner phenomenon)
- 50% associated with nail changes
  - Nail pitting
  - Distal separation of nail plate (onycholysis)
  - Yellow/brown discoloration
  - Subungual hyperkeratosis
  - If severe, loss of nail plate
Flexural psoriasis
- Occurs in older patients
- Patches in:
  - Groin
  - Natal cleft
  - Submammary areas
Guttate psoriasis
- Raindrop-like lesions on trunk
- Occurs in children/young adults 2 weeks after a streptococcal sore throat

Arthritis associated with psoriasis
- See page 270

Management
- Education and explanation
- Emollients
- Avoid irritants
- Topical steroids
- Calcipotriol (vitamin D_3 analogue)
- Coal tar
- Phototherapy, e.g. PUVA (psoralen + UVA)
- Methotrexate, TNF-α inhibitors if severe

Complications
- Erythroderma – see below

Erythroderma

- Widespread inflammation of the skin

Common causes
- Atopic eczema
- Psoriasis
- Drugs, e.g. sulphonamides, gold
- Seborrhoeic dermatitis

Management
- Bed rest
- Liberal i.v. fluids
- Keep warm
- Emollients
- Beware of sepsis
- Treat/remove the cause

Complications
- High-output cardiac failure
- Hypothermia
- Dehydration
- Hypoalbuminaemia
- Increased basal metabolic rate
- Capillary leak syndrome

ACNE VULGARIS

- Affects 85% of adolescents

Cause
- Follicular epidermal hyperproliferation
- Blockage of pilosebaceous unit
- Increased sebum production
- Infection with propiobacterium acnes

Clinical features
- Open comedones – blackheads
- Closed comedones – whiteheads
- Inflammatory papules
- Pustules

Treatment
- Reduce sebum production and reduce bacteria
- Topical retinoids and antibiotics
- Low dose oral antibiotics
- Oral retinoid drugs

SKIN CANCER

- There are three common types, see Table 12.3
- All are related to exposure to sunlight

CUTANEOUS FEATURES OF SYSTEMIC DISEASE

Erythema nodosum

- Painful dusky/purplish nodules
- Commonly on the shins
- Associations – see Table 12.4

Table 12.3 Features of the three common skin cancers

Type	Clinical features	Spread	Management
Basal cell carcinoma (rodent ulcer)	Occur in later life Slow-growing nodule May ulcerate Pearly edge Telangiectasia Can erode local structures	No metastases	Surgical excision Radiotherapy
Squamous cell carcinoma	Rapidly growing nodule which ulcerates More common in immunosuppressed patients, e.g. renal transplant patients Also occurs in areas of chronic inflammation	Metastases occur	Surgical excision
Malignant melanoma	Can occur in young patients Transformation of 'moles' Consider in all bleeding pigmented lesions or 'changing moles'	Early metastases	Wide excision Radiotherapy Immunotherapy Chemotherapy for metastases

Table 12.4 Aetiology of erythema nodosum and erythema multiforme

Erythema nodosum
    Streptococcal infection
    Drugs (e.g. antibiotics, oral contraceptive pill)
    Tuberculosis
    Inflammatory bowel disease
    Sarcoid
    Leprosy
    Fungal infection, e.g. histoplasmosis
    Chlamydia infection
    Idiopathic
Erythema multiforme
    Herpes/Epstein–Barr virus infection
    Drugs (e.g. antibiotics, barbiturates)
    Mycoplasma infections
    Connective tissue disease, e.g. SLE HIV
    Carcinoma/lymphoma

Erythema multiforme

- Erythematous lesion with central pallor (target lesions)
- Symmetrical, particularly on limbs
- May blister
- Mucosal involvement = Stevens–Johnson syndrome
- Associations – see Table 12.4

Pyoderma gangrenosum

- Erythematous nodules with ulceration
- Large areas of ulceration
- Bluish/black edge
- Purulent surface
- Associations
  - Inflammatory bowel disease
  - Rheumatoid arthritis
  - Myeloma/leukaemia/lymphoma
  - Liver disease
  - Idiopathic

Management
- Topical/oral steroids
- Treatment of underlying condition
- Ciclosporin

Acanthosis nigricans

- Thickened hyperpigmented skin in the flexures, e.g. axilla
- Associations
  - Insulin resistance
  - Malignancy (particularly GI tract)

Chronic discoid lupus

- Red scaly atrophic plaques ± telangiectasia
- Face/exposed areas of skin
- May be associated with alopecia
- Triggered/exacerbated by UV light
- 30% antinuclear factor-positive
- 5% develop systemic lupus erythematosus (SLE)

Management
- Topical steroids
- Hydroxychloroquine
- Oral steroids/azathioprine/ciclosporin/thalidomide

Systemic lupus erythematosus (skin manifestations)

- Macular erythema on cheeks/nose/forehead (butterfly rash)

Pruritus (medical conditions associated with itching)

- Iron deficiency
- Malignancy, e.g. lymphoma
- Diabetes mellitus
- Chronic kidney disease
- Cholestasis
- Chronic liver disease

- Thyroid disease
- HIV
- Polycythaemia vera

BULLOUS DISORDERS

Pemphigus vulgaris

- Middle age
- ♀ > ♂

Pathogenesis
- Autoantibodies against desmosomal protein desmoglein 1 and 3

Clinical features
- Mouth ulcers 50%
- Flaccid blisters on trunk
- Rapidly denuding blisters

Treatment
- High dose corticosteroids

Bullous pemphigoid

- Age >60 years
- Mucosal involvement rare
- Deep blisters
- Large tense bullae on hands and feet
- Itchy

Treatment
- Corticosteroids

Dermatitis herpetiformis

- Rare blistering disorder associated with gluten sensitive enteropathy (coeliac disease)
- Young adults
- ♀ > ♂

Treatment
- Gluten free diet
- Dapsone

LEG ULCERS

Aetiology
- Venous hypertension
- Arterial insufficiency
- Neuropathic (e.g. diabetes mellitus)
- Neoplastic (e.g. squamous cell carcinoma)
- Vasculitis

Venous ulcers

- Infection, e.g. syphilis
- Blood disorders, e.g. sickle cell disease
- Trauma
- Most common cause associated with venous hypertension or previous thrombosis

- Often recurrent and chronic
- Usually painless
- Medial aspect of leg
- Exclude arterial insufficiency with Doppler

Management

- Topical therapy to ulcer
- Compression bandaging and elevation of legs
- Antibiotics for overt infection
- Diuretics for oedema
- Analgesia if painful
- Skin grafting if resistant to therapy

Arterial ulcers

- Punched out
- Painful
- Leg cold and pale
- Absent pulses
- History of hypertension, claudication, smoking, angina
- Investigate with Doppler studies/angiogram

Management

- Analgesia
- Topical treatment of ulcer
- Vascular reconstruction

Neuropathic ulcers

- Over pressure areas, e.g. metatarsal heads
- Result of trauma
- Polyneuropathy, e.g. diabetes mellitus
- Painless

Management

- Keep clean
- Avoid trauma including good foot care

SELF-ASSESSMENT QUESTIONS

Multiple choice questions (single best answer)

1. Which of the following is a risk factor for skin malignancy?
   A. Methotrexate
   B. Diabetes mellitus
   C. Steroids
   D. Phenytoin
   E. Sunlight exposure
2. In dermatology:
   A. A bulla is pus-filled
   B. Acral lesions affect the scalp
   C. An ecchymosis is a large bruise
   D. Purpura blanch on pressure
   E. Ringworm is a viral infection
3. In eczema:
   A. The rash is rarely itchy
   B. The rash is often on the extensor surfaces
   C. Stress can be a trigger factor

  D. Ciclosporin is the usual treatment
  E. 10% of the population experience the condition at some time in
     their lives
4. Psoriasis:
  A. Is more common in males
  B. Is not triggered by stress
  C. Most commonly affects extensor surfaces
  D. Is easily cured
  E. Is usually treated with topical antibiotics
5. Basal cell carcinoma:
  A. Is associated with early metastases
  B. May have telangiectasia
  C. Never ulcerates
  D. Is treated with chemotherapy
  E. Is most common in young adults
6. Malignant melanoma:
  A. Is not associated with early metastases
  B. Is rarely life-threatening in young people
  C. Is easily distinguished from benign moles
  D. Is treated by wide excision and adjuvant therapy
  E. Only occurs in the skin
7. Erythema nodosum:
  A. Often occurs on the arms
  B. Is not associated with Crohn's disease
  C. Is associated with use of oral contraceptives
  D. Is common in tuberculosis
  E. Is most commonly associated with a viral infection
8. In erythema multiforme:
  A. Uniform red patches occur
  B. Lesions on the feet occur in Stevens–Johnson syndrome
  C. Is not caused by barbiturates
  D. Disease is less likely in immunosuppressed patients
  E. The rash is usually symmetrical
9. Leg ulcers:
  A. Are most commonly caused by arterial insufficiency
  B. Are always painful if venous
  C. Associated with neuropathy occur over metatarsal heads
  D. May need treatment with steroids
  E. Are rarely recurrent
10. Erythroderma:
  A. Is not a complication of eczema
  B. Is usually treated with fluid restriction
  C. Capillary leak syndrome may require intensive care
  D. Is treated with induced hypothermia
  E. Is localized to the legs

Extended matching questions

Question 1 Theme: Erythematous rash

A. Eczema
 B. Psoriasis
 C. Meningococcal septicaemia
D. Squamous cell carcinoma
 E. Systemic lupus erythematosus

F. Impetigo

G. Erysipelas

H. Erythema multiforme

I. Erythema nodosum

J. Typhoid fever

For each of the following questions, select the best answer from the list above:

I. A 39-year-old female presents with an erythematous rash on her legs. She has just returned from holiday in North Africa. The lesions are purplish, painful and warm to the touch. She has a medical history of Crohn's disease and at present has a flare-up of her symptoms with diarrhoea. What is the most likely diagnosis?

II. A 12-year-old female presents with an erythematous rash on her arms. She has a history of asthma. She also says that she is having difficulty sleeping because of itching. The rash is flexural in distribution and she has nail pitting. What is the most likely diagnosis?

III. A 28-year-old male presents with a rash on his hands. It is weeping fluid and in parts has yellow crusting areas. His girlfriend has a similar rash. It responds to treatment with antibiotics. What is the most likely diagnosis?

Question 2 Theme: Skin ulcers

A. Venous ulcers

B. Squamous cell carcinoma

C. Malignant melanoma

D. Erythema multiforme

E. Erythema nodosum

F. Pyoderma gangrenosum

G. Impetigo

H. Erythrasma

I. Leprosy

For each of the following questions, select the best answer from the list above:

I. A 39-year-old female presents with an ulcer on her right shin. She recently injured this area while on holiday in Africa. She has a medical history of Crohn's disease. She is worried that the ulcer is rapidly increasing in size. What is the most likely diagnosis?

II. An 82-year-old female presents with an ulcer just above the medial malleolus. She has been treated with dressings by the community nurses for 6 weeks without improvement. She has previously had surgery for varicose veins and is on aspirin for angina. The skin around the ulcer is pigmented and brownish. What is the most likely diagnosis?

III. A 48-year-old male presents with an ulcer on his ear. He is a keen gardener. He has had an area of crusting skin there for some time. There is an enlarged hard post-auricular lymph node. What is the most likely diagnosis?

Question 3 Theme: Pruritus

A. Iron deficiency

B. Squamous cell carcinoma

C. Diabetes mellitus

D. Erythema multiforme

E. Erythema nodosum

F. Cholestasis

G. HIV

H. Erythrasma

I. Polycythaemia rubra vera

For each of the following questions, select the best answer from the list above:

I. A 39-year-old male presents with pruritus. A full blood count reveals that he has a low lymphocyte count. What is the most likely cause of his itching?

II. An 82-year-old female presents with itching, weight loss and abdominal pain. Her neighbours have told her that she looks yellow. She has recently been diagnosed with diabetes. An ultrasound suggests a mass in the head of the pancreas. What is the most likely cause of her itching?

III. A 48-year-old male presents with itching. He has also noted a change in his bowel habit and is awaiting colonoscopy. His full blood count shows a haemoglobin of 8.9 g/dL with an MCV of 69 fL. What is the most likely cause of his itching?

Hormones

- Chemical messengers
  - Polypeptide (e.g. insulin)
  - Lipid (e.g. cortisol)
  - Amine (e.g. tyrosine)
  - Glycoprotein (e.g. TSH)
- Signal between cells or organs
- Influence via:
  - Cell membrane receptors (e.g. insulin) → rapid effect
  - Intracellular receptors (e.g. thyroxine) → slow effect
- Allow adjustment to internal and external environment
- Transmitted via:
  - Blood (endocrine)
  - Directly to adjacent cells (paracrine)
- Secretion control
  - Usually negative feedback loop
  - Effect of hormone on release of secretion factor (e.g. thyroxine on TSH)
  - Effect of end substance on secretion (e.g. glucose on insulin)
  - Circadian rhythm (e.g. cortisol)

Endocrine disorders

- Common
  - Type 1 diabetes mellitus (10–30/100 000 per year)
  - Type 2 diabetes mellitus (2% of the population)
  - Thyroid disease (1.5–3 cases/1000 per year)
  - Subfertility (5–10% of all couples)
  - Menstrual disorders
  - Osteoporosis
  - Primary hyperparathyroidism (0.1%)
- Caused by abnormalities in hormone
  - Synthesis
  - Secretion
  - Control
  - Function
- Common disorders are shown in Table 13.1
- Rarer conditions provide classical cases for both written and clinical examinations and will be included in this chapter

Common pathologies

- Affect endocrine glands or their target organs
- Organ-specific autoimmune disorders
- Endocrine tumours

Table 13.1 Common endocrine disorders

Diabetes mellitus	Osteoporosis
Thyroid disease	Primary hyperparathyroidism
Subfertility	Short stature
Menstrual disorders	Delayed puberty
Excess hair growth	

- Drugs affecting endocrine function
  - Direct induction (chlorpromazine → ↑ prolactin)
  - Direct inhibition (amiodarone → hypothyroidism)
  - Simulation (ACE inhibitors → hypoaldosteronism)
  - Toxicity (chemotherapy → gonadal failure)
  - Altered protein binding (anticonvulsants → ↓ T_4)
  - Exogenous hormones (steroids → Cushing syndrome)

CLINICAL HISTORY IN ENDOCRINE DISEASE

See Table 13.2.

EXAMINING THE ENDOCRINE SYSTEM

- Overall appearance (i.e. spot diagnosis), e.g. acromegaly, Graves' disease, should be assessed
- All clinical 'systems' may be involved in endocrine disorders
- Full examination of all systems is expected (Box 13.1)
- Certain parts of the examination may be discriminatory in diagnosis

---

Table 13.2 Points to note in taking an endocrine history

Past medical history
    Diabetes mellitus
    Hypertension
    Previous pregnancies/fertility
    Previous surgery – thyroid/parathyroid, ovarian, testicular
    Childhood milestones and development
    Puberty
    Previous radiation exposure – neck (thyroid), gonads
Family history
    Autoimmune disorders
    Endocrine disorders
    Diabetes mellitus
Social history
    Alcohol or drug abuse
    Diet, e.g. salt/iodine intake
Drug history
    Details of *all* drugs taken at present and previous regular
        medications
    Corticosteroids
    Sex hormones, e.g. HRT, oral contraceptive pill

- Overall appearance
- Height, weight and nutritional status
- Blood pressure (including postural measurements)
- Neck – look for goitre
- Thyroid status (see Box 13.2)
- Eyes – look for exophthalmos, Graves' eye disease
- Visual fields – pituitary tumours
- Secondary sexual characteristics and testicular examination
- Skin and hair – pigmentation, bruising, telangiectasia, acne
- Urine – check for glucose, protein, β-human chorionic gonadotrophin

LABORATORY TESTS IN ENDOCRINOLOGY

- Hormones may be measured in blood/plasma or urine
- Markers of function
  - Glucose in diabetes
  - Calcium in hyperparathyroidism

Basal levels

Blood or plasma levels

- Useful measurements for hormones with a long half-life, e.g. thyroxine (T_4 and T_3)
- Also applied to certain conditions in which normal values are known, e.g.
  - Time of day – cortisol and adrenocorticotropic hormone (ACTH)
  - Period of menstrual cycle – follicle stimulating hormone (FSH), oestrogen, progesterone
  - Posture – aldosterone

24-hour urine collections

- Provide an average of a whole day's secretion of a hormone
- Require normal renal function and accurately timed and complete urine collection

Dynamic tests

- Test ability of a gland to respond appropriately to stimulation or suppression
- Failure of normal negative feedback causing uncontrolled hormone secretion
  - From within the gland
  - From an ectopic source
- Failure of a normal positive response to stimulation of a gland

Examples

Stimulation test – SynACTHen test

- Normal adrenal response to a dose of synthetic ACTH is an increase in plasma cortisol levels
- Primary adrenal failure – a diminished or absent response
- Adrenal failure secondary to lack of pituitary secretion of ACTH – normal or enhanced cortisol response

Suppression test – dexamethasone suppression test
- Normal response to a dose of synthetic steroid is reduction in pituitary release of ACTH and subsequent fall in adrenal cortisol release and plasma levels
- Uncontrolled endogenous production of ACTH from a pituitary tumour or ectopic source leads to inadequate suppression of plasma cortisol level

THYROID DISORDERS

Control of thyroxine secretion

See Figure 13.1 and Table 13.3.

Examination of thyroid gland and status

See Box 13.2 and Chapter 3.

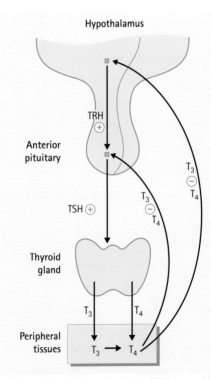

Fig. 13.1 The hypothalamic-pituitary-thyroid axis. TRH, thyrotrophin releasing hormone. TSH, thyroid stimulating hormone.

Table 13.3 Biochemistry of thyroid disorder

	Hormone levels		Dynamic and other tests
	T4 and T3	TSH	
Hyperthyroidism	↑	↓	Autoantibodies
Primary hypothyroidism	↓	↑	Autoantibodies
Secondary hypothyroidism	↓	↓ or normal	

Box 13.2. Examination of thyroid gland and status

General inspection
- Look for signs of thyroid disease

Examine the neck
- Look for a goitre
- Ask the patient to take a sip of water and hold it in the mouth, then ask him or her to swallow while watching the neck – look for movement of goitre with swallowing
- Stand behind the patient and feel the thyroid with both hands, starting in the centre below the thyroid cartilage over the trachea, and moving laterally to the two lobes, which extend behind the sternomastoid muscle. Ask the patient to swallow while palpating. Assess the goitre for size, nodularity or diffuse enlargement, discrete nodules and firmness
- Palpate for lymph nodes
- Auscultate – listen over the thyroid for a bruit

Assess thyroid status
- Pulse – count the rate and note the presence or absence of atrial fibrillation
- Palms – warm and sweaty
- Tremor of outstretched arms

Examine the eyes
- Exophthalmos
- Lid retraction
- Lid lag

Examine the reflexes
- Slow relaxation in hypothyroidism

Goitre

Aetiology in a euthyroid patient
- Simple non-toxic goitre
  - Iodine deficiency
  - Treated Graves' disease
  - Puberty
- Solitary nodule
  - Thyroid adenoma
  - Thyroid cyst
  - Thyroid carcinoma

Aetiology in a hypothyroid patient
- Hashimoto's thyroiditis
- Radioiodine-treated Graves' disease

Aetiology in a hyperthyroid patient
- Graves' disease
- Toxic multinodular goitre

Hypothyroidism

Aetiology
- Atrophic (autoimmune – antithyroid antibodies)
- Hashimoto's thyroiditis (thyroid peroxidase antibodies)
- Iodine deficiency
- Post radioiodine-treated hyperthyroidism
- Thyroidectomy

Clinical features
- Weight gain
- Tiredness
- Depression
- Patient feels the cold
- Constipation
- Poor appetite/libido
- Menstrual disturbances
- Myxoedema facies; thickened skin
- Dry, thin, brittle hair
- Periorbital puffiness
- Bradycardia and hypertension
- Slow relaxing reflexes

Investigations
- Biochemistry (Table 13.3)
- Haematology
  - Anaemia (usually normocytic/normochromic)
  - Macrocytosis (low T_4 or pernicious anaemia)
  - Microcytic (due to menorrhagia)
- Anti-thyroid antibodies
- Hypercholesterolaemia

Management
- Thyroxine replacement
- Caution in cardiac disease
- Monitor TSH

Hyperthyroidism

Common causes
- Graves' disease (anti-TSH receptor antibodies mimic TSH)
- Toxic multinodular goitre
- Single toxic nodule
- Gestational
- Drugs (e.g. amiodarone)

Clinical features
- Heat intolerance
- Weight loss
- Increased appetite

- Diarrhoea
- Irritability
- Sleeplessness, tiredness
- Exertional breathlessness
- Goitre
- Tachycardia/atrial fibrillation
- Tremor
- Hyperkinesia
- Proximal muscle wasting
- Cardiac failure
- Pretibial myxoedema

Eye signs (Graves' disease)
- Exophthalmos
- Lid lag
- Lid retraction
- Ophthalmoplegia

Investigations
- TSH suppressed
- raised T_3 and/or T_4

Management
Medical treatment
- Carbimazole (risk of agranulocytosis)
- Propylthiouracil (risk of agranulocytosis)
- β-blockers
- Radioiodine

Surgical treatment for
- Malignancy
- Pressure symptoms
- Failure of medical treatment

PITUITARY DISORDERS

Functions of the anterior pituitary

See Figure 13.2 and Table 13.4.

Control of growth hormone secretion

See Figure 13.3.

Acromegaly

Aetiology
- Pituitary tumour

Clinical features
- Often insidious nonspecific onset
- Headaches
- Polyuria
- Erectile dysfunction
- Visual field defects, e.g. bitemporal hemianopia
- Nerve compression, e.g. carpal tunnel syndrome
- Typical facies, e.g.
  - Thick greasy skin
  - Protrusion of lower jaw
  - Gaps between teeth

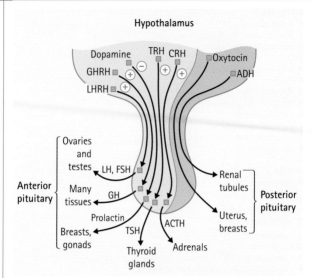

Fig. 13.2 The hypothalamic-pituitary axis. LHRH, luteinizing hormone releasing hormone; TSH, thyroid stimulating hormone; FSH, follicle stimulating hormone; CRH, corticotrophin releasing hormone; GHRH, growth hormone releasing hormone; ACTH, adrenocorticotropic hormone. TRH, thyrotrophin releasing hormone; ADH, antidiuretic hormone.

Table 13.4 Biochemistry of disorders of the hypothalamic-anterior pituitary axis

	Hormone levels	Dynamic and other tests
Acromegaly	Growth hormone ↑	Oral glucose load (growth hormone (GH) fails to suppress)
Prolactinoma	Prolactin ↑	
Panhypopituitarism	Luteinizing hormone (LH)/follicle stimulating hormone (FSH) ↓ GH ↓ TSH ↓ ACTH ↓	Luteinizing hormone releasing hormone (LHRH) test Insulin stress test TRH test SynACTHen test

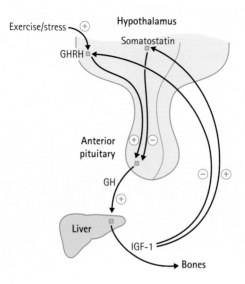

Fig. 13.3 The growth axis. IGF-1, insulin-like growth factor 1.

- Large 'spade-like' hands
- Cardiac failure
- Diabetes mellitus
- Hypertension

Investigations
- Glucose tolerance test – GH not suppressed by glucose
- Insulin like growth factor 1
- Visual fields (bitemporal hemianopia)
- MRI pituitary

Management
- GH antagonists (pegvisomant)
- Dopamine agonists (bromocriptine)
- Somatostatin analogues (octreotide)
- Pituitary radiotherapy (post-surgery)
- Trans-sphenoidal hypophysectomy

Hypopituitarism

Aetiology
Congenital
- Kallmann syndrome (hypogonadism)
Infective
- Basal meningitis (e.g. tuberculosis)
- Encephalitis
- Syphilis
Vascular
- Sheehan syndrome (postpartum necrosis)

Tumours
- Pituitary
- Hypothalamic
- Craniopharyngioma
- Meningioma
- Glioma
- Metastases (especially breast)
- Lymphoma

Infiltration
- Sarcoidosis
- Langerhans histiocytosis
- Haemochromatosis

Others
- Radiation
- Anorexia nervosa
- Trauma or previous surgery

Clinical features
- Due to progressive loss of anterior pituitary hormones (listed in order of frequency)

Growth hormone
- Growth failure
- Short stature

Prolactin
- Failure of lactation

Gonadotrophins
- Delayed puberty
- Infertility
- Amenorrhoea
- Loss of body hair

TSH
- Hypothyroidism

ACTH
- Adrenal failure (without pigmentation)

Investigations
- Determine hormone deficiencies
- Pituitary imaging, e.g. CT scan, MRI scan

Management
- Treat cause
- Hormone replacement

ADRENAL HORMONE ABNORMALITIES

Control of cortisol secretion

See Figure 13.4.

Cushing syndrome

- Overproduction of corticosteroids or excess corticosteroid treatment

Aetiology
ACTH-dependent (Cushing's disease)
- Pituitary adenoma
- Ectopic ACTH-secreting tumours

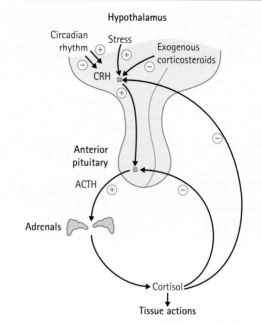

Fig. 13.4 The hypothalamic–pituitary–adrenal axis.

Non-ACTH-dependent
- Adrenal adenoma
- Adrenal carcinoma
- Steroid treatment

Others
- Alcohol-induced pseudo-Cushing syndrome

Clinical features
- Weight gain
- Thin skin
- Striae
- Bruising
- Menstrual disturbances
- Psychosis
- Red face
- Central obesity
- Buffalo hump
- Hirsutism
- Proximal myopathy
- Hypertension
- Diabetes mellitus

Table 13.5 Biochemistry of disorders of the pituitary-adrenal axis

	Hormone levels	Dynamic and other tests
ACTH-secreting pituitary adenoma (Cushing's disease)	24-hour urine cortisol ↑ Midnight cortisol ↑	Dexamethasone suppression test
Ectopic ACTH secretion	24-hour urine cortisol ↑ Midnight cortisol ↑	Dexamethasone suppression test
Adrenal adenoma	24-hour urine cortisol ↑ Midnight cortisol ↑	Dexamethasone suppression test
Pituitary failure	9 a.m. cortisol ↓	Synacthen test (normal response)
Primary adrenal failure	9 a.m. cortisol ↓	Synacthen test (diminished response)

Investigations
- Biochemistry (Table 13.5)
- Serum electrolytes
  - Sodium ↓
  - Potassium ↑
- Pituitary imaging
- Adrenal imaging
- Chest X-ray (ACTH secreting bronchogenic carcinoma)

Management
Pituitary-dependent
- Trans-sphenoidal resection of tumour
Adrenal adenomas
- Medical treatment with metyrapone, to induce remission before adrenalectomy
Ectopic ACTH
- Remove tumour if possible
- Control Cushing's with metyrapone

Primary hypoadrenalism – Addison's disease

- Destruction of adrenal cortex causing reduced production of glucocorticoid, mineralocorticoid and sex steroids

Aetiology
See Table 13.6.

Clinical features
- Tiredness
- Debility
- Nausea, vomiting
- Anorexia, weight loss
- Abdominal pain

Table 13.6 Causes of primary hypoadrenalism

Common
  Autoimmune disease (approx. 90%)
  Tuberculosis (<10% in UK)
  Surgical removal
Uncommon
  Haemorrhage/infarction
  Meningococcal septicaemia
  Venography
  Malignant destruction
  Amyloid

- Diarrhoea
- Depression
- Menstrual disturbance
- Pigmentation – mouth, palmar creases
- Postural hypotension
- Dehydration
- Loss of body hair

Investigations
See Table 13.5.

Management
- Replacement of glucocorticoids and mineralocorticoids with oral hydrocortisone and fludrocortisone

PARATHYROIDS (SEE ALSO CH. 11)

Hyperparathyroidism

Aetiology
Primary
- Adenoma (80% solitary)
- Hyperplasia
- Carcinoma
Secondary
- Hyperplasia in hypocalcaemia
- Chronic kidney disease
- Osteomalacia
Tertiary
- Autonomous secretion after prolonged hypocalcaemia

Clinical features
- Abdominal pain
- Anorexia
- Constipation
- Pain
- Pathological fractures
- Polydipsia and polyuria
- Renal calculi

} Due to hypercalcaemia

Investigations
See Table 13.7.

Table 13.7 Biochemistry of disorders of calcium homeostasis

	Hormone levels	Dynamic and other tests
Osteoporosis	PTH normal	
Primary hyperparathyroidism	PTH ↑	Serum calcium ↑ Serum phosphate ↓
Tertiary hyperparathyroidism	PTH ↑	Serum calcium ↑ Serum phosphate ↑
Primary hypoparathyroidism	PTH undetectable	Serum calcium ↓
Pseudohypoparathyroidism	PTH normal	Serum calcium ↓

Management
- Treat underlying cause
- Parathyroidectomy if Ca^{++} >3 or symptoms
- Treat hypercalcaemia (p. 281)

Hypoparathyroidism

Aetiology
- Post-surgical
- Post-radiotherapy
- Autoimmune
- Pseudohyperparathyroidism = end organ resistance

Clinical features
- Cataracts
- Cramps
- Fits ⎬ Due to hypocalcaemia
- Paraesthesiae
- Tetany

Investigations
See Table 13.7.

Osteoporosis

- Reduction in bone density below normal for age and sex (p. 276)

SEX HORMONE AND REPRODUCTIVE DISORDERS

Amenorrhoea – primary or secondary

Aetiology
Pituitary causes
- Hyperprolactinaemia
- Hypopituitarism
- Thyrotoxicosis
- Anorexia nervosa

Ovarian causes (Table 13.8)
- Surgery
- Primary ovarian failure
- Polycystic ovary syndrome

Table 13.8 Biochemistry of ovarian disorders

	Hormone levels	Dynamic and other tests
Polycystic ovary syndrome	Androgens ↑	
Primary ovarian failure	FSH ↑ LH ↑ Oestrogen ↓	LHRH test Clomiphene stimulation test

- Congenital adrenal hyperplasia
  - Autosomal recessive
  - Enzyme deficiency in cortisol synthesis
  - → Sexual ambiguity/adrenal failure
- Chromosomal abnormalities
  - Turner syndrome (XO)

SALT AND WATER BALANCE DISORDERS

Control of salt and water homeostasis

See Box 13.3 and Figure 13.5.

Diabetes insipidus

- Deficiency of antidiuretic hormone (ADH) or insensitivity to its action

---

Box 13.3. Water deprivation test

- Free fluid overnight

08:00 hours
- No access to fluids
- Record hourly
  - Urine and plasma osmolality
  - Urine volume
  - Body weight
- Stop and allow fluid if body weight loss >3%

16:00 hours
- 2 µg desmopressin injection i.m.
- Continue fluid restriction according to urine output

04:00 hours
- Stop

Normal
- Normal plasma osmolality maintained up to urine concentration >800 mosm/kg

Cranial DI
- Urine fails to concentrate
- Plasma osmolality rises
- Abnormality is corrected with desmopressin

Nephrogenic DI
- As for cranial DI but not corrected by desmopressin

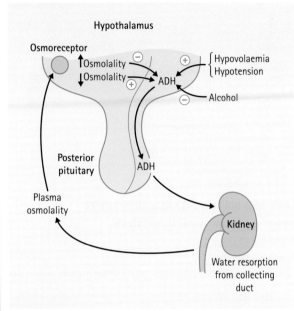

Fig. 13.5 The thirst axis.

Aetiology
- Cranial causes
  - Idiopathic
  - Familial (DIDMOAD – diabetes insipidus, diabetes mellitus, optic atrophy, deafness)
  - Tumours, e.g. craniopharyngioma, glioma, metastases (breast)
  - Infiltration, e.g. sarcoidosis, histiocytosis
  - Sheehan syndrome (pituitary infarction following post- or antepartum haemorrhage)
- Nephrogenic causes
  - Idiopathic
  - Renal tubular acidosis
  - Hypokalaemia
  - Hypercalcaemia
  - Drugs, e.g. lithium, demeclocycline, glibenclamide

Clinical features
- Polyuria urine output (10–15 L/day)
- Thirst
- Nocturia
- Polydipsia
- Dehydration

Differential diagnosis
- Primary polydipsia (excessive water drinking/normal ADH secretion)

Table 13.9 Biochemistry of the hypothalamic-posterior pituitary axis

	Hormone levels	Dynamic and other tests
Cranial diabetes insipidus	ADH ↓ (not measured routinely)	Water deprivation test High plasma osmolality Low urine osmolality Normal response to desmopressin
Nephrogenic diabetes insipidus	ADH ↑ (not measured routinely)	Water deprivation test High plasma osmolality Low urine osmolality No response to DDAVP
Inappropriate ADH	ADH ↑ (not measured routinely)	Plasma osmolality low Urine osmolality high

Investigations
See Table 13.9.

Management
- Treat underlying cause
- Synthetic vasopressin analogue
- Desmopressin
- Carbamazepine
- Chlorpropamide

Syndrome of inappropriate ADH secretion (SIADH)

- Inappropriate ADH secretion → retention of water and hyponatraemia
- Low plasma osmolality with continued urinary sodium secretion

Aetiology
Tumours
- Small cell carcinoma of lung
- Prostate cancer
- Pancreatic cancer

Lungs
- Pneumonia
- TB

CNS
- Meningitis
- Tumours
- Head injury
- Chronic subdural haematoma
- SLE vasculitis

Drugs
- Chlorpropamide
- Carbamazepine
- Phenothiazines

Clinical features
- Confusion
- Nausea

- Fits
- Coma

Management
- Underlying cause
- Fluid restriction
- Demethylchlortetracycline

ENDOCRINE CAUSES OF HYPERTENSION

Control of the renin-angiotensin-aldosterone system

See Figure 13.6.

Primary hyperaldosteronism (Table 13.10)

- Rare (<1% of all hypertension)

Aetiology
- Conn syndrome (adrenal adenoma 60%)
- Bilateral adrenal hyperplasia (40%)

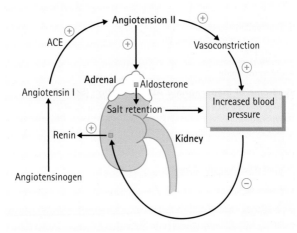

Fig. 13.6 The renin-angiotensin-aldosterone system. ACE, angiotensin-converting enzyme.

Table 13.10 Biochemistry of hyperaldosteronism		
	Hormone levels	**Dynamic and other tests**
Primary hyperaldosteronism (Conn syndrome)	Renin ↓ Aldosterone ↑	Serum K ↓ Aldosterone : renin ratio ↑ Metabolic alkalosis
Secondary hyperaldosteronism	Renin ↑ Aldosterone ↑	Serum K ↓ Metabolic alkalosis

Management
- Surgery for tumours
- Aldosterone antagonists, e.g. spironolactone

Phaeochromocytoma

- Very rare
- Tumour of the sympathetic nervous system (90% adrenal)
- Secretion of norepinephrine and epinephrine leading to
  - Peripheral vasoconstriction
  - Inotropic effects
  - Tachycardia
  - High blood pressure

Clinical features
- Anxiety, panic attacks
- Palpitations
- Tremor
- Sweating
- Headache
- Flushing
- GI upset
- Weight loss
- Hypertension (paroxysmal or continuous)
- Tachycardia
- Arrhythmias
- Fever

Investigations
- Raised 24-hour excretion of urinary catecholamines
- CT or MRI adrenal glands
- MIBG scan ^{131}I metaiodobenzylguanidine is specifically taken up in sites of sympathetic activity
  - Positive in 90% of phaeochromocytomas

Management
- Remove tumour
- α- and β-blockade (α first with phenoxybenzamine, then β with propranolol) prior to surgery to prevent dangerous swings in blood pressure

Multiple endocrine neoplasia (MEN)

- Simultaneous or metachronous occurrence of tumours in a number of endocrine glands with autosomal dominant inheritance

Type 1
- 95% Parathyroid – adenomas, hyperplasia
- 70% Pituitary – adenomas
- 50% Pancreas – islet cell tumours (e.g. insulinoma), gastrinoma
- 40% Adrenal adenoma
- 20% Thyroid adenoma

Type 2a
- 95% Adrenal – phaeochromocytoma
- 90% Thyroid – medullary carcinoma
- 60% Parathyroid – adenomas, adenocarcinoma

Type 2b
- Type 2a plus Marfanoid phenotype plus visceral ganglioneuromas
- No hyperparathyroidism

DIABETES MELLITUS

- Syndrome characterized by chronic hyperglycaemia due to relative insulin deficiency or resistance or both

WHO classification of diabetes

Type 1
- β cell destruction usually leading to absolute insulin deficiency
- Autoimmune or idiopathic

Type 2
- Variable combination of insulin resistance and defects in insulin secretion

Other specific types

Genetic defects
- Defects of β cell function or insulin function
- Maturity onset diabetes of the young (MODY)
- DIDMOAD syndrome

Endocrinopathies
- Cushing syndrome
- Acromegaly

Table 13.11 WHO criteria for the diagnosis of diabetes (glucose mmol/L)

WHO criteria for the diagnosis of diabetes are:
- Fasting plasma glucose >7.0 mmol/L (126 mg/dL)
- Random plasma glucose >11.1 mmol/L (200 mg/dL)
- One abnormal laboratory value is diagnostic in symptomatic individuals; two values are needed in asymptomatic people. The glucose tolerance test is only required for borderline cases and for diagnosis of gestational diabetes.
- HbA_{1c} >6.5 (48 mmol/mol)

The glucose tolerance test – WHO criteria			
	Normal	Impaired glucose tolerance	Diabetes mellitus
Fasting	<7.0 mmol/L	<7.0 mmol/L	>7.0 mmol/L
2 h after glucose	<7.8 mmol/L	7.8–11.0 mmol/L	>11.1 mmol/L

- Adult: 75 g glucose in 300 mL water
- Child: 1.75 g glucose/kg bodyweight
- Only a fasting and a 120-min sample are needed
- Results are for venous plasma – whole blood values are lower.

Note: There is no such thing as mild diabetes. All patients who meet the criteria for diabetes are liable to disabling long-term complications.
(Reproduced from Kumar P, Clark M. Kumar & Clark's Clinical Medicine, 8th edn. Edinburgh: Elsevier; 2012, with permission from Elsevier.)

- Phaeochromocytoma
- Hyperthyroidism

Diseases of the endocrine pancreas

- Trauma
- Pancreatectomy
- Chronic pancreatitis
- Fibrocalculous pancreatic diabetes
- Cystic fibrosis
- Haemochromatosis
- Cancer

Drug-induced

- Corticosteroids
- Thiazides

WHO criteria for diagnosis of diabetes

See Table 13.11 and Figure 13.7.

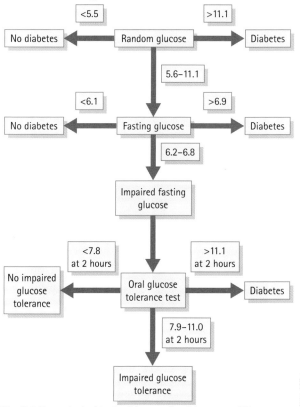

Fig. 13.7 Diagnostic algorithm for diabetes mellitus (glucose mmol/L).

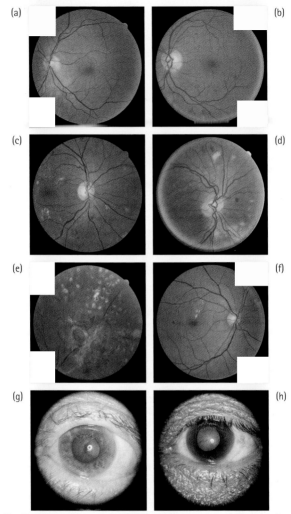

Fig. 13.8 Features of diabetic eye disease. (a) The normal macula (centre) and optic disc. (b) Dot and blot haemorrhages (early background retinopathy). (c) Hard exudates are present in addition in background retinopathy. (d) Multiple cotton-wool spots indicate pre-proliferative retinopathy requiring routine ophthalmic referral. (e) Multiple frond-like new vessels, the hallmark of proliferative retinopathy. White fibrous tissue is forming near the new vessels, a feature of advanced retinopathy. (This eye also illustrates multiple xenon arc laser burns superiorly.) (f) Exudates appearing within a disc width of the macula are a feature of an exudative maculopathy. (g, h) Central and cortical cataracts can be seen against the red reflex with the ophthalmoscope. *(Reproduced from Kumar P, Clark M. Kumar and Clark's Clinical Medicine, 7th edn. Edinburgh: Elsevier; 2009, with permission from Elsevier.)*

Presenting clinical features

Due to hyperglycaemia
- Thirst
- Polyuria
- Weight loss
- Ketoacidosis
- Lack of energy
- Visual blurring
- *Candida* infections
- Asymptomatic, picked up on blood/urine testing

Due to complications
- Skin infections
- Retinopathy
- Polyneuropathy
- Erectile dysfunction
- Arterial disease
- Renal disease

Clinical features of complications

Macrovascular and microvascular disease
- Atheroma
- Strokes
- Myocardial ischaemia
- Renal disease
- Peripheral vascular disease
- Retinopathy

Eyes
See Figure 13.8.

Kidney
- Glomerulosclerosis
- Microalbuminuria
- Persistent proteinuria
- End-stage renal failure (associated with anaemia, raised ESR and hypertension)
- Ischaemia
- Ascending infection (pyelonephritis)

Neuropathy
- Peripheral polyneuropathy (loss of ankle jerks and malleolar vibration sense)
- Glove and stocking sensory neuropathy
- Mononeuritis multiplex
- Peripheral and cranial nerve
- Autonomic neuropathy:
  - Diarrhoea
  - Postural hypotension
  - Erectile dysfunction
  - Gastroparesis
- Diabetic amyotrophy – painful asymmetrical wasting of quadriceps
- Charcot's joints

Diabetic foot (Table 13.12)
- Ischaemic and/or neuropathic ulcers

Table 13.12 The diabetic foot

	Ischaemic	Neuropathic
Symptoms	Claudication Rest pain	Usually painless
Signs	Trophic changes	High arch, clawed toes
	Cold	Warm
	Pulseless	Bounding pulse
	Painful ulcers	Painless ulcers
	Ulcers on heels and toes	Ulcers on sole and where shoes rub

Infections
- Only increased in poor glycaemic control
- Skin sepsis, e.g. *staphylococcal* or *candida*
- Urinary tract infection
- Pneumonia
- TB

Management of diabetes mellitus

- Based on self-monitoring and management by the patient, helped and advised by specialists
- Requires good education and understanding of disease by the patient, including:
  - Monitoring blood sugar
  - Self-injection of insulin
  - Managing hypoglycaemic events

Box 13.4. Hypoglycaemia

Clinical features
- Sweating
- Tremor
- Pounding heart
- Pallor
- Drowsiness
- Confusion
- Coma
- Fits

Management
- Mild
  - Oral rapidly absorbed carbohydrate, e.g. glucose drink, tea with sugar or sweets
- Severe
  - i.v. 50% glucose injection 20–50 mL (after taking blood to confirm hypoglycaemia but before waiting for result)
  - 1 mg i.m. glucagon injection

- How to recognize complications
- When to contact specialists for help

Glycaemic control

Diet
- All patients need education regarding a diabetic diet

Drugs
- Sulphonylureas, e.g. gliclazide
  - May cause hypoglycaemia (Box 13.4) and weight gain
- Biguanides, e.g. metformin; α-glucosidase inhibitors, e.g. acarbose
  - Do not cause hypoglycaemia
  - May aid weight loss
- Incretins, e.g. dipeptyl peptidase-4 inhibitors, e.g. sitagliptin, GLP-1 agonists, e.g. exenatide
- Insulin sensitizers, e.g. pioglitazone
  - May cause hepatotoxicity
  - May cause drop in haemoglobin

Insulin formulations

- Synthetic human insulins are almost exclusively used
- Insulin is given regularly by subcutaneous injection
- Insulin regimes are developed to suit individual patients and may be tailored according to specific needs for certain situations, e.g. missing meals, heavy exercise

Soluble insulin
- Fast-acting and short duration of action
- Good for fine control
- Needs frequent administration

Prolonged acting insulin
- Mixed in varying degrees with soluble insulin to give a prolonged duration of action but with less accuracy and slower onset of action

Insulin analogues
Long acting
- Insulin glargine; longer duration of action and less peaked concentration
Short acting
- Enter and leave circulation more rapidly

Complications of insulin treatment

- Lipoatrophy and lipohypertrophy at injection site
- Weight gain
- Hypoglycaemia

Monitoring diabetic control

Home monitoring
- Urine reagent strips – simple but not very accurate
- Blood glucose reagent strips – more immediately accurate

Hospital blood tests
- HbA_{1c} (glycosylated haemoglobin)
- Fructosamine (glycosylated plasma protein)
- Both give an index of average blood glucose concentration over the past 6 weeks

Diabetes clinic check-up visits
- Every visit
  - Review self-monitoring
  - Review current treatment (including diet)
  - Ongoing patient education

Box 13.5. Diabetic ketoacidosis

Clinical features
- Prostration
- Hyperventilation (Kussmaul's breathing)
- Nausea and vomiting
- Abdominal pain
- Confusion
- Coma
- Dehydration
- Ketones on breath
- Hyperglycaemia
- Ketonuria or ketonaemia
- Acidosis

Principles of management
- Replace fluid loss
- Replace electrolyte loss
- Restore acid-base balance (usually achieved by correcting circulating volume and stopping ketone production with insulin)
- Replace deficient insulin
- Continuous i.v. infusion of soluble insulin
- Monitor blood glucose
- i.v. glucose in i.v. fluids to prevent hypoglycaemia (*Do not stop insulin*)
- Seek underlying cause and treat appropriately

Emergency treatment
- Insulin
  - Intravenous insulin 6 units stat then
  - 6 units/hour by continuous infusion with blood glucose monitoring
- Fluid
  - 0.9% saline
  - 1 L in 30 minutes then
  - 1 L in 1 hour then
  - 1 L in 2 hours then
  - 1 L in 4 hours then
  - 1 L every 6 hours for 24 hours
  - i.e. at least 4 L in first 24 hours
- Check serum potassium hourly initially and add 20 mmol/L of i.v. fluid when <4 mmol
- Monitor central venous pressure if shocked at presentation
- Insert urinary catheter if anuric for >2 hours
- Antibiotics if septic
- Subcutaneous heparin to prevent thrombosis

- Annual review
  - Weight
  - Blood pressure
  - Biochemical assessment of control
  - Visual acuity and retinal examination
  - Check feet for condition, pulses, sensation and ankle jerks
  - Urinalysis for proteinuria
  - Blood lipids
  - Renal function

Diabetic emergencies/diabetic ketoacidosis

- Uncontrolled diabetes with acidosis and ketosis due to insulin deficiency (Box 13.5)

Hyperglycaemic hyperosmolar state

- Severe hyperglycaemia without ketosis usually in type 2 diabetes

Clinical features
- Severe dehydration
- Stupor
- Coma
- Underlying illness (e.g. pneumonia)

Investigations
- High plasma osmolarity
- High serum sodium
- Very high plasma glucose
- High urea
- Normal arterial pH

Management
- Treat underlying cause
- Intravenous insulin to correct hyperglycaemia
- 0.9% saline to correct fluid depletion – beware rapid changes of osmolality due to reducing plasma sodium or glucose levels too fast
- Subcutaneous prophylactic heparin
- Mortality is up to 25%

SELF-ASSESSMENT QUESTIONS

Multiple choice questions (single best answer)

1. TSH:
   - A. Is produced by the parathyroid glands
   - B. Is reduced in primary hypothyroidism
   - C. Is a sensitive marker of under-treatment during thyroxine replacement
   - D. Secretion should be inhibited in a normal TRH stimulation test
   - E. Levels are high in Graves' disease
2. The following are common features of Graves' disease:
   - A. Atrial fibrillation
   - B. Multinodular goitre
   - C. Oedema
   - D. Anorexia
   - E. Weight gain

3. The following are common features of hypothyroidism:
   A. Heat intolerance
   B. Pretibial myxoedema
   C. Hoarse voice
   D. Weight loss
   E. Suicide

4. The following statements about pituitary function are correct:
   A. Suspected diabetes insipidus is investigated with a fluid challenge
   B. Prolactin production, unlike that of other pituitary hormones, is principally controlled by a stimulatory factor
   C. ACTH and cortisol production display a circadian rhythm
   D. Sheehan syndrome is commoner in men than women
   E. TSH is secreted from the posterior pituitary

5. In patients with untreated active acromegaly:
   A. About 25% of patients have impaired glucose tolerance
   B. Arthritis is a common feature
   C. An oral glucose tolerance test is used to confirm the diagnosis
   D. The incidence of carcinoma of the colon is increased
   E. All of the above

6. The following are common features of panhypopituitarism:
   A. Diabetes mellitus
   B. Galactorrhoea
   C. Infertility
   D. Pigmentation
   E. Increased urinary catecholamines

7. The following biochemical findings are often seen in an acutely unwell patient presenting with an Addisonian crisis:
   A. Hypernatraemia
   B. Hyperkalaemia
   C. A low ACTH
   D. Hypocalcaemia
   E. A raised glucose

8. The following statements about Cushing syndrome are correct:
   A. The commonest cause is an ACTH-secreting tumour of the pituitary
   B. There is impaired glucose tolerance in 75% of cases
   C. Severe hypokalaemia may be indicative of ectopic ACTH production
   D. Proximal myopathy is a common feature
   E. C and D

9. The following are true of ectopic ACTH secretion:
   A. There is failure of suppression of cortisol secretion during a high-dose dexamethasone suppression test
   B. It may be caused by a bronchial carcinoma
   C. It may cause increased skin pigmentation
   D. It is associated with small atrophic adrenal glands
   E. A, B and C

10. The following are features of cranial diabetes insipidus:
    A. It may be associated with acanthosis nigricans
    B. It may be associated with postpartum haemorrhage
    C. It is caused by treatment with lithium
    D. It responds to treatment with DDT
    E. It is treated with fluid restriction

11. The following are causes of nephrogenic diabetes insipidus:
    A. Sheehan syndrome
    B. Pancreatic islet cell antibodies
    C. Excessive water drinking
    D. Hypocalcaemia
    E. Hypokalaemia

12. The following are features of SIADH:
    A. Hypernatraemia
    B. Low urine osmolality
    C. Diagnosis requires serum ADH measurement
    D. It often presents with fits
    E. Treatment includes fluid restriction

13. The following are true of phaeochromocytoma:
    A. It is the cause of 10% of all hypertension
    B. It is caused by a tumour of adrenal cortex in 90% of cases
    C. α- and β-Adrenergic blockers are used prior to surgery to prevent swings in blood pressure
    D. It is seen in MEN type 1
    E. It is associated with coarctation of the aorta

14. The following are seen in MEN type 2a:
    A. Marfanoid phenotype
    B. Phaeochromocytoma
    C. Pancreatic islet cell tumours
    D. Pituitary tumours
    E. Papillary carcinoma of the thyroid

15. The following statements about diabetes mellitus are correct:
    A. The diagnosis is made on the basis of a fasting glucose >7.8 mmol/L
    B. When it presents in pregnancy (gestational diabetes) it usually continues after delivery
    C. In patients with proliferative diabetic nephropathy, thrombolysis is contraindicated in the event of a myocardial infarction
    D. The glycated haemoglobin (HbA$_{1c}$) level is used to diagnose diabetes
    E. The mortality following anterior myocardial infarction is twice as high in diabetic as in non-diabetic patients

16. Regarding type 2 diabetes:
    A. Treatment with metformin works by increasing pancreatic insulin production
    B. Retinopathy is much rarer than in type 1 diabetes
    C. The thiazolidinediones are a new class of drug for treatment
    D. It only affects adults over the age of 40
    E. The incidence in the UK is falling

17. In type 1 diabetes:
    A. Patients control their blood glucose by regular self-injection of i.m. insulin
    B. There is a strong genetic association with HLA-B27
    C. The average life expectancy is less than in type 2 diabetes
    D. There is an association with coeliac disease
    E. Patients on insulin are unable to hold a UK driving licence

18. The following statements about diabetic ketoacidosis are correct:
    A. It does not occur in patients with type 2 diabetes
    B. The plasma potassium is usually raised at presentation

C. When treatment is started the arterial pH falls

D. The plasma anion gap is normal

E. It can result in a low plasma phosphate level

19. In diabetic ketoacidosis:

    A. Patients should be treated immediately with subcutaneous insulin

    B. Acid reflux usually corrects with insulin and fluid replacement

    C. Patients should eat normally as soon as possible

    D. A fast respiratory rate indicates concurrent pneumonia

    E. Insulin therapy is no longer needed when the blood glucose returns to normal

Extended matching questions

Question 1 Theme: Polyuria

A. Diabetes mellitus

B. Diabetes insipidus

C. Chronic kidney disease

D. Primary hyperparathyroidism

E. Chronic hypokalaemia

F. Urinary tract infection

G. Diuretic therapy

H. Compulsive water drinking

I. Supraventricular tachycardia

For each of the following questions, select the best answer from the list above:

I. A 48-year-old female with a previous Whipple's operation (pancreatoduodenectomy) for Zollinger–Ellison syndrome presents with a 3-month history of polyuria and constipation. What is the most likely diagnosis?

II. A 27-year-old female presents with polyuria 2 months after home delivery of a healthy 3.2 kg son. She needed urgent hospital admission after the birth for blood transfusion for postpartum haemorrhage. What is the most likely diagnosis?

III. A 16-year-old male presents with a 4-week history of thirst, polyuria, malaise and loss of appetite. Serum urea and electrolytes are normal apart from $HCO_3 = 19$ mmol/L. What is the most likely diagnosis?

Question 2 Theme: Weight loss

A. Thyrotoxicosis

B. Coeliac disease

C. Carcinoma of the stomach

D. Diabetes mellitus

E. Addison's disease

F. Anorexia nervosa

G. Breast cancer

H. Crohn's disease

I. Amphetamine abuse

For each of the following questions, select the best answer from the list above:

I. A 57-year-old female on B_{12} injections for pernicious anaemia presents with anxiety, palpitations, intermittent diarrhoea and weight loss of 6 kg over 3 months. What is the most likely diagnosis?

II. A 29-year-old male presents with night sweats, fever, abdominal pain and weight loss of 10 kg since he returned from Bangladesh 3 months ago. Examination shows increased pigmentation in the palmar creases and postural hypotension. What is the most likely diagnosis?

III. A 36-year-old female from Galway presents with a 6-month history of weight loss and abdominal cramps. Blood tests show iron deficiency and folate deficiency. What is the most likely diagnosis?

Short answer questions

1. Describe the clinical features of the following:
   A. Hyperthyroidism
   B. Acromegaly
   C. Primary hypoadrenalism
2. Write short notes on the following:
   A. Multiple endocrine neoplasia
   B. Phaeochromocytoma
   C. Goitre
3. Briefly discuss the causes of the following:
   A. Cushing syndrome
   B. Adrenal failure
   C. Diabetes insipidus
4. Write short notes on the following:
   A. Thyroid-related eye abnormalities
   B. SIADH
   C. Causes of polyuria
5. List the following:
   A. The hormones secreted by the anterior pituitary and their functions
   B. The causes of hypopituitarism
   C. The biochemical changes seen in primary hyperaldosteronism

FUNCTIONS OF THE KIDNEY

Excretory

- Waste products of metabolism

Regulatory

- Control of body fluid volume and composition

Endocrine

- Erythropoietin → haemoglobin synthesis
- Renin-angiotensin → blood pressure control

Autocrine

- Prostaglandins → renal blood flow
- Renal natriuretic peptide → sodium and chloride transport
- Nitric oxide → sodium excretion
- Protein catabolism

Metabolic

- Vitamin D → calcium metabolism

Functional structure

Cortex
- Glomerulus
  - Hydrostatic and oncotic pressure
  - → Ultrafiltration of blood
  - → 120 mL/min protein- and fat-free fluid
- Proximal convoluted tubule
  - Resorption of 60–80% water and Na^+
  - Resorption of >99% $K^+/HCO_3^-/glucose/amino acids$
- Distal convoluted tubule
  - Water and NaCl control
  - Via action of ADH
  - K^+ excretion

Medulla
- Loop of Henle
  - 15% long loops
  - Active transport of $Na^+/K^+/Cl^-$
  - Interstitium is hypertonic (urea recycling)
    - → Water resorption and urine concentration

EXAMINING THE RENAL SYSTEM

- All systems need to be examined but pay special attention to the following:

- Place one hand posteriorly on the flank with the other hand anteriorly
- Gently push up from below aiming to 'ballot' the kidney
- Differences between kidney and spleen
  - Kidneys are ballotable
  - Spleen has a notch
  - You cannot get above the spleen
  - Spleen is dull to percussion

Kidneys (Box 14.1)

- Position
  - Usually impalpable
  - Usual location: superior tip level with 11th rib
  - Transplanted kidneys in the iliac fossae
- Size: Normally 3×6×11 cm
- Shape
- Scars from previous surgery
- Auscultate 5 cm above and lateral to umbilicus for renal artery stenosis

Urine

Urinalysis
- Chemical (Stix) testing
  - Blood
  - Protein
  - Glucose
  - Bacterial nitrites plus leucocyte esterases
  - pH
  - Specific gravity and osmolality

Microscopy
- White cells >10/mm^3: inflammation or infection
- Red cells >10/mm^3: bleeding
- Bacteria
- Casts: tubular deposits
  - Red cell casts always indicate disease
  - White cell casts in pyelonephritis
  - Coarse granular casts in proteinuria
  - Fine granular casts after exercise
  - Cell casts in acute tubular necrosis

Volume
- Oliguria
- Polyuria

INVESTIGATIONS IN NEPHROLOGY

Imaging: Plain X-rays

- Renal calcification
- Renal calculi

Excretory urography

- Intravenous contrast excreted by kidneys
  - Anatomy of renal tract
  - Excretion of contrast

Ultrasound

- Masses
- Cysts
- Dilatation of renal tract – obstruction
- Renal size
- Bladder emptying
- Renal vessel Doppler

CT and MRI

- Detection of calculi/urography
- Renal masses
- Staging tumours
- Renal vessel imaging
- Retroperitoneal masses

Arteriography

- Extrarenal arterial imaging

Dynamic scintigraphy

- DPTA/MAG3/Hippuran – show perfusion
- Two phases:
  - Glomerular filtration
  - Outflow of urine from collecting system

Static scintigraphy

- DMSA – uptake proportional to renal function
- Allows comparison of two kidneys
- Visualization of kidney

Renal biopsy

- Transcutaneous under ultrasound control

Indications

- Nephrotic syndrome
- Unexplained renal failure
- Diagnosis of systemic disease

Contraindications

- Single kidney
- Small kidneys
- Haemorrhagic disorders
- Uncontrolled hypertension

Biochemical renal function tests

Serum urea and creatinine
- Urea
  - Byproduct of hepatic protein metabolism
  - Rapidly reflects changes in renal perfusion and nephron function

- Creatinine
  - Byproduct of muscle function
  - Synthesis constant over time
  - Used to compare renal function over long time periods
- Increase when glomerular filtration rate (GFR) is reduced by 50–60% (i.e. may be normal in the presence of significant decrease in renal function)

Creatinine clearance

$$\text{Estimates GFR} = \frac{V \text{ (urine volume)} \times U \text{ (urine creatinine concentration)}}{P \text{ (plasma creatinine concentration)}} \times 100$$

(eGFR can be estimated from a formula requiring serum creatinine only.)

Arterial blood gases

- Metabolic acidosis in renal failure due to failure to excrete fixed acid and to renal bicarbonate wasting

GLOMERULAR DISEASES

Glomerulopathy

- A group of disorders
  - With immunologically mediated injury to glomerulus
  - Involving both kidneys
  - With secondary injury after initial immune insult
  - May be part of generalized disease (e.g. SLE)
- Classification by histology
  - Focal: <75% glomeruli affected
  - Diffuse: >75% glomeruli affected
  - Segmental: only part of the glomerulus affected
  - Proliferative: glomerular cell hyperplasia
  - Crescents: lymphocyte infiltration of Bowman's space
  - Membranous: Capillary wall thickening
- Classification by clinical features
  - Asymptomatic proteinuria ± microscopic haematuria
  - Acute nephritic syndrome (Fig. 14.1)
  - Nephrotic syndrome (Fig. 14.2)
  - Rapidly progressive glomerulonephritis

Pathogenesis

- Deposition of immune complexes
- Deposition of anti-glomerular basement membrane (anti-GBM) antibody

Aetiology

Immune complex nephritis

- Unknown antigen
- Viruses
  - Mumps
  - Measles
  - Hepatitis B and C
  - Epstein–Barr virus (EBV)
  - Coxsackie
  - Varicella
  - HIV
- Bacteria
  - Group A β-haemolytic streptococci
  - *Streptococcus viridans*

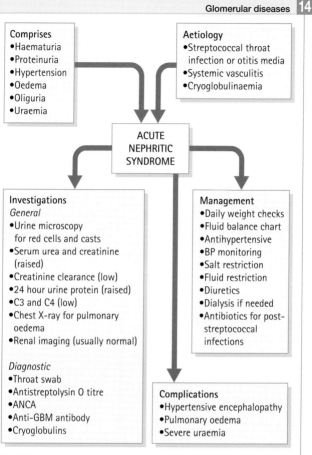

Comprises
- Haematuria
- Proteinuria
- Hypertension
- Oedema
- Oliguria
- Uraemia

Aetiology
- Streptococcal throat infection or otitis media
- Systemic vasculitis
- Cryoglobulinaemia

ACUTE NEPHRITIC SYNDROME

Investigations
General
- Urine microscopy for red cells and casts
- Serum urea and creatinine (raised)
- Creatinine clearance (low)
- 24 hour urine protein (raised)
- C3 and C4 (low)
- Chest X-ray for pulmonary oedema
- Renal imaging (usually normal)

Diagnostic
- Throat swab
- Antistreptolysin O titre
- ANCA
- Anti-GBM antibody
- Cryoglobulins

Management
- Daily weight checks
- Fluid balance chart
- Antihypertensive
- BP monitoring
- Salt restriction
- Fluid restriction
- Diuretics
- Dialysis if needed
- Antibiotics for post-streptococcal infections

Complications
- Hypertensive encephalopathy
- Pulmonary oedema
- Severe uraemia

Fig. 14.1 Acute nephritic syndrome.

- Staphylococci
- *Treponema pallidum*
- Gonococci
- Salmonellae
- Parasites
  - *Plasmodium malariae*
  - *Schistosoma*
  - Filariasis
- Host antigens
  - DNA (systemic lupus erythematosus – SLE)
  - Cryoglobulins
  - Malignant tumours

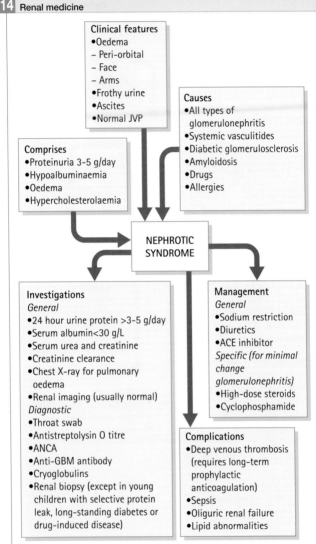

Clinical features
- Oedema
  - Peri-orbital
  - Face
  - Arms
- Frothy urine
- Ascites
- Normal JVP

Causes
- All types of glomerulonephritis
- Systemic vasculitides
- Diabetic glomerulosclerosis
- Amyloidosis
- Drugs
- Allergies

Comprises
- Proteinuria 3–5 g/day
- Hypoalbuminaemia
- Oedema
- Hypercholesterolaemia

NEPHROTIC SYNDROME

Investigations
General
- 24 hour urine protein >3–5 g/day
- Serum albumin <30 g/L
- Serum urea and creatinine
- Creatinine clearance
- Chest X-ray for pulmonary oedema
- Renal imaging (usually normal)
Diagnostic
- Throat swab
- Antistreptolysin O titre
- ANCA
- Anti-GBM antibody
- Cryoglobulins
- Renal biopsy (except in young children with selective protein leak, long-standing diabetes or drug-induced disease)

Management
General
- Sodium restriction
- Diuretics
- ACE inhibitor
Specific (for minimal change glomerulonephritis)
- High-dose steroids
- Cyclophosphamide

Complications
- Deep venous thrombosis (requires long-term prophylactic anticoagulation)
- Sepsis
- Oliguric renal failure
- Lipid abnormalities

Fig. 14.2 Nephrotic syndrome.

- Drugs
  - Penicillamine
  - Hydralazine

Anti-GBM antibody
- Antibodies to type IV collagen

Secondary mechanisms
- Complement activation
- Fibrin deposition
- Platelet aggregation
- Neutrophil-driven inflammation
- Kinin activation

Clinical features
- GN presents in one of four ways (see above)

Investigations
- 24-hour urinary protein (measure twice)
  - Nephrotic >3.5 g/day
- Urine microscopy
  - Red cell casts/haematuria
- Renal function
- Autoantibodies
  - ANCA: vasculitis
  - ANA: SLE
  - Anti-glomerular basement membrane: Goodpasture's
- Renal biopsy

Specific types of GN (Table 14.1)

IgA nephropathy
Pathology
- Focal proliferative GN
- Mesangial deposits of IgA
Clinical features
- Microscopic haematuria
- Children and young adults
Prognosis
- Usually good
- 20% eventually develop renal failure

Henoch–Schönlein purpura
Pathology
- Focal segmental GN
Clinical features
- Purpuric rash
- Abdominal colic ± GI bleeding
- Joint pain
- ♂ > ♀ (2:1)
- May follow recent respiratory infection
Prognosis
- Usually good

Goodpasture syndrome
Pathology
- Severe proliferative crescentic GN

Table 14.1 Glomerulonephritis

Histology	Example of causes	Clinical presentation
Proliferative glomerulonephritis		
Diffuse	Post-streptococcal	Acute nephritic syndrome
Focal segmental	SLE	Haematuria
	Henoch–Schönlein purpura	Proteinuria
Crescentic	Wegener's granulomatosis Goodpasture syndrome	Progressive renal failure
Mesangiocapillary		
Type 1	Hepatitis B and C	Haematuria Proteinuria
Type 2	Measles	Nephrotic syndrome
Membranous	Unknown Malaria	Nephrotic syndrome
Minimal change	Unknown	Nephrotic syndrome (especially in children)
IgA nephropathy	Henoch–Schönlein purpura	Asymptomatic haematuria
Focal glomerulosclerosis	Diabetes mellitus	Proteinuria Nephrotic syndrome

Clinical features
- Lung involvement → haemoptysis
- Progressive renal failure

Prognosis
- Usually progresses to renal failure

Acute nephritic syndrome
Classically occurs 3 weeks after streptococcal throat infection or otitis media (see Fig. 14.1).

Nephrotic syndrome
See Figure 14.2.

RENAL INVOLVEMENT IN SYSTEMIC DISEASE

Systemic vasculitis

- SLE – all types of glomerulonephritis
- Polyarteritis nodosa (PAN) – renal failure
- Microscopic polyarteritis – crescentic glomerulonephritis

- Wegener's granulomatosis – glomerulonephritis
- Antiphospholipid syndrome

Cryoglobulinaemia

- Monoclonal or polyclonal expansion of abnormal immunoglobulins which precipitate reversibly in the cold (cryoglobulins)

Aetiology
- Viral infections, e.g. hepatitis B and C, cytomegalovirus (CMV), EBV
- Fungal infections
- Malaria
- Infective endocarditis
- Autoimmune diseases

Clinical features
- Glomerulonephritis
- Purpura
- Raynaud's phenomenon
- Systemic vasculitis
- Polyneuropathy
- Hepatic involvement

Multiple myeloma

- 20–30% → acute kidney injury
  - Light chain deposition
  - AL amyloidosis
  - Hypercalcaemic nephropathy

Diabetes mellitus

See Chapter 13.

Amyloidosis

- A disorder of protein metabolism with extracellular deposition of insoluble fibrillar proteins in organs and tissues

Types
- AL amyloidosis
- Familial amyloidosis
- Secondary amyloidosis

AL amyloidosis

Pathology
- Plasma cell production of amyloidogenic immunoglobulin light chains (AL)
- AL chains are excreted in urine (Bence Jones proteins)
- Associated with myeloma and Waldenström's macroglobulinaemia

Clinical features
- Nephrotic syndrome
- Cardiomyopathy
- Autonomic neuropathy
- Sensory neuropathy
- Carpal tunnel syndrome
- Hepatomegaly
- Splenomegaly

- Bruising
- Macroglossia

Familial amyloidosis

Pathology
- Autosomal dominant inherited mutant protein formation
- Mutant protein forms amyloid fibrils

Mutant proteins
- Transthyretin (commonest)
- Apolipoprotein A-1
- Fibrinogen
- Lysozyme

Clinical features
- Peripheral sensorimotor neuropathy
- Autonomic neuropathy
- Conduction defects in heart

Secondary amyloidosis

Pathology
- Amyloid is formed from acute phase protein serum amyloid A (SAA)

Aetiology
- Rheumatoid arthritis
- Inflammatory bowel disease
- Familial Mediterranean fever
- Tuberculosis
- Bronchiectasis
- Osteomyelitis

Clinical features
- Renal disease
- Hepatosplenomegaly

Diagnosis of amyloidosis

- Rectal or gum biopsy
- Amyloid stains with Congo red with green birefringence in polarized light

Management of amyloidosis

- Treat associated disorder
- Treat nephrotic syndrome or cardiac failure
- Chemotherapy for AL
- Liver transplant for transthyretin-associated amyloidosis

HIV-associated nephropathy (HIVAN)

- Focal glomerulosclerosis
  - Proteinuria → nephrotic syndrome
  - → Rapidly progressive renal failure
- 90% of patients are black
- HAART may slow/halt progression

Pre-eclampsia

- Proteinuria can → nephrotic syndrome – usually settles after delivery

Haemolytic-uraemic syndrome (HUS)

- Follows gastroenteritis or respiratory tract infection, *E. coli* O157
- Comprises
  - Intravascular haemolysis
  - Thrombocytopenia
  - Acute kidney injury

Thrombotic thrombocytopenic purpura

- Microangiopathic haemolysis
- Renal failure
- Neurological disturbance

TUBULOINTERSTITIAL NEPHRITIS (TIN)

Acute TIN

- Drugs
  - Penicillin/cephalosporins
  - Sulphonamides
  - NSAIDs
  - Allopurinol
  - Phenytoin
  - Diuretics: furosemide
- Infections

Chronic TIN

- Drugs: NSAIDs
- Sickle cell disease/trait
- Reflux nephropathy
- Diabetes mellitus

HYPERTENSION AND THE KIDNEY

- Benign essential hypertension
  - Intimal thickening of small vessels
  - Reduction in kidney size
  - Increased glomerular damage → CRF
  - Requires careful control of BP <140/85
- Renal hypertension
  - Complicates bilateral renal disease
  - → Activation of renin-angiotensin system
  - → Salt and water retention → hypertension
- Renovascular disease
  - Renal artery stenosis → reduced renal blood flow
  - → Activation of renin-angiotensin system
  - → Salt and water retention → hypertension
  - May be exacerbated by ACE inhibitors

URINARY TRACT INFECTION

- 50 000/million per year
- Common in women; 90% of attacks are isolated
- Uncommon in men

Bacterial infections

Causative organisms
- Usually from patient's own bowel flora
- *E. coli* – 68%
- *Proteus mirabilis* – 12%
- *Staphylococcus saprophyticus* or *epidermidis* – 10%
- *Klebsiella aerogenes* – 4%
- *Enterococcus faecalis* – 6%

Associated diseases
- Diabetes mellitus
- Sickle cell disease or trait
- Analgesic misuse
- Stones
- Obstruction
- Polycystic kidneys
- Vesico-ureteric reflux

Clinical features
- Cystitis
  - Frequency of micturition
  - Dysuria
  - Suprapubic pain/tenderness
  - Haematuria
  - Smelly urine
- Pyelonephritis
  - Loin pain/tenderness
  - Fever
  - Systemic upset

Investigations
- Symptomatic women
  - Dipstix + for nitrites and leucocytes
  - $>10^2$ coliforms/mL + pyuria ($>10\,WCC/mm^3$) *or* ⎫
  - $>10^5$ any pathogenic organism/mL *or* ⎬ MSU
  - Any growth from suprapubic bladder aspiration ⎭
- Symptomatic men
  - $>10^3$ pathogenic organisms/mL
- Asymptomatic patients
  - $>10^5$ pathogenic organisms/mL (on two occasions)
- Causes of sterile pyuria
  - *Chlamydia*
  - TB
  - Partially treated bacterial UTI

Radiology
- Excretory urography is now seldom performed; CT/MRI is more appropriate
  - Women with ≥3 attacks
  - All men
  - All children
- Abdominal X-ray and ultrasound
  - Acute pyelonephritis

Management
- Oral antibiotics
  - Amoxicillin
  - Nitrofurantoin

- Trimethoprim
- Oral cephalosporin
- Intravenous antibiotics
  - For acute pyelonephritis with high fever, vomiting or systemic upset
  - Cefuroxime
  - Gentamicin
  - Ciprofloxacin

Tuberculosis of the renal tract

- Affects the renal cortex spreading to the papillae and into the urine, ureters and bladder
- May cause ureteric obstruction and hydronephrosis

Investigations
- Culture of acid-fast bacillae from early morning urine (EMU) samples

RENAL CALCULI

Prevalence
- 2% of UK population

Types of urinary stone
See Table 14.2.

Aetiology
- Dehydration
- Specific chemical abnormalities
  - Hypercalcaemia
  - Hypercalciuria
  - Hyperoxaluria
  - Hyperuricaemia
  - Cystinuria
- Infection
- Renal tubular acidosis
- Primary renal disease
- Drugs → calcium stones:
  - Loop diuretics
  - Vitamins D and E
  - Glucocorticoids
  - Antacids
- Drugs → uric acid stones
  - Thiazide diuretics
  - Salicylates

Table 14.2 Types of urinary stone	
Type	Frequency (%)
Calcium oxalate	65
Calcium phosphate	15
Magnesium ammonium phosphate	10–15
Uric acid	3–5
Cystine	1–2

- Drugs that precipitate
  - Indinavir

Clinical features
- Asymptomatic
- Renal colic
- Haematuria
- Urinary tract infection
- Obstruction

Investigations
- Midstream urine (MSU) and culture
- Serum urea and electrolytes, creatinine, eGFR
- Serum calcium
- Serum urate
- Plain abdominal X-ray
- Spiral CT
- Excretion urography
- Urinary calcium, oxalate and uric acid
- Sieve urine to trap stones for analysis

Management
- Analgesia (opiates, NSAIDs)
- High fluid intake
- Stones <0.5 cm pass spontaneously
- Stones >1 cm require intervention
- Obstruction or infection requires intervention

Intervention

Percutaneous nephrolithotomy
- Endoscopic extraction of renal pelvis stones through a percutaneous tract

Extracorporeal shock-wave lithotripsy (ESWL)
- Fragmentation of stones with shock waves focused in from an external source

URINARY TRACT OBSTRUCTION

See Table 14.3.

Hydronephrosis

- Dilatation of renal pelvis above obstruction

Clinical features
- Loin pain/tenderness
- Anuria – bilateral obstruction
- Polyuria
- Bladder outflow obstruction (hesitancy, poor stream, terminal dribbling)
- Palpable enlarged kidney(s)

Investigations
- Urea and electrolytes
- Ultrasound
- Excretion urography
- Cystoscopy

Table 14.3 Causes of urinary tract obstruction

Within lumen	Neuropathic bladder
Calculus	Urethral stricture
Blood clot	Calculus
Sloughed papilla	Gonococcal infection
Tumour	Outside pressure
Within wall	Tumours
Ureteric stricture	Aortic aneurysm
TB	Prostatic obstruction
Calculus	Retroperitoneal fibrosis
Post-surgical	Accidental ligation of ureter
Schistosomiasis	Phimosis

Management
- Relieve obstruction by temporary drainage via nephrostomy or urethral or suprapubic catheter
- Treat underlying cause
- Prevent and/or treat infection

Surgical drainage
- Urinary diversion
- Ureteric stents

ACUTE KIDNEY INJURY

- Abrupt deterioration in renal function which is usually reversible

Pre-renal uraemia

- Impaired perfusion of kidneys

Aetiology
- Hypovolaemia (acute blood loss, dehydration, sepsis)
- Hypotension
- Cardiac failure
- Renal artery stenosis (± ACE inhibitors)
- NSAIDs → reduced renal prostaglandins

Management
- Correct hypovolaemia or hypotension
- Monitor central venous pressure to maintain adequate vascular volume
- Stop causative agents

Acute uraemia due to renal causes

Aetiology
- Acute tubular necrosis (Fig. 14.3)
- Vasculitis
- Pre-eclampsia
- Haemolytic-uraemic syndrome
- Rhabdomyolysis

Post-renal uraemia

- Urinary tract obstruction

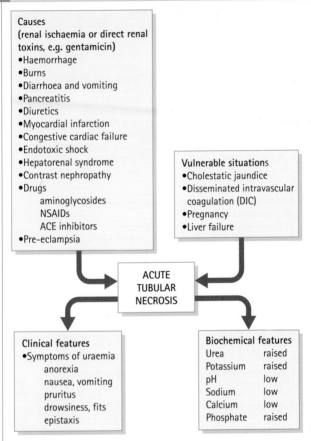

Causes
(renal ischaemia or direct renal toxins, e.g. gentamicin)
- Haemorrhage
- Burns
- Diarrhoea and vomiting
- Pancreatitis
- Diuretics
- Myocardial infarction
- Congestive cardiac failure
- Endotoxic shock
- Hepatorenal syndrome
- Contrast nephropathy
- Drugs
  aminoglycosides
  NSAIDs
  ACE inhibitors
- Pre-eclampsia

Vulnerable situations
- Cholestatic jaundice
- Disseminated intravascular coagulation (DIC)
- Pregnancy
- Liver failure

ACUTE TUBULAR NECROSIS

Clinical features
- Symptoms of uraemia
  anorexia
  nausea, vomiting
  pruritus
  drowsiness, fits
  epistaxis

Biochemical features
Urea   raised
Potassium   raised
pH   low
Sodium   low
Calcium   low
Phosphate   raised

Fig. 14.3 Acute tubular necrosis.

Investigations in acute kidney injury

Determine whether pre-renal, renal or post-renal
- Exclude bladder outflow obstruction – insert urinary catheter
- Ultrasound – to exclude upper urinary tract obstruction
- Fluid challenge – increased urine output will differentiate pre-renal from renal

Urinalysis
- Dipstick for protein and blood
- Myoglobin

Serum biochemistry
- Urea and electrolytes
  - Urea ↑, K$^+$ ↑, Na$^+$ ↓

- Metabolic acidosis (pH $\downarrow$/HCO_3^- $\downarrow$/negative base excess)
- Creatinine $\uparrow$, eGFR down
- Calcium $\downarrow$ and phosphate $\uparrow$
- Albumin
- Alkaline phosphatase
- Urate
- Drug levels

Haematology
- Full blood count and blood film
  - Normal Hb
- ESR
- Coagulation studies

Microbiology
- Urine microscopy and culture
- Blood cultures

Management of acute uraemia

General management
- Admit to renal unit or ITU for support of all systems, with the aim of keeping the patient alive while waiting for renal function to recover

Diet
- Sodium and potassium restriction
- Protein restriction only if trying to avoid dialysis

Fluid balance
- Assessment of input–output chart
- Signs of fluid overload
- Serum electrolytes
- Daily weight check

Treat sepsis
- Avoid nephrotoxic drugs and alter dose for renally excreted drugs

Dialysis and haemofiltration in acute kidney injury

Indications
- Symptomatic uraemia
- Complications of uraemia, e.g. pericarditis
- Severe biochemical derangement
- Uncontrolled hyperkalaemia (Box 14.2)
- Pulmonary oedema
- Acidosis
- Removal of toxic drugs, e.g. aspirin overdose, gentamicin

Options
- Peritoneal dialysis
- Continuous haemofiltration

Prognosis
- Up to 50% mortality

Contrast nephropathy
- Caused by iodinated radiological contrast media
- Dose-dependent effect

> ### Box 14.2. Hyperkalaemia
>
> - Check result is compatible with patient's clinical condition (if not repeat sample)
> - ECG to look for changes of hyperkalaemia (peaked T waves, widened QRS complexes – Fig. 14.4) and put patient on cardiac monitor
> - K^+ >6.0 or with symptoms or ECG changes, give:
>   - i.v. calcium gluconate 10 mL 10%
>   - i.v. 50 mL 50% dextrose plus 10 units soluble rapid-acting insulin over 30 minutes, monitoring blood glucose for hypoglycaemia
>   - Nebulized salbutamol 10 mg
>   - Oral calcium resonium 15–30 g 2–3 times daily *or*
>   - Rectal calcium resonium retention enema 50 g daily
>   - Dialysis or haemofiltration if no correction

- Risk increased with
  - Pre-existing renal impairment
  - Hypovolaemia
  - Low cardiac output
  - Diabetes mellitus
  - Hyperviscosity
- Risk reduced by
  - *n*-Acetyl cysteine
  - Pre-hydration with saline

CHRONIC KIDNEY DISEASE

- Long-standing progressive impairment of renal function

Prevalence
- 600/million per year in UK
- End-stage renal failure – 200/million per year in UK

Aetiology
See Table 14.4.

Clinical features
History
- Duration of symptoms
- Drug ingestion, e.g. NSAIDs, analgesics and herbal therapies
- Past surgical history
- Previous chemotherapy
- Family history of renal disease

Symptoms
- Asymptomatic
- Malaise, loss of energy
- Insomnia
- Nocturia, polyuria
- Itching
- Nausea, vomiting, diarrhoea
- Paraesthesiae
- 'Restless legs' syndrome

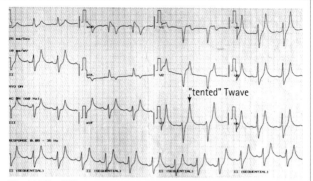

Fig. 14.4 The ECG in hyperkalaemia.

Table 14.4 Causes of chronic kidney disease	
Congenital	Tubulo-interstitial disease
Polycystic kidney	Nephritis
disease	Idiopathic
Glomerular disease	Drugs
Primary glomerulonephritis	Reflux nephropathy
Secondary glomerulonephritis	TB
(SLE, diabetes,	Schistosomiasis
amyloidosis)	Diabetes
Vascular disease	Obstruction
Atherosclerosis	Stones
Vasculitis	Prostate disease
SLE	Pelvic tumours
Hypertension	Retroperitoneal fibrosis

- Bone pain
- Peripheral or pulmonary oedema
- Anaemia
- Amenorrhoea and erectile dysfunction

Signs

- Short stature
- Anaemia
- Pigmentation on sun-exposed areas
- Brown nails
- Fluid overload
- Signs of underlying disease

Investigations

Urine

- Urinalysis
- Microscopy
- Culture
- 24-hour creatinine clearance or eGFR

Biochemistry
- Urea and electrolytes
  - Urea ↑
  - Normal K^+ or ↑
- Creatinine ↑ or eGFR ↓
- Calcium ↓ and phosphate ↑

Haematology
- Full blood count
  - Anaemia

Radiology
- Renal tract ultrasound
- Plain abdominal X-ray
- CT scan of abdomen and pelvis

Immunology
- Urinary Bence Jones proteins
- Serum electrophoresis and immunoglobulins
- Autoantibodies
- Complement levels

Microbiology
- Antistreptolysin O titre – post-*Strep*. infection
- Malaria film
- Hepatitis B and C serology

Histology
- Renal biopsy

Complications
- Anaemia (erythropoietin)
- Renal osteodystrophy (osteomalacia, rickets, hyperparathyroidism, osteoporosis, osteosclerosis)
- Pruritus
- Delayed gastric emptying
- Peptic ulceration (↑ gastrin)
- Pancreatitis
- Constipation
- Gout
- Hyperlipidaemia
- Hyperprolactinaemia
- Erectile dysfunction and male infertility
- Amenorrhoea and female infertility
- Short stature
- Cardiovascular disease
- Cardiac failure
- Sudden death
- Pericarditis
- Stroke

Management
General
- Treat underlying disease if possible
- Control hypertension
- Early referral to nephrologist when serum creatinine >350 µmol/L *or* in diabetics >250 µmol/L

Diet
- Calcium supplements
- Low phosphate diet
- Sodium and potassium restriction
- Protein restriction
- Fluid restriction

Anaemia
- Erythropoietin
- Iron therapy

RENAL REPLACEMENT THERAPY

Haemodialysis

- Blood from the patient is pumped through semipermeable membranes against a dialysate fluid allowing diffusion of molecules along concentration gradients
- Requires rapid blood flow through a large-bore double-lumen central venous catheter or arteriovenous fistula

Frequency
- Usually 4–5 hours 3 times per week

Complications
- Hypotension while on dialysis

Haemofiltration

- Removal of plasma water and dissolved electrolytes (potassium, sodium, urea and phosphate) by flow across a semipermeable membrane and replacement with a solution of desired biochemical composition
- Mostly used in acute kidney injury

Frequency
- Usually continuous

Peritoneal dialysis

- Uses peritoneum as semipermeable membrane
- Dialysis fluid is run into peritoneal cavity through a tube in the anterior abdominal wall
- Urea, creatinine and phosphate pass into the dialysate from the blood in peritoneal capillaries along a diffusion gradient
- Water and electrolytes go in through osmosis

Frequency
- Dialysis fluid is exchanged usually 3–5 times per day
- Fluid exchange takes about 40 minutes

Renal transplantation

- A kidney, explanted from either a cadaveric or living related donor, is anastomosed to the iliac vessels of the recipient
- The ureter is placed into the bladder
- Immunosuppression is required for the rest of the patient's life

Prognosis
- 80% of grafts survive 5–10 years
- 60% of grafts survive for 10–30 years

CYSTIC RENAL DISEASES

- Solitary or multiple simple renal cysts are common, affecting
- 50% of the population >50 years old
- Usually asymptomatic

Autosomal dominant polycystic kidney disease

- Inherited disorder
- Presents in adulthood
- Multiple bilateral renal cysts
- Associated with hepatic cysts

Prevalence
- 1:400–1000

Responsible genes
- PKD 1 on chromosome 16
- PKD 2 on chromosome 4

Clinical features
- Acute loin pain ± haematuria (due to haemorrhage, infection or stone formation)
- Loin discomfort (due to large kidneys)
- Subarachnoid haemorrhage (secondary to berry aneurysm rupture)
- Hypertension
- Liver cysts
- Chronic kidney disease
- Large irregular palpable kidneys
- Hepatomegaly
- Ultrasound shows multiple renal cysts

Complications
- Progression to chronic kidney disease ~70% by age 70
- Pain
- Cyst infection
- Renal stones
- Hypertension
- Liver cysts
- Berry aneurysms (10%) → sub-arachnoid haemorrhage

Screening
- Children and siblings of patients should have renal ultrasound after age 20

TUMOURS OF THE UROGENITAL TRACT AND PROSTATE

Renal cell carcinoma

- Average age at presentation – 55 years
- ♂ > ♀ (2:1)

Clinical features
- Haematuria
- Loin pain
- Mass in flank
- Malaise
- Weight loss
- Polycythaemia (excess erythropoietin)

Investigations
- Ultrasound or CT
- MRI (for tumour staging)
- Raised ESR

Management
- Nephrectomy
- α-interferon/interleukin-2
- Tyrosine kinase inhibitors, e.g. sunitinib

Prognosis
- 60–70% 5-year survival for localized tumour
- 15–35% 5-year survival for lymph node involvement
- 5% 5-year survival for distant metastases

Urothelial tumours

- Transitional cell carcinoma, most common in the bladder
- ♂ > ♀ (4:1)
- Present most commonly after 40 years

Risk factors
- Cigarette smoking
- Industrial carcinogen exposure (β-naphthylamine, benzidine)
- Drugs (phenacetin, cyclophosphamide)
- Chronic inflammation (schistosomiasis causes squamous cell carcinoma)

Clinical features
- Painless haematuria
- Clot retention

Investigations
- Urine cytology
- CT/MRI
- Cystoscopy

Management
- Local tumour ablation – endoscopic diathermy
- Local tumour resection – endoscopic transurethral bladder tumour resection (TURBT)
- Cystectomy
- Radiotherapy
- Local or systemic chemotherapy

Prognosis
- 80% 5-year survival (T1 N0 M0)
- 5% 5-year survival (distant metastases)

Prostate cancer

- Sixth commonest cause of cancer death in men
- Malignant change in prostate gland is very common in older men
- About 80% >80 years
- Usually dormant or asymptomatic

Clinical features
- Bladder outflow obstruction
- Distant metastases to bone, lung or brain

Investigations
- Cystoscopy
- Transrectal ultrasound
- Prostatic biopsy
- Prostate-specific antigen (PSA)
- Bone scan

Management

Local disease
- Radical prostatectomy
- Radiotherapy

Metastatic disease
- Orchidectomy
- LHRH analogues (buserelin, goserelin)

Prognosis
- Variable

Testicular tumours

- Commonest in young men aged 30–35
- Seminomas 30%
- Teratomas 70%
- Higher risk in undescended testes and history of orchidopexy

Clinical features
- Testicular swelling (painless or painful)
- Distant metastases

Investigations
- Testicular ultrasound
- Surgical exploration and biopsy via the groin

Staging
- Chest X-ray
- α-fetoprotein
- β-human chorionic gonadotrophin
- Abdominal CT scan

Management

Seminomas
- Radiotherapy
- Chemotherapy

Teratomas
- Orchidectomy
- Chemotherapy

DISEASES OF THE PROSTATE

Benign prostatic enlargement

- Common over 60 years

Clinical features
- Bladder outflow obstruction
- Urinary tract infection
- Stones
- Acute urinary retention (Box 14.3)
- Chronic retention with overflow incontinence
- Bilateral hydronephrosis
- Smooth enlarged prostate on rectal exam

Box 14.3. Acute urinary retention

Clinical features
- Anuria
- Pain
- Urgency
- Palpable bladder

Management
- Urethral catheterization
- Suprapubic catheterization
- Look for a cause

Investigations
- Urine culture
- Assessment of renal function
- PSA
- Cystoscopy

Management
- Observation

Medical
- α-receptor blockers
- Finasteride

Surgical
- Transurethral resection of prostate (TURP)
- Prostatic stents

SELF-ASSESSMENT QUESTIONS

Multiple choice questions (single best answer)

1. IgA nephropathy:
    A. Is associated with carcinoma of the bronchus
    B. Presents after streptococcal infections
    C. Presents with a purpuric rash
    D. Is caused by anti-GBM antibody
    E. Usually progresses to chronic kidney disease
2. Goodpasture syndrome:
    A. May present with haemoptysis
    B. Is caused by immune complex deposition
    C. Causes membranous glomerulonephritis
    D. Rarely progresses to chronic kidney disease
    E. Is treated by nephrectomy
3. Acute nephritic syndrome:
    A. Occurs after *E. coli* infections
    B. Comprises oedema and low albumin
    C. Does not progress to acute kidney injury
    D. Urine microscopy shows red cell casts
    E. Is commonly complicated by hypercholesterolaemia
4. In nephrotic syndrome:
    A. Urine protein excretion is >3 g/day
    B. The renal lesion is always proliferative glomerulonephritis
    C. The urine may be fatty

D. The JVP is raised
E. Renal biopsy is contraindicated

5. Urinary tract infection:
   A. Is commoner in males
   B. Is always symptomatic
   C. Usually indicates an abnormal renal tract in females
   D. May be treated with oral gentamicin
   E. Is most commonly caused by *E. coli* infection

6. Pyelonephritis:
   A. Is associated with a low urine leucocyte count
   B. Is usually secondary to urinary tract obstruction
   C. Is associated with diabetes insipidus
   D. Causes infertility
   E. May be complicated by septicaemia

7. Renal calculi:
   A. Are most commonly composed of uric acid
   B. May be asymptomatic
   C. May be caused by hyperkalaemia
   D. Are usually radiolucent
   E. Larger than 2 cm pass spontaneously

8. Management of bladder outflow obstruction should include:
   A. Fluid restriction
   B. External beam shock wave lithotripsy
   C. Ventriculo-peritoneal shunt
   D. Urethral catheter
   E. Orchidectomy

9. Pre-renal uraemia:
   A. Is caused by hypertension
   B. May be due to gastrointestinal bleeding
   C. Does not correct with fluid replacement
   D. Usually requires emergency dialysis
   E. Presents with pericarditis

10. Complications of acute kidney injury include:
    A. Subarachnoid haemorrhage
    B. Encephalitis
    C. Hypokalaemia
    D. Pericarditis
    E. Contrast nephropathy

11. Acute tubular necrosis:
    A. Is the renal lesion of amyloidosis
    B. May be part of multisystem failure
    C. May be caused by a reaction to oral radiological contrast
    D. Rarely requires dialysis
    F. Has a good overall prognosis

12. Causes of chronic kidney disease include:
    A. Paracetamol toxicity
    B. Sarcoidosis
    C. Cirrhosis of the liver
    D. Herbal therapies
    E. Gilbert syndrome

13. Management of chronic kidney disease commonly includes:
    A. Emergency urography
    B. Bone marrow transplant

    C. Abdominal paracentesis
    D. Total dental extraction
    E. Phosphate restriction

14. Complications of chronic kidney disease commonly include:
    A. Anaemia
    B. Pseudogout
    C. Paget's disease
    D. Haematuria
    E. AV fistula formation

15. A 66-year-old woman was found to be hypertensive and was commenced on ramipril. Ten days later she felt unwell and blood tests revealed: Urea 38 mmol/L (2.5–6.7), creatinine 420 µmol/L (79–118), potassium 6.9 mmol/L (3.5–5.0). What is the most likely underlying diagnosis?
    A. IgA nephropathy
    B. Chronic tubulointerstitial nephritis
    C. Chronic NSAID misuse
    D. Renal sarcoidosis
    E. Bilateral renal artery stenosis

16. A 77-year-old man was admitted with a pneumonia. His blood tests revealed: Urea 25 mmol/L (2.5–6.7), creatinine 280 µmol/L (79–118), potassium 7.2 mmol/L (3.5–5.0). What is the first step in his management?
    A. Oral calcium resonium
    B. Intravenous calcium gluconate
    C. Subcutaneous enoxaparin
    D. Intravenous insulin and dextrose
    E. Inhaled salbutamol

17. The glomerulus is responsible for the synthesis of an ultrafiltrate from blood. Which of the following is most important in this function?
    A. Na^+/K^+ transmembrane pump
    B. Capillary hydrostatic pressure
    C. Osmotic pressure in Bowman's capsule
    D. Proximal loop amino acid resorption
    E. Urea recycling in the loop of Henle

18. A 64-year-old man presented with nocturia and hesitancy with a poor flow when urinating. What is the most likely diagnosis?
    A. Benign prostatic hypertrophy
    B. Bladder stone
    C. Transitional cell carcinoma of the bladder
    D. Prostatic adenocarcinoma
    E. Nonspecific urethritis

19. A 34-year-old woman is found to have multiple cysts on both kidneys and in the liver at ultrasound. A diagnosis of autosomal dominant polycystic kidney disease is made. What is the likelihood of her developing chronic kidney disease requiring renal replacement therapy?
    A. 5%
    B. 20%
    C. 50%
    D. 70%
    E. 90%

20. A 13-year-old girl was referred with peripheral oedema. Her urinary protein was 5 g/L. Which one of the following is most commonly associated with this diagnosis?
    A. Hypokalaemia
    B. Hyperamylasaemia
    C. Achlorhydria
    D. Hyperproteinaemia
    E. Hypercholesterolaemia

Extended matching questions

Question 1 Theme: Right-sided abdominal pain

A. Pyelonephritis
B. Right ovarian cyst
C. Renal calculi
D. Appendicitis
E. Polycystic kidney disease
F. Crohn's disease
G. Gallstones
H. Right lower lobe pneumonia
I. Pancreatitis
J. Renal cell carcinoma
K. Hydronephrosis
L. Hepatitis
M. Irritable bowel syndrome

For each of the following questions, select the best answer from the list above:

I. A 39-year-old advertising executive, who suffers with gout, presents with sudden onset of excruciating colicky pain in the right loin. On examination he is distressed and tender in the right flank. He is apyrexial. Urinalysis shows blood^{+++} and no nitrite. What is the most likely diagnosis?

II. A 49-year-old woman with chronic multiple sclerosis, confined to a wheelchair, presents with fever, confusion and vomiting. She is incontinent of urine with a permanent indwelling catheter. She is pyrexial with a temperature of 39°C. There is reduced air entry to the right lung base. Her PO_2 is 7.6 and urinalysis shows protein^{++}, blood^{+}, nitrite^{+}. What is the most likely diagnosis?

III. A 39-year-old man presents with a 6-month history of a chronic dull ache in the right flank with a feeling of fullness on that side. Eighteen months ago he had emergency neurosurgical clipping of a berry aneurysm after suffering a subarachnoid haemorrhage. What is the most likely diagnosis?

Question 2 Theme: Acute kidney injury

A. Hepatorenal syndrome
B. Contrast nephropathy
C. Gentamicin toxicity
D. Acute GI haemorrhage
E. Hypertensive nephropathy
F. Haemolytic-uraemic syndrome
G. Goodpasture syndrome
H. Wegener's granulomatosis
I. Prostatic obstruction
J. Retroperitoneal fibrosis
K. Renal artery stenosis

For each of the following questions, select the best answer from the list above:

 I. A 48-year-old alcoholic cirrhotic female was admitted 2 days ago with constipation and confusion. She has become pyrexial with low blood pressure and oliguria. Her blood tests show acute kidney injury. What is the most likely diagnosis?

 II. A 90-year-old man is admitted in a dehydrated, febrile and confused state. He was seen by his GP for a 'stomach upset' 2 days ago. His full blood count shows anaemia and thrombocytopenia with red-cell fragments on the blood film. His biochemistry shows acute kidney injury. What is the most likely diagnosis?

III. A 74-year-old male is admitted with symptoms of a urinary tract infection. In the past 2 days he has developed increasing abdominal pain, fever and anuria. On examination he has a mass in the pelvis which is tender and dull to percussion. His blood tests show acute kidney injury. What is the most likely diagnosis?

Haematology 15

Haematology comprises the study of the components of the blood and the bone marrow, along with disorders of the lymphoreticular system. Common disorders include the anaemias and haematological malignancy.

BASIC SCIENCE IN HAEMATOLOGY

Components of blood

Cellular
- Erythrocytes (red cells)
- Reticulocytes (immature red cells)
- Leucocytes (white cells)
  - Lymphocytes
  - Monocytes
  - Eosinophils
  - Basophils
  - Neutrophils
- Platelets

Non-cellular
Plasma
- Liquid component of blood
- Includes
  - Fibrinogen
  - Clotting factors
  - Immunoglobulins
  - Albumin
  - Other plasma proteins
  - Electrolytes

Serum
- Fluid remaining after the formation of a fibrin clot (i.e. no fibrinogen)

Stem cells
- Progenitor cells for blood cells
- Proliferation and differentiation
- → Mature blood cells
- Self-renewal, so source cells not depleted (Fig. 15.1)

Growth factors
- Glycoproteins, e.g. granulocyte colony-stimulating factor (G-CSF)
- Regulate proliferation and differentiation of progenitor cells and mature cell functions
- Used to increase number of cell lines in response to stress, e.g. infection, blood loss, chemotherapy

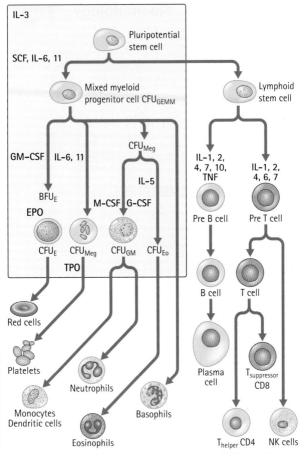

Fig. 15.1 Normal haemopoiesis. *(Reproduced from Kumar P, Clark M. Kumar and Clark's Clinical Medicine, 8th edn. Edinburgh: Elsevier; 2012, with permission from Elsevier.)*

Laboratory values (Table 15.1)

Red cell indices
- Size, number and haemoglobin content of erythrocytes
- Important in the classification of anaemia

Erythrocyte sedimentation rate (ESR)
- Rate of fall of red cells in a column of blood
- Measure of acute phase proteins and therefore of inflammation
- Increases with age
- ♀ > ♂

Table 15.1 Normal values for peripheral blood

	Male	Female
Hb (g/L)	135–175	115–160
PCV (haematocrit; L/L)	0.4–0.54	0.37–0.47
RCC (10^{12}/L)	4.5–6.0	3.9–5.0
MCV (fL)	80–96	
MCH (pg)	27–32	
MCHC (g/L)	320–360	
RDW (%)	11–15	
WBC (10^9/L)	4.0–11.0	
Platelets (10^9/L)	150–400	
ESR (mm/h)	<20	
Reticulocytes	0.5–2.5% (50–100 × 10^9/L)	

ESR, erythrocyte sedimentation rate; Hb, haemoglobin; MCH, mean corpuscular haemoglobin; MCHC, mean corpuscular haemoglobin concentration; MCV, mean corpuscular volume of red cells; PCV, packed cell volume; RCC, red cell count; RDW, red blood cell distribution width; WBC, white blood count.

(Reproduced from Kumar P, Clark M. Kumar and Clark's Clinical Medicine, 8th edn. Edinburgh: Elsevier; 2012, with permission from Elsevier.)

Plasma viscosity
- Measure of acute phase proteins
- No sex and little age variation

Reticulocyte count
- Immature red cells
- Measure of erythropoiesis
- Normally <2%
- Increased by high marrow activity, e.g.
  - After bleeding
  - Anaemia
  - Haemolysis

Haemoglobin

Structure
- Four globin (protein) chains
- Four haem (iron-containing) molecules
- Molecular weight 68 000

Function
- Haem moiety binds and transports oxygen and CO_2

Genetics
- Adult Hb (HbA) consists of two α and two β globins
- HbA_2 consists of two α and two β globins (2% of adult Hb)
- Fetal Hb consists of two α and two γ globins

Table 15.2 Iron indices in anaemia

	Iron deficiency	Anaemia of chronic disease	Macrocytic anaemia
Hb	↓	↓	↓
MCV	↓	↓ or ↔	↑
Ferritin	↓	↑, ↓ or ↔	↑ or ↔
Serum iron	↓	↓	↔
Total iron binding capacity	↑	↓	↔
Transferrin saturation	↓	↓	↔

ANAEMIA

Anaemia (haemoglobin below the reference range) is not a diagnosis and a cause must be found.

Classification (Table 15.2)

- By erythrocyte volume (MCV)

Macrocytic – large red cells
- B_{12} deficiency
- Folate deficiency
- Chronic alcohol misuse
- Chronic liver disease
- ↑ Reticulocytes
- Hypothyroidism
- Drugs, e.g. azathioprine

Microcytic – small red cells
- Iron deficiency
- Thalassaemia
- Sideroblastic anaemia
- Anaemia of chronic disease
- Myelodysplasia

Normocytic – normal red cells
- Acute blood loss
- Anaemia of chronic disease
- Haemolysis
- Infection
- Pregnancy
- Hypopituitarism
- Hypothyroidism (may be macrocytic)
- Renal failure

Clinical features
Symptoms
- Fatigue ⎫
- Headache ⎬ Common in normal population
- Faintness ⎭
- Breathlessness
- Angina
- Intermittent claudication
- Palpitations

Signs
- Pallor
- Tachycardia
- Systolic flow murmur
- Cardiac failure
- Koilonychia – spoon-shaped nails in iron deficiency
- Jaundice – haemolytic anaemia
- Bone deformity – thalassaemia major
- Leg ulcers – sickle cell disease

Investigations
- White cell count – if low, may be dilutional or bone marrow failure
- Reticulocyte count – measures bone marrow activity
- Blood film for erythrocyte morphology – may show dimorphic picture (both large and small red cells); seen in combined iron and folate deficiency

Iron deficiency anaemia

Iron metabolism
- Iron requirements
  - ♂ 0.5–1 mg/day
  - ♀ 1.2–1.7 mg/day (2–3 mg/day in pregnancy)
- Dietary iron 15–20 mg/day
- 10% absorbed
- Absorption is in duodenum and jejunum (Fig. 15.2)
- Transported in blood bound to transferrin
- Stored as ferritin and haemosiderin

Causes of iron deficiency
- Blood loss (commonly menstrual)
- Growth or pregnancy (↑ requirement)
- Decreased absorption (e.g. gastrectomy)
- Low dietary intake

Clinical features
- Koilonychia and brittle nails/hair
- Angular stomatitis
- Dysphagia
- Glossitis } Plummer–Vinson or Paterson–Brown–Kelly syndrome

Investigations
- Blood count and film
- ↓ Serum ferritin
- ↓ Serum iron and ↑ iron-binding capacity ↓ transferrin saturation
- ↑ Serum soluble transferrin receptors

Management
- Identify and treat cause
- Oral iron – ferrous sulphate (first choice preparation) or gluconate
- Parenteral iron, severe malabsorption or chronic disease, e.g. inflammatory bowel disease if unable to tolerate oral

Anaemia of chronic disease

Aetiology
- Reduced erythropoiesis
- Reduced red cell survival

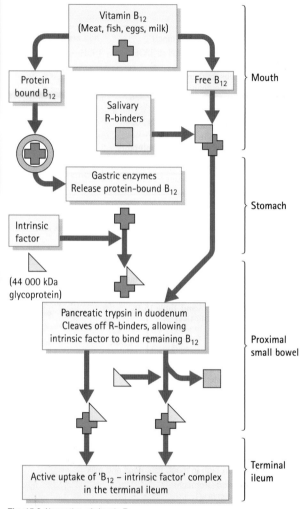

Fig. 15.3 Absorption of vitamin B₁₂.

Table 15.4 Causes of folate deficiency	
Nutritional	*Pathological*
Poor intake	Increased red cell synthesis, e.g.
Old age	haemolysis
Poor diet	Inhibited metabolism
Starvation	Drugs
Alcohol abuse	Anticonvulsants, e.g. phenytoin
Malabsorption	Methotrexate
Coeliac disease	Trimethoprim
Crohn's disease	Increased cell turnover, e.g.
Anorexia	malignancy
Malignancy	Inflammatory disease
GI disease	Metabolic disease, e.g.
↑ Utilization	homocystinuria
Physiological	Haemodialysis
Pregnancy	
Lactation	

Pernicious anaemia

- → Megaloblastic anaemia

Aetiology
- Autoimmune disease
- Common (esp. in elderly)
- Anti-intrinsic factor antibodies in 50%
- Anti-parietal cell antibodies in 90%
- → Intrinsic factor deficiency due to autoimmune gastritis
- → B_{12} malabsorption

Disease associations
- Autoimmune thyroid disease
- Addison's disease
- Vitiligo
- Blond hair and blue eyes
- Blood group A
- Higher risk of gastric cancer in males

Pathology
- Gastric mucosal atrophy
- Achlorhydria (loss of gastric acid synthesis)

Clinical features
- Pallor and mild jaundice
- Glossitis (sore red tongue)
- Angular stomatitis
- Progressive polyneuropathy
  - Subacute combined degeneration of the cord
  - → Paraesthesia, weakness and ataxia
  - → Paraplegia
  - Rarely, optic atrophy or dementia

Management

- 1 mg vitamin B_{12} per day for 7 days i.m.
- Then 1 mg every 3 months for life
- Oral high dose (e.g. 2 mg a day) vitamin B_{12} can be prescribed as an alternative but requires good compliance

Folate deficiency

- $\rightarrow$ Megaloblastic anaemia

Folate absorption

- Found in spinach, broccoli, liver and kidney
- Cooking destroys folate
- Daily requirement 100 mg
- B_{12} required for folate metabolism

Clinical features

- Anaemia
- Glossitis
- No neuropathy

Management

- Oral folate 5 mg/day

Prophylaxis

- Advised prior to and during pregnancy
- Reduces risk of neural tube defects

Sickle cell disease

Aetiology

- Mutation $\rightarrow$ abnormal β globin (HbS)
- $\rightarrow$ Sickle cell trait (heterozygote HbAS)
- Or sickle cell disease (homozygote HbSS)
- HbS is insoluble when deoxygenated
- $\rightarrow$ Hb forms crystals and deforms red cells
- $\rightarrow$ Sickle shape
- $\rightarrow$ Reduced red cell survival and microvascular obstruction

Epidemiology

- 25% of Africans carry abnormal gene
- Also India, Middle East and southern Europe

Precipitation of crisis

- Infection
  - Chest $\rightarrow$ hypoxia
  - Parvovirus $\rightarrow$ marrow aplasia $\rightarrow$ pancytopenia
  - Haemolysis due to sepsis
- Sequestration of red cells in liver and spleen
- Dehydration $\rightarrow$ increased plasma viscosity

Clinical features

- Onset after 6 months (as HbF level drops)
- Chronic haemolytic anaemia
- Recurrent painful crises
- Bone pain
- Chest – pleuritic pain (common cause of death – acute chest syndrome)
- Cerebral – fits, neurological signs
- Kidneys – papillary necrosis, inability to concentrate urine

- Spleen – splenic infarcts → hyposplenism
- Liver – pain and abnormal liver function
- Penis – priapism

Long term
- Hyposplenism → risk of infection
- Chronic leg ulcers
- Gallstones
- Necrosis of femoral heads
- Chronic kidney disease
- Chronic respiratory disease
- Stroke
- Retinopathy

Investigations
- Full blood count
  - Anaemia
  - Infection (leucocytosis)
- Blood film
  - Sickling
  - Hyposplenism
- Hb electrophoresis demonstrates HbS

Management
Acute (Box 15.1)
- i.v. fluids
- Oxygen
- Antibiotics if evidence of infection
- Adequate analgesia
- Exchange transfusions if severe crisis

Long term
- Pneumococcal and *Haemophilus influenzae* vaccines
- Folic acid
- Transfusions for clear indications and complications only
- Hydroxyurea increases Hb F production
- Bone marrow transplantation

Thalassaemia

Aetiology
- Inherited failure of synthesis of one globin type
- Accumulation of remaining globin type
- → Haemolysis and ineffective erythropoiesis

β-thalassaemia
Minor (trait)
- Carrier state (heterozygote)
- Asymptomatic
- Low MCV and MCH

Major
- Homozygote
- Severe anaemia requiring transfusions
- Onset 3–6 months old
- Infections
- Extramedullary haemopoiesis
  → Skull expansion and bossing

> **BOX 15.1.** Management of acute painful crisis in opioid naive adults with sickle cell disease
>
> ### Morphine/diamorphine
> - 0.1 mg/kg i.v./s.c. every 20 minutes until pain controlled, then
> - 0.05–0.1 mg/kg i.v./s.c. (or oral morphine) every 2–4 hours
>
> ### Patient controlled analgesia (PCA) (example for adults >50 kg)
> *Diamorphine*
> - Continuous infusion: 0–10 mg/hour
> - PCA bolus dose: 2–10 mg
> - Dose duration: 1 minute
> - Lockout time: 20–30 minutes
>
> ### Adjuvant oral analgesia
> - Paracetamol 1 g 6 hourly
>   – ± Ibuprofen[a] 400 mg 8 hourly
> - Or diclofenac[a] 50 mg 8 hourly
>
> ### Laxatives (all patients)
> For example:
> - Lactulose 10 ml×2 daily
> - Senna 2–4 tablets daily
> - Sodium docusate 100 mg×2 daily
> - Macrogol 1 sachet daily
> - Lubiprostone
>
> ### Other adjuvants
> *Anti-pruritics*
> - Hydroxyzine 25 mg×2 as required
> *Antiemetics*
> - Prochlorperazine 5–10 mg×3 as required
> - Cyclizine 50 mg×3 as required
> *Anxiolytic*
> - Haloperidol 1–3 mg oral/i.m.×2 as required

[a]Caution advised with NSAIDs in renal impairment. *(Adapted from Rees DC, Olujohungbe AD, Parker NE et al. Guidelines for the management of the acute painful crisis in sickle cell disease. Br J Haematol 2003; 120(5):744–752. Reproduced from Kumar P, Clark M, Kumar and Clark's Clinical Medicine, 8th edn. Edinburgh: Elsevier; 2012, with permission from Elsevier.)*

Treatment
- Folic acid
- Regular transfusions to suppress haemopoiesis and avoid deformity and anaemia
- Iron chelation to reduce overload
- Bone marrow transplantation

α-thalassaemia
- Deletion in one to four of the four α globin genes
- All four deleted → fetal death (hydrops fetalis)
- Three of four → moderate anaemia
- Two of four → carrier state, no anaemia

Haemolytic anaemia

- Anaemia due to the premature breakdown of erythrocytes, resulting in reduced red cell survival
- If haemolysis is acute, anaemia, jaundice and haemoglobinuria are seen

Aetiology

Inherited

- Sickle cell disease
- Thalassaemia
- Hereditary spherocytosis
- Hereditary elliptocytosis
- Glucose-6-phosphate dehydrogenase deficiency
  - X-linked recessive
  - → Haemolysis due to drugs, e.g. aspirin
  - Favism (fava beans → haemolysis)
  - Haemolysis due to infection
- Pyruvate kinase deficiency
  - Autosomal recessive
  - → Anaemia and splenomegaly

Acquired

- Autoimmune haemolytic anaemia (Table 15.5)
  - Autoantibodies against red cell membrane
  - Positive direct Coombs' test (Fig. 15.4)
- Drug-induced autoimmune haemolysis
  - Quinine
  - Penicillin
  - Methyldopa
- Haemolytic disease of the newborn
  - Maternal anti-red cell IgG crosses placenta
  - → Fetal red cell destruction (Rhesus disease)
- Paroxysmal nocturnal haemoglobinuria
  - Red cell destruction by complement
  - → Haemolysis due to infection or surgery
  - → Early morning haemoglobinuria
  - Increased risk of venous thrombosis
- Mechanical haemolysis
  - Cardiac prosthetic valves
  - Marching
  - Microangiopathic haemolytic anaemia
- Others
  - Extensive burns
  - Renal and liver disease
  - Malaria

BLOOD GROUPS AND BLOOD TRANSFUSION

- Blood group of a particular patient is determined by red cell surface antigens
- The two common and most important groupings are ABO and Rhesus status
- The process of typing blood is based on a series of indirect Coombs' tests to analyse the blood for the presence of these antigens

Table 15.5 Causes and major features of autoimmune haemolytic anaemias

	Warm	Cold
Temperature at which antibody attaches best to red cells	37°C	Lower than 37°C
Type of antibody	IgG	IgM
Direct Coombs' test	Strongly positive	Positive
Causes of primary conditions	Idiopathic	Idiopathic
Causes of secondary condition	Autoimmune disorders, e.g. systemic lupus erythematosus Chronic lymphocytic leukaemia Lymphomas Hodgkin's lymphoma Carcinomas Drugs, many including methyldopa, penicillins, cephalosporins, NSAIDs, quinine, interferon	Infections, e.g. infectious mononucleosis, *Mycoplasma pneumoniae*, other viral infections (rare) Lymphomas Paroxysmal cold haemoglobinuria (IgG)

(Reproduced from Kumar P, Clark M. Kumar and Clark's Clinical Medicine, 8th edn. Edinburgh: Elsevier; 2012, with permission from Elsevier.)

- Cross-matching blood for transfusion is carried out by looking for agglutination when blood cells to be donated are mixed with the patient's serum (Fig. 15.4)

ABO blood group (Table 15.6)

- Presence of A or B antigens on red cells
- Presence of anti-A or anti-B in serum
- Mixing incompatible blood → haemolysis

Rh blood group

- Presence or absence of D antigen
- Antibodies form if a D-negative patient is given D-positive blood

Fetal Rhesus D syndrome
- RhD-negative mother with a D-positive child will be sensitized at the first delivery
- Subsequent D-positive fetuses will be subjected to anti-D antibodies → hydrops fetalis
- Prophylaxis with anti-D antibodies given to the mother at each delivery suppresses the mother's own antibody production, protecting future fetuses

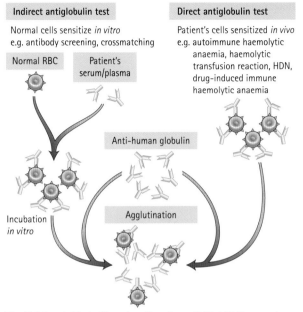

Indirect antiglobulin test

Normal cells sensitize *in vitro*
e.g. antibody screening, crossmatching

Normal RBC

Patient's serum/plasma

Incubation *in vitro*

Direct antiglobulin test

Patient's cells sensitized *in vivo*
e.g. autoimmune haemolytic anaemia, haemolytic transfusion reaction, HDN, drug-induced immune haemolytic anaemia

Anti-human globulin

Agglutination

Fig. 15.4 Coombs' tests. *(Reproduced from Kumar P, Clark M. Kumar and Clark's Clinical Medicine, 8th edn. Edinburgh: Elsevier; 2012, with permission from Elsevier.)*

Table 15.6 The ABO and Rhesus blood groups

Group	Genotype antigens	Red cell	Antibodies	Frequency	Notes
O	OO	None	Anti-A and anti-B	44%	Universal donor
A	AO or AA	A	Anti-B	45%	
B	BO or BB	B	Anti-B	8%	
AB	AB	A and B	None	3%	Universal recipient
D +ve	C or D or E	D	None		Three genes determine genotype: C, D and E
D −ve	CDE	None	Anti-D[a]		[a]After exposure

Blood products

- Whole blood ~500 mL
- Packed cells – 250 mL of plasma removed
- Red cell concentrate – all plasma removed
- Platelet concentrates
- Granulocyte concentrates
- Fresh frozen plasma – replacement of clotting factors
- Cryoprecipitate – factor VIII, fibrinogen and von Willebrand factor
- Human albumin
- Normal immunoglobulin

Procedure for blood transfusion

- Type patient's blood
- Cross-match donor blood with patient serum
- Donor blood is coded and labelled with the patient's name; a record sheet with the unit number of the donor blood and the patient's name and identification number is produced

When administering blood

- Two members of staff check the following:

Between the patient and record sheet
- Name of the patient
- Date of birth of the patient
- Identification number of the patient

Between the blood and record sheet
- Blood unit number
- Blood group
- Name, age and date of birth of the patient

Complications of blood transfusion

- Incompatibility → poor red cell survival

Transfusion reactions
- Usually ABO incompatibility
- Haemolysis and haemoglobinuria
- Rigors
- Dyspnoea
- Hypotension
- Renal failure
- Disseminated intravascular coagulation

Febrile transfusion reactions
- Mild fever and flushing
- Rarely due to haemolysis

Transmission of infection
- Viruses, parasites, bacteria and prions
- All blood screened for known infections

BLOOD COAGULATION (FIG. 15.5)

Vessel wall injury leads to:

- Vasoconstriction → reduced blood flow
- Platelet activation → serotonin and thromboxane
- Coagulation → fibrin clot formation

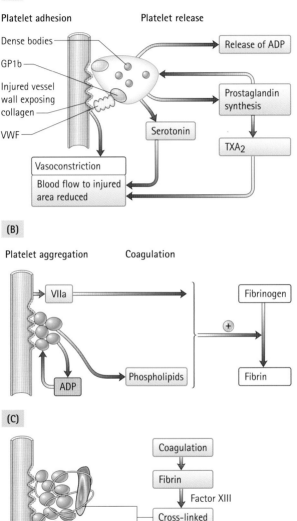

(A)

Platelet adhesion   Platelet release

- Dense bodies
- GP1b
- Injured vessel wall exposing collagen
- VWF

Release of ADP

Prostaglandin synthesis

Serotonin

TXA₂

Vasoconstriction

Blood flow to injured area reduced

(B)

Platelet aggregation   Coagulation

VIIa

ADP

Phospholipids

Fibrinogen

Fibrin

(C)

Coagulation

Fibrin

Factor XIII

Cross-linked fibrin

Fig. 15.5 Formation of the haemostatic plug. *(Reproduced from Kumar P, Clark M. Kumar and Clark's Clinical Medicine, 8th edn. Edinburgh: Elsevier; 2012, with permission from Elsevier.)*

Platelet adhesion

- Adhesion to collagen exposed by vessel damage via glycoprotein Ia receptor on platelets and in combination with von Willebrand factor via glycoprotein Ib receptors
- Fibrinogen then binds to platelets, is converted to fibrin and forms cross-links, producing a platelet plug

Platelet prostaglandin

- Prostaglandin metabolism → thromboxane production
- → Vasoconstriction and platelet activation
- Process is inhibited by aspirin

Coagulation cascade (Fig. 15.5)

- Enzymatic reactions
- → Activation of coagulation proteins
- → Conversion of fibrinogen to fibrin

Coagulation factors

- Synthesized in the liver
- Enzyme precursors (XII, XI, X, IX)
- Enzyme co-factors (V, VIII)

Coagulation inhibitors

- Antithrombin inactivates clotting factors
- Activated protein C destroys factors V and VIII and initiates fibrinolysis
- Protein S – co-factor for protein C

Fibrinolysis (Fig. 15.6)

- Plasminogen converted to plasmin by tissue plasminogen activator (t-PA)
- Converts fibrin to fibrin degradation products and D-dimer fragments

Measurements of coagulation (Table 15.7)

- Prothrombin time (PT, normal 10–16 seconds)
  - Lengthened by factor VII, X, V or II abnormality
  - Increased by warfarin
- International normalized ratio (INR, normal = 1–1.3)
  - Comparison of prothrombin time to a known standard
  - Used to monitor warfarin
- Activated partial thromboplastin time (APTT, normal 23–31 seconds)
  - Abnormalities of factors XI, IX, VIII, X, V, II or I
  - Increased by heparin
- Thrombin time (TT, normal 12 seconds)
  - Prolonged by fibrinogen deficiencies and heparin
- Bleeding time
  - Standard cut made and time taken for bleeding to stop is measured

Correction tests – addition of normal plasma

- If this corrects an abnormal test, then a factor deficiency is the cause of the coagulopathy
- If no correction occurs, it suggests the presence of an inhibitor in the patient's plasma

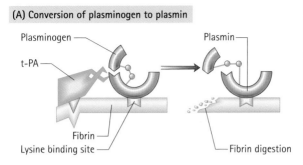

(A) Conversion of plasminogen to plasmin

Plasminogen

t-PA

Plasmin

Fibrin

Lysine binding site

Fibrin digestion

(B) Plasmin α₂–antiplasmin complex

Plasmin

α₂–antiplasmin

Fig. 15.6 Fibrinolysis. *(Reproduced from Kumar P, Clark M. Kumar and Clark's Clinical Medicine, 8th edn. Edinburgh: Elsevier; 2012, with permission from Elsevier.)*

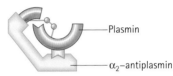

Table 15.7 Blood results in coagulopathy					
	Prothrombin time (PT)	Activated partial thromboplastin time (APTT)	Bleeding time	Factor VIII: C level	Von Willebrand factor (vWF)
Platelet disorders	Normal	Normal	↑	Normal	Normal
Vitamin K deficiency	↑	↑	Normal	Normal	Normal
Haemophilia A and B	Normal	↑	Normal	↓	Normal
Von Willebrand's disease	Normal	↑	↑	↓	↓

D-dimer assay
- Increased during fibrinolysis, e.g. after pulmonary embolus
- If negative, PE is very unlikely

Fibrin degradation products (FDPs)
- Increased by fibrinolysis, e.g. pulmonary embolus

Inherited coagulation defects: Haemophilia A

- X-linked inheritance found in 1:5000 men
- Factor VIII deficiency

Factor VIII <1% of normal
- Frequent spontaneous bleeding
- Joint bleeds → deformity

Factor VIII <5% of normal
- Severe bleeding after injury

Factor VIII >5% of normal
- Mild disease
- Prolonged bleeding after trauma

Investigations
See Table 15.7.

Management
- Factor VIII:Concentrate (C) i.v.
- Desmopressin intranasal spray (increases factor VIII:C levels)
- Minor bleeding – aim for 30% of normal
- Major bleeding – aim for 50% of normal
- Surgery – aim for 100% preoperatively

Complications of treatment
- Antibodies against factor VIII:C
- Complications of blood transfusion

Haemophilia B (Christmas disease)

- X-linked inheritance found in 1:30000 men
- Factor IX deficiency
- Clinically identical to haemophilia A

Management
- i.v. factor IX

Von Willebrand's disease

- Three types (all chromosome 12)
  - Type 1: mild disease, autosomal dominant
  - Type 2: mild disease, autosomal dominant
  - Type 3: severe disease, autosomal recessive
- Bleeding follows trauma and surgery
- Spontaneous epistaxis
- Defect of platelet adhesion combined with factor VIII:C deficiency

Management
- Intranasal desmopressin
- Factor VIII/von Willebrand factor if required

Acquired coagulation defects: Vitamin K deficiency

- Failure of synthesis of vitamin K-dependent factors
- Reduced factors II, VII, IX and X
- Reduced protein C and S

Aetiology
- Inadequate stores (newborn children)
- Malabsorption (fat-soluble vitamin)
- Oral anticoagulants, e.g. warfarin

Investigations
- Elevated prothrombin time and APTT

Management
- Intravenous vitamin K

Chronic liver disease

- Vitamin K deficiency
- Reduced clotting factor synthesis
- Thrombocytopenia
- Abnormal platelet function

Disseminated intravascular coagulation (DIC)

- Uncontrolled fibrin production in blood vessels
  - Malignancy
  - Septicaemia
  - Transfusion reactions
  - Placental abruption and amniotic fluid embolism
  - Trauma, burns, surgery
  - Infections, e.g. Falciparum malaria
  - Liver disease
  - Snake bites

Investigations
- Elevated PT, APPT and TT if severe
- Low platelets and fragmented red cells
- Elevated FDPs and D-dimers

Clinical features
- Haemorrhage
- Shock
- Epistaxis, bleeding gums

Management
- Diagnose and treat cause
- Platelets
- Fresh frozen plasma (FFP)
- Cryoprecipitate
- Blood if required

Massive blood transfusion

- Lack of factors VIII and V in transfusion blood
- Few platelets
- Citrate in transfusions lowers serum calcium
- If giving >10 units, check clotting and platelets
- Consider platelets and fresh frozen plasma
- Calcium i.v.

Clotting factor autoantibodies

- 10% of haemophiliacs – antibodies against factor VIII
- SLE
- Post-childbirth

Anticoagulant drugs

Warfarin (Box 15.2)
- Oral vitamin K antagonist
- Increases prothrombin time

Heparin
- Parenteral administration
- Potentiates antithrombin III
- Elevates APTT

BOX 15.2. Uncontrolled bleeding due to anticoagulation with warfarin

Severe bleeding
- Stop warfarin immediately
- i.v. access
- Give 5 mg of i.v. vitamin K by slow infusion
- Prothrombin complex concentrate 50u/kg
- Blood transfusion if required

Less severe bleeding
- e.g. Epistaxis or haematuria or INR >8
- Withhold warfarin
- Consider vitamin K 0.5 mg i.v.

Low molecular weight heparin
- Subcutaneous administration
- Predictable anticoagulant effect dosed by weight

Fibrinolytics
- Activate plasmin
- Recombinant t-Pa
- Streptokinase

Anti-platelet drugs
- Aspirin
- Clopidogrel
- Dipyridamole
- Glycoprotein IIb/IIIa receptor antagonists
- Epoprostenol

New oral anticoagulants
- Direct thrombin inhibitors, e.g. dabigatron
- Factor Xa inhibitor, e.g. rivaroxaban

Thromboembolic disease

Thromboembolic disease is a very common cause of death; just under 50% of adult deaths result from its manifestations.
- Coronary artery thrombosis
- Cerebral artery thrombosis
- Pulmonary embolism (PE)

Thrombus

- Formation of solid clot in a vessel

Embolus

- Fragment of clot carried to a distant site
- → Obstruction of a vessel

Arterial thrombus

- Associated with atheroma
- → Platelet attachment
- → Propagation of thrombus

Table 15.8 Risk factors for venous thromboembolism	
Patient factors	**Disease or surgical procedure**
Age BMI >30 kg/m^2 Varicose veins Continuous travel more than 3 h in preceding 4 weeks Immobility (bed rest ≥3 days) Pregnancy and puerperium Previous deep vein thrombosis or pulmonary embolism Thrombophilia Antithrombin deficiency Protein C or S deficiency Factor V Leiden Resistance to activated protein C (caused by factor V Leiden variant) Prothrombin gene variant Hyperhomocysteinaemia Antiphospholipid antibody/lupus anticoagulant Oestrogen therapy including HRT Dysfibrinogenaemia Plasminogen deficiency	Trauma or surgery, especially of pelvis, hip or lower limb Malignancy Cardiac or respiratory failure Recent myocardial infarction or stroke Acute medical illness/severe infection Inflammatory bowel disease Behçet's disease Nephrotic syndrome Myeloproliferative disorders Paroxysmal nocturnal haemoglobinuria Paraproteinaemia Sickle cell anaemia Central venous catheter *in situ*

(Reproduced from Kumar P, Clark M. Kumar and Clark's Clinical Medicine, 8th edn. Edinburgh: Elsevier; 2012, with permission from Elsevier.)

Venous thrombus

- Occurs in normal vessels
- Commonly deep leg veins
- Risk factors (Table 15.8)

Thrombophilia

- Recurrent venous thrombosis
- Venous thrombosis under the age of 40
- Often a family history

Aetiology

- Factor V Leiden syndrome
- Antithrombin deficiency
- Protein C and S deficiency
- Antiphospholipid syndrome

Deep vein thrombosis (DVT)

Formation of thrombus in:
- Deep calf vein
- Axillary vein

Clinical features
- Pain and tenderness
- Swelling of the limb
- Redness of overlying skin
- Pulmonary embolism

Investigations
- Doppler ultrasound of the vein
- Venography (intravenous contrast)

Management
- Low molecular weight heparin *or*
- IV heparin
- Warfarin
- Bed rest until anticoagulated
- Graduated pressure stockings

Complications
- Phlebitis
- Venous eczema

Pulmonary embolism

- Obstruction of a branch of the pulmonary artery by clot from a DVT

Clinical features
Small or medium PE
- Pleuritic chest pain
- Shortness of breath
- Haemoptysis in 30%
- Tachypnoea
- Pleural rub
- Coarse crackles
- Pleural effusion

Massive PE
- Collapse
- Shock
- Cardiac arrest electromechanical dissociation
- Elevated JVP ('a' wave)
- Gallop rhythm

Recurrent PE
- Breathlessness
- Weakness
- Syncope
- Gradual deterioration

Diagnosis
Clinical scoring to predict probability e.g., Wells or Geneva Score.

Investigations
- Chest X-ray – oligaemic area
- ECG often normal except for sinus tachycardia
  - S wave in lead I, Q wave and inverted T in lead III
  - Right axis deviation
  - Right bundle branch block
- Plasma D-dimers are elevated (high negative predictive value)
- CT pulmonary angiogram (first choice investigation)

- $\dot{V}/\dot{Q}$ scan (see Fig. 5.51)
  - Radionucleotide scan
  - Demonstrates defects in perfusion of the lung in areas with normal ventilation
- Blood gases – hypoxia and low $PaCO_2$

Management
- High-flow oxygen
- Analgesia
- Low molecular weight heparin
- Warfarin
- Consider thrombolysis in massive PE

HAEMATOLOGICAL MALIGNANCY

These are malignant proliferations of:
- Lymphocytes
  - Hodgkin's disease
  - Non-Hodgkin's lymphoma
  - Chronic lymphocytic leukaemia
  - Myeloma (plasma cells)
- Immature lymphocytes
  - Acute lymphoblastic leukaemia
  - Hairy cell leukaemia
- Myeloid cells
  - Acute myelogenous leukaemia
  - Chronic myeloid leukaemia

Lymphomas: Hodgkin's disease

- B cell malignant clone

Clinical features (Table 15.9)
- Lymphadenopathy
- B symptoms: fever, drenching sweats, weight loss
- Pruritis, fatigue
- Alcohol-induced pain
- Hepatomegaly
- Splenomegaly

Investigations
- Blood count – normal or anaemia, eosinophilia (Table 15.11)
- ESR ↑
- Uric acid sometimes ↑
- Chest X-ray – mediastinal mass or hilar lymph nodes
- CT scan
  - Lymphadenopathy
  - Liver or spleen enlargement or infiltration
- Lymph node biopsy and histology
- PET scan
- Bone marrow biopsy (shows Sternberg–Reed cells)

Management
- Depends on
  - Stage and histology
  - Site of tumour
  - Presence of B symptoms (Table 15.9)

Table 15.9 Cotswolds modification of Ann Arbor staging classification

Stage	Description
I	Involvement of a single lymph-node region or lymphoid structure (e.g. spleen, thymus, Waldeyer's ring) or involvement of a single extralymphatic site
II	Involvement of two or more lymph-node regions on the same side of the diaphragm (hilar nodes, when involved on both sides, constitute stage II disease); localized contiguous involvement of only one extranodal organ or site and lymph-node region(s) on the same side of the diaphragm (IIE). The number of anatomic regions involved should be indicated by a subscript (e.g. II_3)
III	Involvement of lymph-node regions on both sides of the diaphragm (III), which may also be accompanied by involvement of the spleen (IIIS) or by localized involvement of only one extranodal organ site (IIIE) or both (IIISE)
III-1	With or without involvement of splenic, hilar, coeliac or portal nodes
III-2	With involvement of para-aortic, iliac and mesenteric nodes
IV	Diffuse or disseminated involvement of one or more extranodal organs or tissues, with or without associated lymph-node involvement
Designations applicable to any disease state	
A	No symptoms
B	Fever (temperature >38°C), drenching night sweats, unexplained loss of more than 10% of body weight within the previous 6 months
X	Bulky disease (a widening of the mediastinum by more than one-third of the presence of a nodal mass with a maximal dimension greater than 10 cm)
E	Involvement of a single extranodal site that is contiguous or proximal to the known nodal site

(Adapted from Diehl V, Thomas RK, Re D et al. Hodgkin's lymphoma–diagnosis and treatment. Lancet Oncology 2004; 5:19–26, with permission. Reproduced from Kumar P, Clark M. Kumar and Clark's Clinical Medicine, 8th edn. Edinburgh: Elsevier; 2012, with permission from Elsevier.)

- Radiotherapy
- Chemotherapy
- Myeloablation and stem cell support

Prognosis
- 40–70% survival at 20 years
- Depends on stage of original tumour

Non-Hodgkin's lymphoma

Aetiology
- 80% B cell
- Associated with EBV, HTLV and HIV infection

Clinical features
- Lymphadenopathy
- Symptoms due to site of tumour
- May involve GI tract, lungs, brain

Investigations
- Blood count
  - Anaemia
  - Thrombocytopenia
- Liver chemistry
- Chest X-ray
- CT scan of abdomen and thorax
- Bone marrow biopsy
- Lymph node biopsy

Management
- Depends on grade
- Radiotherapy
- Chemotherapy

Burkitt's lymphoma

- Associated with Epstein–Barr virus
- Endemic in West Africa
- Jaw, abdominal and ovarian tumours
- Curable

Acute leukaemias

Aetiology
- Unknown in most cases
- T-cell leukaemia – retrovirus (HTLV-1)
- Specific genetic mutations
- Chromosome translocations, e.g. t (15; 17)
- Environmental factors
- Ionizing radiation

Clinical features
- Bone marrow failure
- → Weakness and tiredness due to anaemia
- → Bruising due to thrombocytopenia
- → Repeated infections

Investigations
- Blood count
- Blood film – leukaemic blast cells
- Bone marrow – blast cells

Management
- Correct anaemia and thrombocytopenia
- Treat any infection
- Chemotherapy to achieve remission
- Myeloablation with stem cell support to clear marrow of malignant cells

Table 15.10 WHO classification of acute leukaemia

(a) Acute myeloid leukaemia

AML with recurrent genetic abnormalities
AML with t(8;21)(q22;q22) (RUNX1/RUNX1T1)
AML with inv(16)(p13q22) or t(16;16)(p13;q22) (CBFβ/MYH11)
Acute promyelocytic leukaemia with t(15;17)(q22;q12) PML/RAR-α and variants
AML with t(9;11)(p22;q23) (MLLT3/MLL)
AML with t(6;9)(p23;q34) (DEK/NUP214)
AML with inv(3)(q21q26) or t(3;3)(q21;q26) (RPN1/EVI1)
AML with CEBPA mutation
AML with NPM mutation
AML with MDS related changes
  Therapy related myeloid neoplasm
  Alkylating agent
  Radiation-related type
  Topoisomerase II inhibitor-related type
  Other
AML, not otherwise categorized[a]
  AML, minimally differentiated
  AML without maturation
  AML with maturation
  Acute myelomonocytic leukaemia
  Acute monoblastic/acute monocytic leukaemia
  Acute erythroid leukaemia (erythroid/myeloid and pure
    erythroleukaemia variants)
  Acute megakaryoblastic leukaemia
  Acute basophilic leukaemia
  Acute panmyelosis with myelofibrosis
  Myeloid sarcoma

(b) Acute lymphoid leukaemia – precursor lymphoid neoplasm

B-cell lymphoblastic leukaemia/lymphoma with recurrent genetic
  abnormality
  t(9;22)(q34;q11) (BCR/ABL)
  t(v;11q23) (MLL rearranged)
  t(1;19)(q23;p13) (E2A/PBX1)
  t(12;21)(p13;q22) (TEL/RUNX1)
Hyperdiploidy
Hypodiploidy
B-cell lymphoblastic leukaemia/lymphoma not otherwise specified
T-cell lymphoblastic leukaemia/lymphoma

[a]The entities included in this group are defined almost identically to the corresponding entity in the French–American–British (FAB) classification.
(Modified from Jaffe ES, Harris NL, Stein H, Vardiman JW, eds. World Health Organization Classification of Tumours. Pathology and genetics of tumours of haematopoietic and lymphoid tissues. Lyon: IARC Press; 2008, with permission of the World Health Organization.)

Table 15.11 Causes of eosinophilia	
Parasites	Lung disease
Ascaris	Asthma
Hookworm	Allergic bronchopulmonary aspergillosis
Strongyloides	Churg–Strauss syndrome
Allergy	Skin disorders
Allergic rhinitis	Urticaria
Drug reactions	Pemphigus
Malignancy	Eczema
Hodgkin's disease	Others
Carcinoma	Sarcoidosis

Acute myeloid leukaemia (AML)

- Classified by cell type (Table 15.10)
- 70% alive at 1 year → 30% alive at 5 years
- Treatment aims for complete remission
- Followed by bone marrow ablation

Acute lymphoblastic leukaemia (ALL)

- Predominantly a disease of children
- Cure rate 50–60% in children, 30% in adults
- Central nervous system involvement common
- → Prophylactic intrathecal chemotherapy

Chronic leukaemias

- Chronic leukaemias occur in older patients, most of whom die within 5 years of diagnosis
- Clinical course consists of a chronic illness lasting 3–4 years, followed by transformation into an acute leukaemia or sometimes myelofibrosis in the case of chronic myeloid leukaemia

Chronic myeloid leukaemia (CML)

Clinical features
- Anaemia
- Night sweats and fever
- Weight loss
- Splenomegaly → pain

Investigations
- Blood count – raised white count
- Multiple myeloid precursors
- Bone marrow biopsy
- Genetic testing for the Philadelphia chromosome (9:22 translocation) (positive in 90–95%)

Management
- Imatinib – tyrosine kinase inhibitor – 95% response rates
- Myeloablation with bone marrow transplant

Chronic lymphocytic leukaemia (CLL)

Clinical features
- Often an incidental finding
- Infections due to neutropenia
- Anaemia (may be due to haemolysis)
- Lymphadenopathy
- Hepatosplenomegaly

Investigations
- Haemoglobin low or normal
- White count $>15 \times 10^9/L$
- 40% lymphocytes
- Platelets low or normal
- Serum immunoglobulins may be low

Management
- Nothing if asymptomatic
- Steroids for haemolysis
- Chemotherapy

Hairy cell leukaemia

- Rare
- Usually a B cell tumour
- Cells have filament-like projections
- Cladribine produces a 90% remission

Myeloproliferative disorders

- Uncontrolled proliferation of a blood cell line
- Can transform into acute leukaemias or from one myeloproliferation to another

Polycythaemia vera

- Red cell proliferation
- Patients usually >60 years old

Clinical features
- Tiredness
- Depression
- Tinnitus
- Vertigo
- Visual disturbance
- Itching after a hot bath
- Gout (due to increased cell turnover)
- Thrombosis or haemorrhage
- Plethora and cyanosis
- Splenomegaly

Investigations
- Haemoglobin raised
- Packed cell volume (haematocrit) ↑
- Acquired JAK2 genetic mutations in 95%
- 50% have ↑ platelets
- 75% have ↑ white cells
- Uric acid ↑
- Leucocyte alkaline phosphatase ↑

Management
- Venesection
- Chemotherapy
- Allopurinol to avoid gout, low dose aspirin for recurrent thrombosis

Prognosis
- 30% → myelofibrosis
- 5% → AML

Essential thrombocythaemia

- Platelet count >1000×10^9/L
- → Bruising and bleeding (poor platelet function)
- Increased risk of thrombosis

Myelofibrosis

- Stem cell proliferation
- Bone marrow fibrosis

Clinical features
- Anaemia
- Weight
- Splenomegaly
- Bone pain
- Gout

Investigations
- Anaemia
- High platelets
- 'Dry' bone marrow aspirate
- High uric acid

Management
- Blood transfusion
- Folic acid, allopurinol, analgesia
- Chemotherapy and radiotherapy
- Splenectomy may be required

Prognosis
- 10–20% → AML

Myelodysplasia

- Stem cell defects
- → Bone marrow failure
- Abnormal red cells, leucocytes and platelets

Management
- Supportive therapy
- Chemotherapy

Multiple myeloma and hyperglobulinaemia

- Clonal expansion of plasma cells resulting in very high production of a single immunoglobulin (paraprotein) or an immunoglobulin component

Myeloma

Clinical features
- Elderly patients
- Bone lesions → pain and fractures

- Hypercalcaemia
- Bone marrow infiltration
- → Anaemia, neutropenia
- Renal impairment
- Hyperviscosity syndrome (headache, stroke, retinal vein and artery occlusion)

Investigations

- Blood count (anaemia, low white cells)
- Elevated ESR and CRP
- Elevated calcium, urea and creatinine
- Protein electrophoresis – monoclonal band
- Skeletal X-ray survey – lytic lesions, e.g. skull (see Fig. 5.17)
- 24-hour urine for light chain proteins
- Bone marrow aspirate – plasma cells

Management

- Supportive treatment and treatment of complications, e.g. for fractures
- Steroids and radiotherapy for bone lesions
- Chemotherapy + stem cell transplantation

Waldenström's macroglobulinaemia

- Older males
- IgM paraprotein
- → Hyperviscosity syndrome
- Lymphadenopathy
- Malaise and weight loss

PLATELET DISORDERS

Platelets, derived from megakaryocytes, are involved in the formation of clots.

Thrombocytopenia

- Low platelet count
- Low production in bone marrow
- High destruction in circulation
- Causes (Table 15.12)

Autoimmune thrombocytopenic purpura

- Follows viral infection in children (acute)
- Idiopathic in adult women (chronic)
- 60% have antiplatelet antibodies
- → Purpuric rash
- Epistaxis and menorrhagia
- Treat with steroids/splenectomy

Thrombocytosis

- High platelet count
- Haemorrhage
- Inflammation (any site)
- Essential thrombocythaemia

Table 15.12 Causes of thrombocytopenia

Impaired production
  Selective megakaryocyte depression:
    Rare congenital defects
    Drugs, chemicals and viruses
  As part of a general bone marrow failure:
    Cytotoxic drugs and chemicals
    Radiation
    Megaloblastic anaemia
    Leukaemia
  Myelodysplastic syndromes
  Myeloma
  Myelofibrosis
  Solid tumour infiltration
  Aplastic anaemia
  HIV infection
Excessive destruction or increased consumption
  Immune
    Autoimmune – ITP
    Drug induced, e.g. GP IIb/IIIa inhibitors, penicillins, thiazides
    Secondary immune (SLE, CLL, viruses, drugs, e.g. heparin,
      bivalirudin)
    Alloimmune neonatal thrombocytopenia
    Post-transfusion purpura
  Disseminated intravascular coagulation
  Thrombotic thrombocytopenic purpura
Sequestration
  Splenomegaly
  Hypersplenism
Dilutional
  Massive transfusion

(Reproduced from Kumar P, Clark M. Kumar and Clark's Clinical Medicine, 8th edn. Edinburgh: Elsevier; 2012, with permission from Elsevier.)

SELF-ASSESSMENT QUESTIONS

Multiple choice questions (true or false)

1. Which of the following statements about haemoglobin are correct?
   A. Adult haemoglobin comprises two α and two γ chains
   B. Each haemoglobin molecule comprises four globin chains and one haem group
   C. Deoxyhaemoglobin is insoluble in water
   D. β-thalassaemia is an inherited inability to synthesize β globin chains
   E. Each haemoglobin molecule can carry four oxygen molecules
2. The following are true of vitamin B_{12} absorption:
   A. Active absorption requires the presence of intrinsic factor
   B. Intrinsic factor is produced by gastric G cells
   C. Active absorption takes place in the jejunum

    D. Chronic pancreatic insufficiency is a cause of vitamin B_{12} deficiency

    E. Oral B_{12} given once a month is useful in the treatment of pernicious anaemia

3. In autoimmune haemolytic anaemia:
   A. The direct Coombs' (globulin) test will be positive
   B. The autoantibody is always IgG class
   C. Haemoglobinuria may occur
   D. *Mycoplasma* pneumonia is a recognized cause
   E. Jaundice is a recognized symptom

4. Regarding pernicious anaemia:
   A. Anti-parietal cell or anti-intrinsic factor antibodies are detectable
   B. Chronic hyperplastic gastritis results
   C. There is an increased risk of gastric cancer
   D. Oral intrinsic factor will reverse the vitamin B_{12} deficiency
   E. Men are as commonly affected as women

5. The following are appropriate blood transfusion options:
   A. Group O donor to group A recipient
   B. Group A Rhesus-positive donor to group A Rhesus-negative recipient
   C. Group AB Rhesus-negative donor to group O Rhesus-negative recipient
   D. Group B Rhesus-positive donor to group A Rhesus-positive recipient
   E. Group A donor to group AB recipient

6. The following are recognized complications of blood transfusions:
   A. Urticarial rash
   B. Hepatitis C infection
   C. Fever
   D. Anaphylactic shock
   E. Disseminated intravascular coagulation

Multiple choice questions (single best answer)

7. A 36-year-old woman has the following full blood count: Hb 101 g/L, MCV 76 fl, MCH 24, WCC 9.4, platelets 187. Which one of the following is the most likely diagnosis?
   A. Megaloblastic anaemia
   B. Iron deficiency anaemia
   C. Aplastic anaemia
   D. Folate deficiency
   E. Polycythaemia rubra vera

8. A 25-year-old man presents with a fever, night sweats and abdominal pain. Which one of the following is the most likely diagnosis?
   A. Polycythaemia rubra vera
   B. Acute myeloid leukaemia
   C. Non-Hodgkin's lymphoma
   D. Chronic lymphocytic leukaemia
   E. Acute lymphoblastic leukaemia

9. A 78-year-old man is found to have a white cell count of 32×10^9/L, 95% lymphocytes. What is the most likely diagnosis?
   A. Chronic myeloid leukaemia
   B. Chronic lymphocytic leukaemia

C. Acute lymphoblastic leukaemia

D. Malignant myeloma

E. Myelodysplasia

10. Which one of the following is the best test for measuring the anticoagulant effect of warfarin?

   A. Activated partial thromboplastin time

   B. Bleeding time

   C. Prothrombin time

   D. Whole blood clotting time

   E. Thrombin time

Extended matching questions

Question 1

A. Iron deficiency

B. Vitamin B_{12} deficiency

C. Folic acid deficiency

D. Sickle cell disease

E. α-thalassaemia

F. Hereditary spherocytosis

G. Haemolytic anaemia

H. Anaemia of chronic disease

I. Acute haemorrhage

J. Hypersplenism

For each of the following select the most appropriate diagnosis from the list:

   I. A 43-year-old woman with a microcytic, hypochromic blood film

   II. A 17-year-old man with severe joint pain and abnormal red blood cells

   III. An 87-year-old woman with a macrocytosis following a gastrectomy

Question 2

A. Erythrocytes

B. Platelets

C. Monocytes

D. Neutrophils

E. Basophils

F. Eosinophils

G. Lymphocytes

H. Reticulocytes

I. Megakaryocytes

J. Plasma cells

For each of the following choose the correct answer from the list above:

   I. The cell type from which platelets derive

   II. Cell type responsible for antibody production

   III. A nucleated cell that increases in numbers after acute blood loss

Question 3

A. Blood group O

B. Blood Group A

C. Blood Group B

D. Blood Group AD

E. D-Rhesus positive

F. D-Rhesus negative

For each of the following choose the correct answer from the list above:

I. Blood group with a frequency of 8% in the population

II. Blood group characterized by the presence of anti-A and anti-B antibodies in the blood

III. Blood group of a mother whose fetus suffers Rhesus D syndrome

Oncology and genetic disease 16

Oncology studies the management of 'malignant disease' illness arising from the uncontrolled proliferation of a cell clone. The clone characteristically is able to invade adjacent tissues (local spread) and seed to distant sites via the vascular or lymphatic circulation (metastasis). Malignancy is an important cause of death worldwide, most notably in the developed world (Fig. 16.1). Specific malignancies are discussed in the appropriate system chapter.

CANCER EPIDEMIOLOGY

Sex differences (Table 16.1)

- Sex-specific tumours (e.g. prostate)
- Risk factors (e.g. smoking, diet, alcohol intake)
- Genetic variation
- Hormonal variation (tumours dependent on hormones for growth)

Age differences

Childhood cancers (age 3–13 years)
- Hereditary, e.g. retinoblastoma
- Haematological, e.g. acute leukaemia

Adult cancers
- Frequency increases with age

Geographical differences

- Variation in population genotype distribution
- Variation in environmental factors, e.g.
  - Diet in gastric cancer (Fig. 16.2)
  - Hepatocellular carcinoma secondary to chronic viral hepatitis

CANCER AETIOLOGY

Smoking

- Associated with 30% of cancer deaths in the UK
- Implicated in several cancers
  - Lung carcinoma
  - Oral cavity cancers
  - Oesophageal carcinoma
  - Bladder (transitional cell carcinoma)

Alcohol

- Oral cavity cancers
- Oesophageal carcinoma
- Colorectal carcinoma
- Hepatocellular carcinoma

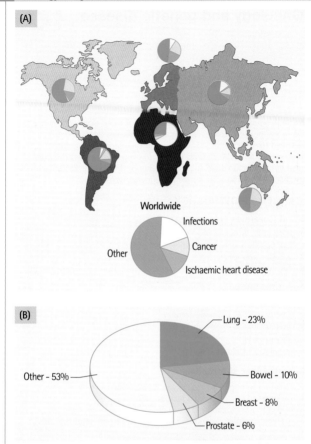

Fig. 16.1 (A) Causes of mortality by continent, demonstrating the relative importance of infection, malignancy and heart disease. Malignancy is responsible for roughly 13.5% of all male and 11.7% of all female deaths worldwide. (Data from the World Health Organization, 2008.) (B) CRC UK 2010 Cancer Mortality by tumour site.

Table 16.1 Age-standardized mortality for the 10 highest causes of malignancy-related death in the UK in 2000

Rank	Male		Female	
	Site	Mortality	Site	Mortality
1	Lung	48.6	Breast	26.8
2	Colon and rectum	18.7	Lung*	21.1
3	Prostate	18.5	Colon and rectum	13.8
4	Stomach	10.1	Ovarian	8.3
5	Oesophagus	8.7	Pancreas	5.3
6	Bladder	7.0	Stomach	4.8
7	Pancreas	6.6	Oesophagus	4.0
8	Lymphoma	5.8	Lymphoma	3.9
9	Leukaemia	4.9	Leukaemia	3.3
10	Brain	4.5	Brain	3.0

*Lung cancer is now more common tan breast cancer.
(Source: Ferlay J, Bray F, Pisani P et al. Globocan 2000, International Agency for Research on Cancer. Lyon: IARC Press; 2001.)

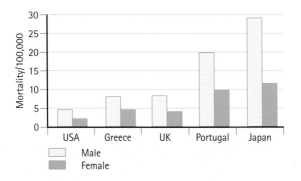

Fig. 16.2 Geographical variation in the mortality from gastric cancer. (Data from the World Health Organization, 1997.)

Environmental risks

Asbestos
- Mesothelioma
- Lung carcinoma

Hydrocarbons
- Lung carcinoma
- Skin cancers

UV light
- Melanoma
- Basal cell carcinoma
- Squamous cell carcinoma

Drugs

Oestrogens
- Vaginal carcinoma
- Endometrial carcinoma

Alkylating agents
- Acute myeloid leukaemia

Infections

- Viral hepatitis – hepatocellular carcinoma
- *Schistosoma* – bladder cancer
- *Helicobacter pylori* – gastric cancer
- Epstein–Barr virus – Burkitt's lymphoma
- Papillomavirus – cervical cancer

CANCER GENETICS

- Malignancy results from genetic mutations that lead to uncontrolled proliferation of a cell clone
- These mutations and abnormalities can arise in several ways

Chromosome abnormalities

- Chronic myeloid leukaemia – 9:22 translocation (Philadelphia chromosome) positive in 95%
- Acute promyelocytic leukaemia – 15:17 translocation positive in >90%
- Burkitt's lymphoma 8:14 translocation → *myc* gene over-expressed

Failure of DNA repair

- Mutation of DNA repair systems → hereditary cancer syndromes, e.g.
  - Xeroderma pigmentosum
  - Ataxia telangiectasia
  - *BCRA 1* and *2* in breast cancer
  - Mismatch repair mutations in colon cancer

Tumour suppressors

- Mutation of tumour suppressor genes → over-expression of mutated gene product
- Failure of control of cell cycle → uncontrolled proliferation
- e.g. *p53* mutations in GI cancers

Inherited cancers

- Specific mutations increase the risk of malignancy if inherited, e.g.
  - *apc* gene: familial adenomatous polyposis
  - *BCRA* genes: breast and ovarian cancer
  - *Rb* gene: hereditary retinoblastoma

Oncogenes

- Genes which, if activated inappropriately by a mutation, →
  malignancy, e.g.
  - *C-Myc*: cervical cancer, Burkitt's lymphoma, breast cancer
  - *K-Ras*: colorectal cancer
- The gene may have a cell cycle regulatory role
  - *bcl-2* expression → resistance of apoptosis → a proliferating clone
    that is open to further mutations → malignant transformation

CANCER BIOLOGY

Cell proliferation

- Uncontrolled proliferation
- Often loss of cell differentiation
- → Exponential growth curve
- 'Doubling time' describes the growth rate
- → Very variable between tumour types
- As tumour enlarges, growth may slow due to:
  - Limitation of blood supply
  - Local production of growth inhibitors

Local invasion

- Penetration of malignant cells into other tissues
- Associated with loss of intercellular adhesion
- Increased production of proteolytic enzymes

Lymphatic spread

- Tumours seed to locally draining lymph nodes

Dissemination (Table 16.2)

- Invasion into blood vessels or lymphatics
- Allows seeding of cells to distant sites
- Metastases → organs with a dense vasculature, e.g.
  - Liver
  - Lungs
  - Bone marrow
- Tumour cells express ligands for endothelial receptors
- → Increased adhesion and invasion
- → Specific metastatic patterns, e.g. breast cancer → long bones

DIAGNOSIS OF CANCER

Clinical features

- Specific combinations of symptoms and signs can suggest particular
  malignancies

Table 16.2 Common sites of metastasis

Site	Origin	Site	Origin
Bone	Breast	Liver	GI tract
	Bronchus		Breast
	Thyroid		Bronchus
	Prostate	Adrenal	Bronchus
	Kidney	Lung	Kidney
Intracerebral	Bronchus		Prostate
	Breast		Breast
	Stomach		Bone
	Prostate		GI tract
	Thyroid		Cervix
	Kidney		Ovary
			Testicular

- For example, painless jaundice and weight loss → pancreatic cancer, dysphagia → oesophageal carcinoma
- Personality change with complex focal neurology → intracerebral tumour
- Cough, haemoptysis and weight loss → bronchogenic carcinoma
- Characteristics of a palpable mass suggesting malignancy:
  - Fixed to deep tissues
  - Fixed to overlying skin
  - Hard/'craggy' texture
  - Overlying ulceration
  - Lymphadenopathy
- Family history of malignancy
  - Colorectal carcinoma
- Exposure to specific risks (see above)
- Associated diseases that increase risk
  - Hepatitis B or C (hepatocellular carcinoma)
  - Pernicious anaemia (gastric cancer)
  - Barrett's oesophagus (oesophageal carcinoma)
  - Asbestosis (bronchogenic carcinoma)

Imaging
- Can be highly suggestive of malignancy
- For example, chest X-ray in lung cancer

Tissue diagnosis
- Vital for confirmation of diagnosis and guiding treatment
- Tumour type
- Degree of differentiation (tumour grade)

Methods

- CT- or ultrasound-guided biopsy
- Endoscopic biopsy

T		Extent of primary tumour
N	N0	No involved lymph nodes
	N1–4	Lymph node groups involved
M	M0	No metastases
	M1	Metastases present

Table 16.3 The TNM system

- Laparoscopic/open surgical biopsy
- Fine needle aspiration (FNA) of subcutaneous mass

Tumour staging (Table 16.3)
- Assessment of distribution of tumour
- Classification varies with tumour
- Staging investigations required, e.g.
  - CT scanning
  - Lymph node sampling
  - PET
  - Laparoscopy

Tumour markers
- Serum markers for the presence of malignancy
- Useful in following response to treatment
- Can help demonstrate relapse post-therapy
- Rarely useful in initial diagnosis
- Examples:
  - Ca-125 – pancreatic/ovarian/GI cancer
  - Ca-19–9 – GI and pancreatic cancers
  - α-fetoprotein – hepatocellular carcinoma
  - β-human chorionic gonadotrophin (HCG) – choriocarcinomas, testicular carcinoma
  - Chorioembronic antigen (CEA) – colorectal carcinoma

Screening
- Investigations used to detect premalignant tissue or malignancy in those in whom cancer has not been diagnosed
- Examples:
  - Mammograms for breast cancer
  - Smears for cervical cancer
  - Faecal occult blood and colonoscopy for colorectal carcinoma

Surveillance
- Investigations to detect recurrence of malignancy following treatment for a previous cancer
- Examples:
  - Mammography after breast cancer
  - Prostate-specific antigen (PSA) for progression of prostatic cancer

TREATMENT OF MALIGNANCY

- Therapeutic efforts in oncology are aimed at:
  - Complete destruction of the tumour (curative therapy)
  - Reduction of the tumour mass in order to improve life expectancy
  - Reduction of symptoms of the cancer (palliative care)

Surgical resection

- May be curative (complete tumour removal)
- May be palliative (symptomatic relief but not curative)

Radiotherapy

- High-energy electromagnetic radiation
- Targeted at specific site
- Useful adjuvant therapy to reduce relapse rate as well as curative intent

Chemotherapy

- Drug therapy aimed at killing tumour cells
- Also kills normal cells
- Given in cycles to allow normal cells to recover

Antimetabolites

- Block cell metabolism
  - Folic acid antagonists: methotrexate
  - Nucleic acid analogues: 5-fluorouracil

Plant alkaloids

- Inhibit microtubule formation
- → Block cell replication
  - Vincristine

Taxanes

- Inhibit microtubule formation
- Useful in breast and ovarian cancers
  - Docetaxel

Cytotoxic antibiotics

- Block DNA replication
  - Doxorubicin

Platinum analogues

- Cross-link DNA strands
- → Block DNA replication
  - Cisplatin

Alkylating agents

- Block DNA synthesis
  - Cyclophosphamide

Endocrine therapy

- Hormonal manipulation of tumour cells that express hormone receptors on their surface
  - Tamoxifen – blocks oestrogen receptor

Biological therapy

- Use of immunologically active substances
  - e.g. α-interferon in melanoma/myeloma
- Targeted therapy, e.g. anti-TNFs

Adjuvant therapy

- Specific therapy after a primary therapy modality
- Used to treat undetected metastases
  - Breast and colon cancers

Neoadjuvant therapy

- Given before primary therapy to reduce the risk of metastasis

Myeloablation with stem cell support

- High-dose chemotherapy and radiotherapy
- Aims to kill all dividing cells
- Haemopoietic stem cells then given
- → Reverses resultant bone marrow failure
- Stem cells may be
  - Allogenic: from a matched donor
  - Autologous: taken from patient before therapy
- Collection of stem cells may be via
  - Bone marrow sampling
  - Peripheral blood sampling

COMPLICATIONS OF TREATMENT

Failure of therapy

- Incomplete surgical resection
- Tumour resistance to chemotherapy
- Failure of response to radiotherapy

Nausea and vomiting

- Common
- Treat with antiemetics (Fig. 16.3)
  - Metoclopramide
  - Domperidone
  - $5HT_3$ antagonists (ondansetron)

Hair loss

- Difficult to avoid, but regrows after therapy

Bone marrow suppression

- Dose-dependent effect of therapy

Neutropenia

- ↑ Bacteria, viral and fungal infection
- Treat with antibiotics
- Stem cell stimulating factors, e.g. GM-CSF

Thrombocytopenia

- → Bleeding
- Treat with platelet transfusion

Anaemia

- Treat with blood transfusion

Cardiotoxicity

- Dose-dependent effect of doxorubicin

Neurotoxicity

- Occurs with vincristine
- Must never be given intrathecally

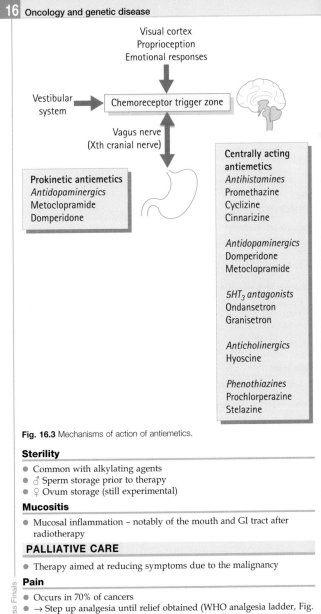

Fig. 16.3 Mechanisms of action of antiemetics.

Sterility

- Common with alkylating agents
- ♂ Sperm storage prior to therapy
- ♀ Ovum storage (still experimental)

Mucositis

- Mucosal inflammation – notably of the mouth and GI tract after radiotherapy

PALLIATIVE CARE

- Therapy aimed at reducing symptoms due to the malignancy

Pain

- Occurs in 70% of cancers
- → Step up analgesia until relief obtained (WHO analgesia ladder, Fig. 16.4)

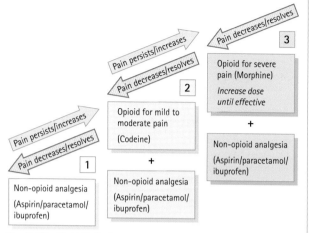

Fig. 16.4 The World Health Organization's Analgesia Ladder.

- Paracetamol and non-steroidal anti-inflammatory drugs (NSAIDs)
- Weak opioids – codeine ± paracetamol
- Strong opioids – morphine or diamorphine

Specific analgesics
- Naproxen for bone pain
- Amitriptyline/gabapentin for pain due to nerve damage
- Carbamazepine/gabapentin for neuropathic pain

Continuous subcutaneous infusions
- Allow continuous delivery of analgesia, antiemetics and sometimes anxiolytics

Patient-controlled analgesia
- Continuous analgesia with the ability for the patient to give limited extra doses

Complications of analgesics
Opioids
- Constipation, nausea, vomiting
- Respiratory and CNS depression
- Drowsiness, hallucinations
NSAIDs
- GI ulceration
- GI bleeding
- Renal failure

Non-drug approaches
- Surgery to reduce tumour mass
- Radiotherapy
- Nerve blocks
- Steroids to reduce local inflammation

Gastrointestinal symptoms

Anorexia
- → Nasogastric feeding if appropriate

Nausea and vomiting
- → Appropriate antiemetic therapy

Bowel obstruction
- → Surgical bypass
- Antispasmodics – hyoscine
- Antiemetics
- Nasogastric tube to reduce vomiting

Psychological support

- Effective communication with the patient
- Honesty about diagnosis and prognosis
- Support for emotional crisis
- Full explanations of symptoms
- Human genetics and inherited disease

HUMAN GENETICS

Chromosomal disorders

- Majority → spontaneous abortion

Abnormal chromosome numbers
- Down syndrome: trisomy 21, 1:650 live births
- Edward syndrome: trisomy 18, 1:3000
- Pataú syndrome: trisomy 13, 1:5000
- Klinefelter syndrome: XXY, 1:1000 males
- Turner syndrome: XO, 1:2500 girls

Abnormal chromosome structure
- Deletion of chromosome segment
  - Prader–Willi syndrome
- Duplication of chromosome segment
  - Charcot–Marie–Tooth syndrome

Mitochondrial DNA abnormalities
- Inherited mitochondrial DNA mutations
- Passed via maternal line (sperm do not donate mitochondria)
- → Myopathies and neuropathies
- e.g. DIDMOAD syndrome (diabetes insipidus, diabetes mellitus, optic atrophy and deafness)

Gene defects (Table 16.4)

- Result in abnormal protein being synthesized
- Homozygous: both gene copies abnormal
- Heterozygous: one gene copy abnormal

Autosomal dominant disorders (Fig. 16.5)

- One of the two gene copies is mutated
- Normal gene not sufficient to compensate
- Or mutated protein is toxic
- Effect may vary in each generation

Table 16.4 Autosomal dominant, autosomal recessive and X-linked recessive disorders

Autosomal dominant	Autosomal recessive	X-linked recessive
Achondroplasia	Albinism	Duchenne muscular
Adult polycystic kidney	Cystic fibrosis	dystrophy
disease	β-thalassaemia	Haemophilia A
Familial Alzheimer's	Friedreich's ataxia	Haemophilia B
disease	Haemochromatosis	Red–green colour
Familial	Phenylketonuria	blindness
hypercholesterolaemia	Sickle cell disease	Wiskott–Aldrich
Huntington's chorea	Wilson's disease	syndrome
Marfan syndrome		
Neurofibromatosis type I		
Von Willebrand's disease		

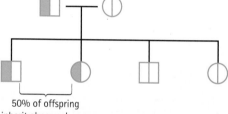

One parent with one copy of abnormal gene

50% of offspring
inherit abnormal gene

Fig. 16.5 Autosomal dominant inheritance.

- Varying penetrance
- → Disease skipping generations
- New cases arise due to germ-line mutations

Autosomal recessive disorders (Fig. 16.6)
- Both gene copies have mutation (homozygous)
- No functioning protein synthesized
- Carrier state exists if only one copy affected (usually no clinical significance)
- → Inborn errors of metabolism

Sex-linked inheritance
- Mutations of genes on the X chromosome
- Vast majority are recessive (Fig. 16.7) *but*
  - Males only have one X chromosome, therefore are affected by mutation
  - Females act as carriers if heterozygotes

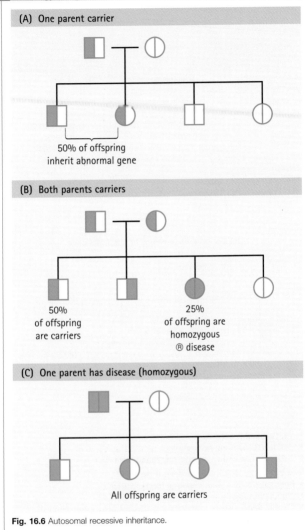

(A) One parent carrier

50% of offspring
inherit abnormal gene

(B) Both parents carriers

50%
of offspring
are carriers

25%
of offspring are
homozygous
® disease

(C) One parent has disease (homozygous)

All offspring are carriers

Fig. 16.6 Autosomal recessive inheritance.

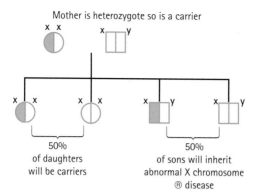

Mother is heterozygote so is a carrier

50%
of daughters
will be carriers

50%
of sons will inherit
abnormal X chromosome
℞ disease

Fig. 16.7 X-linked recessive inheritance.

X-linked dominant
● Heterozygote female has the disease
● Rare
● e.g. Vitamin D-resistant rickets

Trinucleotide repeats
● Multiple repeats of three nucleotides
● Severity of the disease α number of repeats
● Number of repeats increases with each generation
● Therefore severity increases with each generation = genetic
  anticipation
  • Myotonic dystrophy (CTG triplets)
  • Huntington's chorea (CAG triplets)

Genetic imprinting
● Disease phenotype varies
● Depends on origin of mutant gene
● e.g. Deletion of long arm of chromosome 15
  • If inherited from mother → Prader–Willi syndrome
  • If inherited from father → Angelman syndrome

Multifactorial inheritance
● Encoded for by multiple genetic loci (polygenic)
  • Height
  • Hair colour
  • Hypertension
  • Pyloric stenosis
  • Ankylosing spondilitis

Genetic screening and counselling

Provision of information to prospective parents who are carriers of an
inherited disease is vital for informed decisions to be made.
Determination of these risks is important and requires screening.

Screening

- Detection of carrier of a mutation, e.g.
  - Thalassaemia
  - Sickle cell disease
  - Tay–Sachs disease
  - Haemophilia
  - Cystic fibrosis

Prenatal diagnosis

Maternal serum

- Maternal α-fetoprotein – neural tube defects
- Bart's triple test on maternal serum assesses risk of fetal trisomy 21
  - α-fetoprotein (low)
  - β-human chorionic gonadotrophin (high)
  - Unconjugated oestriol (low)

Imaging

- Ultrasound for anatomical abnormalities
- Nuchal fold translucency for Down syndrome

Amniocentesis

- Sampling amniotic fluid for fetal cells
- α-fetoprotein and biochemical analysis
- Risk to fetus <1%

Chorionic villus sampling

- Chromosome/DNA analysis
- Risk to fetus 1–2%

Cordocentesis

- Fetal blood sampling
- Chromosome and DNA analysis
- Risk to fetus 1–2%

Counselling

- Risk of passing on genetic abnormality to child depends on inheritance and parental genome

SELF-ASSESSMENT QUESTIONS

Multiple choice questions (true or false)

1. Smoking has been associated with an increased risk of the following:
   - A. Bronchial cancer
   - B. Oesophageal cancer
   - C. Transitional cell carcinoma
   - D. Pharyngeal cancer
   - E. Breast cancer
2. Regarding malignancy:
   - A. A translocation between chromosomes 9 and 22 is seen in 10% of chronic myeloid leukaemia
   - B. *p53* mutations are common in gastrointestinal malignancy
   - C. *Helicobacter pylori* is associated with a decreased risk of gastric cancer
   - D. Kaposi's sarcoma is only seen in immunocompromised patients
   - E. Family history is important in determining the risk of breast cancer

3. The following are common sites of metastasis for the named primary cancer:
   A. Intracerebral: breast carcinoma
   B. Long bones: osteosarcoma
   C. Vertebral column: prostatic carcinoma
   D. Liver: bronchial carcinoma
   E. Liver: cutaneous basal cell carcinoma

4. The following are autosomal dominant:
   A. Haemophilia A
   B. Achondroplasia
   C. Haemochromatosis
   D. Red–green colour blindness
   E. Leprosy

5. The following genetic abnormalities result in the named condition:
   A. Trisomy 19 – Down syndrome
   B. XO – Turner syndrome
   C. XXY – Klinefelter syndrome
   D. Trisomy 21 – Pataú syndrome
   E. XXO – Smith syndrome

6. The following are inherited in an X-linked recessive manner:
   A. Down syndrome
   B. Polycystic kidney disease
   C. Wiskott–Aldrich syndrome
   D. Haemophilia A
   E. Acute intermittent porphyria

Multiple choice questions (single best answer)

7. Which one of the following is a $5HT_3$ antagonist antiemetic?
   A. Metoclopramide
   B. Cyclizine
   C. Granisetron
   D. Prochlorperazine
   E. Diazepam

8. A 55-year-old man presents with abdominal distension. He has a long history of chronic hepatitis C infection. Which one of the following is he at an increased risk of suffering?
   A. Pancreatic adenocarcinoma
   B. Cholangiocarcinoma
   C. Gallbladder carcinoma
   D. Hepatocellular carcinoma
   E. Gastric adenocarcinoma

9. A 29-year-old man requests information about his risk of colonic carcinoma. His father has just died of the disease at the age of 54. What is the man's risk of developing a colonic carcinoma?
   A. 1 in 250
   B. 1 in 100
   C. 1 in 50
   D. 1 in 20
   E. 1 in 3

10. A 45-year-old woman was seen with a palpable mass in her left breast. What is the most appropriate way of confirming the diagnosis?
   A. Bilateral mammography
   B. Ultrasound guided fine needle aspiration

    C. Breast lumpectomy
    D. Whole body PET scan
    E. Local lymph node excision

11. A 66-year-old man with a previous history of a bronchogenic carcinoma is admitted with confusion, nausea and diplopia. Which one of the following may provide most effective symptom control?
    A. Diazepam
    B. Metoclopramide
    C. Dexamethasone
    D. Odansetron
    E. Domperidone

12. In the treatment of malignancy:
    A. Surgery is always carried out with the aim of a cure
    B. Nausea is a rare side-effect of chemotherapy
    C. Combination chemotherapy is rarely more efficacious than single therapy
    D. Methotrexate is a folate metabolism antagonist
    E. Vincristine can be given intrathecally

EXAMINING THE NERVOUS SYSTEM

General rules

- Explain carefully to patients what you want them to do for each part of the examination and why
- Ask the patient to copy your actions, rather than trying to explain a complicated manoeuvre
- Always compare one side with the other
- Organize your examination into categories:
  - Mental state
  - Cranial nerves
  - Motor function
  - Reflexes
  - Coordination and gait
  - Sensation

Equipment

- Pen torch
- Snellen eye chart or pocket vision card
- Ophthalmoscope
- Tendon hammer
- 128 and 512 Hz tuning forks
- Cotton wool
- 'Neuropins'
- Orange stick

Abbreviated mental test score

Ten questions give an indication of cerebral function, including orientation in time, place, long- and short-term memory; mark correct responses out of 10.

- Name?
- Age?
- Address?
- Where are you now?
- Name of the monarch?
- Name of the prime minister?
- Dates of the Second World War? (or another major event – relevant to the age of the patient)
- Remember the following address and repeat it when asked: 42 West Street, Edinburgh (ask the patient to recall this after asking the rest of the questions)
- What time of day is it now?
- Count backwards from 20 to 10

Cranial nerves

General observations suggesting nerve palsies:

- Ptosis (III)
- Facial droop or asymmetry (VII)
- Hoarse voice (X)
- Articulation of words, dysarthria (V, VII, X, XII)
- Abnormal eye position (III, IV, VI)
- Abnormal or asymmetrical pupils (II, III)

I Olfactory

- Supplies: sense of smell
- Ask the patient about changes in or absence of sense of smell
  - Use things that are close at hand, e.g. coffee/soap

II Optic

- Supplies: visual fields/acuity/field of vision
- Examine the fundi for:
  - Papilloedema
  - Optic atrophy
  - Maculopathy
  - Hypertensive or diabetic retinopathy

Test visual acuity

- Allow the patient to use glasses
- Ask the patient to read a Snellen eye chart with each eye
- Record the smallest line the patient can read for each eye
- Visual acuity is reported as a pair of numbers (20/20), where the first number represents how far the patient is from the chart and the second number is the distance from which the 'normal' eye can read a line of letters. For example, 20/40 means that at 20 feet, the patient can only read letters a 'normal' person can read from twice that distance

Test visual fields

- Position yourself at eye level, 1 metre or so in front of the patient and ask him/her to look into your eyes
- Hold your hands out to the sides halfway between you and the patient and wiggle a finger on both hands asking the patient to indicate which side he/she sees the finger move; if the patient only sees one side this indicates a lateral field defect or sensory neglect on that side
- Test the four quadrants of each eye while asking the patient to cover the opposite eye comparing with your own fields of vision for the appropriate eye

Test pupillary reactions

- Ask the patient to look into the distance
- Shine a bright light obliquely into each pupil in turn
- Look for both the direct (same eye) and consensual (other eye) reactions
- Test accommodation
  - Hold your finger about 10 cm from the patient's nose
  - Ask him/her to look into the distance and then at your finger
  - Look for constriction of the pupil and convergence of the eyes to near vision

III Oculomotor (tested with IV and VI)

- Supplies: superior, medial and inferior rectus and inferior oblique muscles, pupillary muscles, eye)

- Look for ptosis
- Test extraocular movements
  - Holding your finger about 1 metre in front of the patient, ask him/her to follow your finger with the eyes without moving the head
  - Check horizontal, vertical and oblique gaze using a cross or 'H' pattern; ask about diplopia
  - Pause during upward and lateral gaze to check for nystagmus
- Test pupillary reactions to light

IV Trochlear (superior oblique muscle)

- Inward and downward movement of eyes (see above)

VI Abducens (lateral rectus muscle)

- Lateral eye movement (see above)

V Trigeminal

Motor

- Ask the patient to first open the mouth and then clench the teeth
- Palpate the temporal and masseter muscles as this is done

Sensory

- On both sides, use cotton wool to test
  - The forehead (olfactory division)
  - The cheeks (maxillary division)
  - The jaw (mandibular division)

Corneal reflex

- Ask the patient to look up and away
- From the other side, touch the cornea (not sclera) lightly with a fine wisp of cotton wool
- Look for the normal blink reaction of both eyes
- Repeat on the other side

VII Facial

- Observe for any facial droop or asymmetry
- Ask the patient to do the following, noting any weakness or asymmetry
  - Raise eyebrows
  - Close both eyes tightly
  - Smile or show the teeth
  - Puff out the cheeks
- Upper vs lower motor neurone injury
  - With an upper motor neurone lesion (stroke), crossover of innervation means function is preserved over the upper part of the face (forehead, eyebrows, eyelids)
  - With a lower motor neurone lesion (Bell's palsy), the entire side of the face is paralysed

VIII Vestibulocochlear

- Rub your fingers together next to one ear, while whispering a number in the other and ask the patient to tell you the number
- Repeat for the other side

Weber's test

- Use a 512 Hz tuning fork
- Place the base of the vibrating tuning fork firmly on top of the patient's head

- Ask the patient where the sound appears to be coming from (normally in the midline)
  - In sensorineural deafness there will be deafness in the affected ear
  - In conductive deafness, the sound will be heard better in the deaf ear

Rinne's test (to compare air and bone conduction)
- Use a 512 Hz tuning fork
- Place the base of the vibrating tuning fork against the mastoid bone behind the ear
- When the patient no longer hears the sound, hold the end of the fork near the patient's ear and ask if he or she can hear it now (air conduction is normally greater than bone conduction)
  - In conductive deafness bone conduction is better than air conduction

IX and X   Glossopharyngeal and vagus (tested together)
- Ask the patient to swallow a sip of water, look for choking or dribbling
- Ask patient to say 'Agh', watching the movements of the soft palate and the pharynx. The uvula deviates away from the affected side
- Test the gag reflex (unconscious patient)
  - Touch the back of the throat on the soft palate with an orange stick on each side
  - It is normal to gag after each stimulus

XI   Accessory
- From behind, look for wasting of the trapezius muscles
- Ask the patient to shrug the shoulders against resistance
- Ask the patient to turn the head against resistance. Watch and palpate the sternomastoid muscle on the opposite side

XII   Hypoglossal
- Look at the tongue for wasting or fasciculation (lower motor neurone lesion)
- Ask the patient to
  - Protrude the tongue
  - Move the tongue from side to side
- The tongue moves towards the side of any lesion

Motor function (corticospinal or pyramidal tracts)

Observation
- Involuntary movements (e.g. tremor, tics, fasciculation)
- Wasting and asymmetry (pay particular attention to the hands, and shoulder and thigh girdles)

Muscle tone
- Ask the patient to relax
- Holding the patient's hand, flex and extend his/her wrist and elbow
- Place both your hands on the thigh and gently roll the leg from side to side watching for corresponding movement of the foot
- There is normally a small, continuous resistance to passive movement
- Observe for decreased (flaccid) or increased (rigid/cogwheeling/spastic) tone

Power
Pronator drift
- This is a short screening test for muscle strength
- Ask the patient to hold both arms straight out in front, palms up and eyes closed
- With an upper motor neurone lesion, the patient will not be able to maintain extension and supination (and 'drifts' into pronation and flexion)

Muscle strength
- Test strength by asking the patient to move against your resistance
- Always compare one side to the other

Other tests of power
- Flexion (C5, C6, biceps) and extension (C6, C7, C8, triceps) at the elbow
- Extension at the wrist (C6, C7, C8, radial nerve)
- Squeeze two of your fingers as hard as possible ('grip', C7, C8, T1)
- Finger abduction (C8, T1, ulnar nerve)
- Opposition of the thumb (C8, T1, median nerve)
- Flexion (L2, L3, L4, iliopsoas) and extension at the hip (S1, gluteus maximus)
- Adduction (L2, L3, L4, adductors) and abduction at the hips (L4, L5, S1, gluteus medius and minimus)
- Extension (L2, L3, L4, quadriceps) and flexion (L4, L5, S1, S2, hamstrings) at the knee
- Dorsiflexion (L4, L5) and plantar flexion (S1) at the ankle
- Grade strength on a scale from 0 to 5 (Table 17.1)

Tendon reflexes
- Use a tendon hammer with as little force as needed to provoke a response
- Reinforcement
  - If the reflexes are not elicited as above then ask the patient to clench the teeth or grasp the hands together and then pull apart
  - Retest reflexes as this task is performed
- Reflexes should be graded on a 0 to 4 'plus' scale (Table 17.2)

Biceps (C5, C6)
- Position the patient with the arms relaxed across the lap and partially flexed at the elbow with the palm down
- Place your thumb or finger on the biceps tendon

Table 17.1 Muscle strength grading scale	
Grade	**Description**
0/5	No muscle movement
1/5	Visible muscle movement, but no movement at the joint
2/5	Movement at the joint, but not against gravity
3/5	Movement against gravity, but not against added resistance
4/5	Movement against resistance, but less than normal
5/5	Normal strength

Table 17.2 Tendon reflex grading scale

Grade	Description
0	Absent
1+ or +	Hypoactive
2+ or + +	'Normal'
3+ or + + +	Hyperactive without clonus
4+ or + + + +	Hyperactive with clonus

- Tap your finger with the reflex hammer
- Watch for flexion of the elbow

Triceps (C6, C7)
- Hold the patient's hand across the chest
- Tap the triceps tendon above the elbow with the reflex hammer
- Watch for extension of the elbow

Brachioradialis (C5, C6)
- Rest the forearm on the abdomen or lap
- Tap the radius about 3–5 cm above the wrist
- Watch for flexion and supination of the forearm

Knee (L2, L3, L4)
- Hold your arm under the patient's flexed knees, taking the weight of the legs on your forearm
- Tap the patellar tendon just below the patella
- Note contraction of the quadriceps and extension of the knee

Ankle (S1, S2)
- Dorsiflex the foot at the ankle with your hand, with the knee slightly bent and the leg rotated laterally
- Tap the Achilles tendon
- Watch and feel for plantar flexion at the ankle

Clonus
- Support the knee in a partly flexed position
- With the patient relaxed, quickly pull the foot into dorsiflexion
- Observe for sustained rhythmic beats of dorsiflexion

Plantar response (Babinski)
- Run a key or orange stick firmly along the lateral aspect of the sole of each foot
- Flexion of the big toe is normal
- Extension of the big toe with fanning of the other toes is abnormal and indicates an upper motor neurone lesion

Coordination and gait (cerebellospinal connections)

Coordination

Rapid alternating movements (dys-diadochokinesis)
- Ask the patient to tap the back of one hand with, alternately, the palmar and dorsal aspects of the other hand as accurately and quickly as possible

Point-to-point movements (finger–nose and heel–shin)
- Ask the patient to touch your index finger and his/her nose alternately several times. Move your finger about slowly as the

patient performs this task. Holding your finger still, ask the patient to touch his/her nose and then your finger with the eyes closed. Repeat for the other side

● Ask the patient to place one heel on the opposite knee and run it down the shin to the big toe and back again. Repeat with the patient's eyes closed

● Look for past-pointing, intention tremor and clumsiness

Romberg's test (cerebellar connections and dorsal columns)

● Ask the patient to stand with the feet together and eyes closed for 5–10 seconds without support (be prepared to catch the patient if unstable)

● The test is positive if the patient becomes unstable (indicating a vestibular or proprioceptive problem)

Gait

● Ask the patient to walk across the room, turn and come back and then walk heel-to-toe in a straight line

Sensation

General

● Compare symmetrical areas on the two sides of the body and distal and proximal areas of the extremities

● When you detect an area of sensory loss map out its boundaries in detail

● Test the following areas
  ● Shoulders (C4)
  ● Inner and outer aspects of the forearms (C6 and T1)
  ● Thumbs and little fingers (C6 and C8)
  ● Front of both thighs (L2)
  ● Medial and lateral aspect of both calves (L4 and L5)
  ● Little toes (S1)

Light touch (dorsal columns)

● Use a piece of cotton wool to touch the skin lightly

● Touch rather than brush the skin

● Ask the patient to respond whenever a touch is felt

Pain (spinothalamic tracts)

● Use a suitable sharp object (e.g. Neuropin) to test 'sharp' or 'dull' sensation

Temperature (spinothalamic tracts)

● This can be left out if pain sensation is normal

● Use a tuning fork heated or cooled by water and ask the patient to identify 'hot' or 'cold'

Vibration (dorsal columns)

● Use a low-pitched tuning fork (128 Hz)

● Place the stem of the fork over the radial head or medial malleolus, and ask the patient to tell you if he/she feels the vibration

Position sense (dorsal columns)

● Hold the patient's big toe away from the other toes with your fingers on each side of the toe

● Show the patient 'up' and 'down'

● Ask the patient to close the eyes and to identify the direction in which you move the toe

● Test the fingers in a similar fashion

Dermatomes See Figure 17.1.

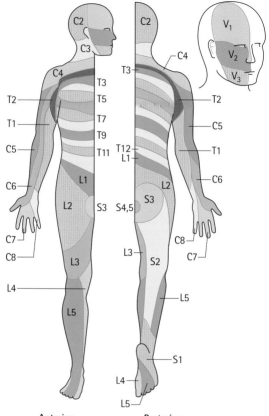

Fig. 17.1 Dermatomes of spinal roots and ophthalmic (V_1), maxillary (V_2) and mandibular (V_3) divisions of the trigeminal nerve.

NEUROLOGICAL INVESTIGATIONS

Routine investigations

See Table 17.3.

Neuroradiology

Skull X-ray
- Skull fracture
- Paget's disease
- Myeloma
- Intracranial calcification
- Intrasellar tumour

Table 17.3 Abnormalities in routine investigations and possible causes

Test	Result	Potential cause/effect
Urinalysis	Glycosuria	Diabetes → Polyneuropathy
	Bence Jones protein	Myeloma → Cord compression
Blood count	Macrocytosis	Vitamin B_{12} deficiency Chronic liver disease Hypothyroidism
ESR	Elevated	Vasculitis
Serum electrolytes	Hypokalaemia	Muscle weakness
	Hyponatraemia	Confusion/coma Central pontine demyelinolysis
Serum calcium	Hypocalcaemia	Tetany/spasms
Serum creatine phosphokinase (CPK)	Raised	Myositis
Chest X-ray	Tumour	Cerebral metastases Osmotic demyelination syndrome
	COPD	CO_2 retention
Thyroid function	Hypothyroidism	Confusion/dementia
Vitamin B_{12}	Low	Polyneuropathy Confusion/dementia Subacute combined degeneration of the cord

Pituitary fossa X-ray
- Enlargement with pituitary tumours

Spinal X-rays
- Fractures/vertebral collapse
- Metastases
- Spondylosis
- Tuberculosis

Computed tomography (CT)

Brain
- Cerebral tumours
- Intracranial haemorrhage
- Infarction
- Subarachnoid haemorrhage
- Midline shift (mass effect)
- Hydrocephalus

- Cerebral atrophy
- Pituitary lesions

Spine
- Cord/bone lesions

Magnetic resonance imaging (MRI)

- Greater resolution than CT for small lesions and does not require contrast injection
- No radiation
- High differentiation of white and grey matter
- Contraindicated in patients with metal implants, e.g. aneurysm clips
- Nerve root compression
- Spinal cord lesions
- Blood vessel imaging without contrast

Cerebral angiography (seldom used)

- Intra-arterial or intravenous contrast is injected to demonstrate arterial or venous systems, e.g. berry aneurysms, arteriovenous malformations

Positron electron tomography (PET)

- Maps function of specific areas of brain
- Based on metabolic activity

Electroencephalography (EEG)

- Records electrical brain activity from scalp electrodes on 16 channels
- Used in:
  - Epilepsy (spikes or spike and wave abnormalities)
  - Diffuse brain disorders (slow waves, e.g. hepatic encephalopathy)

Electromyelography (EMG)

- Demonstrates abnormal muscle innervation and myopathies

Nerve conduction studies

- Neuropathies
- Differentiate axonal and demyelinating pathologies

Visual evoked potentials (VEP)

- Record time for visual stimulus to reach the visual cortex
- Document previous retrobulbar neuritis

Lumbar puncture (LP) and cerebrospinal fluid (CSF) examination

Indications for lumbar puncture
- Diagnosis of meningitis or encephalitis
- Intrathecal injection of contrast or drugs
- Diagnosis of subarachnoid haemorrhage
- Measurement of CSF pressure (Table 17.4)
- Therapeutic removal of CSF
- Detection of CSF abnormalities, e.g. oligoclonal bands in MS
- Cytology

Table 17.4 Normal CSF

Appearance	Protein
Crystal clear, colourless	0.2–0.4 g/L
Pressure	Glucose
60–150 mmH$_2$O	$\frac{2}{3}$–$\frac{1}{2}$ blood glucose level
Cell count	Microbiology
5/mm^3	Sterile
No polymorphs	
No red blood cells	

Contraindications for lumbar puncture
- Raised intracranial pressure
- Suspected intracranial or spinal cord mass lesion
- *Note*: Unconscious patients and those with papilloedema *must* have a CT scan to exclude raised intracranial pressure or mass lesion before LP
- Platelet count <40×10^9/L
- Abnormal coagulation

Brain biopsy

- Inflammatory and degenerative brain diseases
- CT-guided sampling of mass lesions

UNCONSCIOUSNESS AND COMA

- Coma is a state of unrousable unresponsiveness (Box 17.1)
- Consciousness is graded using the Glasgow Coma Scale (GCS, Table 17.5)

Aetiology of coma (Table 17.6)
- Diffuse brain dysfunction
- Brainstem lesion → damage of the lenticular activating system
- Brainstem compression/displacement through foramen magnum

EPILEPSY

- A continuing tendency to suffer epileptic seizures, a seizure being a convulsion or transient abnormal event resulting from paroxysmal discharge of cerebral neurones (Box 17.2)

Prevalence
- 2% of the population has two or more seizures
- 0.5% have ongoing seizures

Classification
- By clinical pattern of seizures (Table 17.7)
Generalized
- Absence (petit mal)
- Myoclonic
- Tonic-clonic (grand mal)
- Tonic
- Akinetic

BOX 17.1. Coma

- Check A B C D E (Airways, Breathing, Circulation, Disability, Exposure)
- Immobilize cervical spine if head or spinal injury suspected
- Look for warning cards/bracelets, etc., e.g. diabetics, epileptics

Examination
- Glasgow Coma Score
- Rectal temperature
- Smell breath for alcohol/ketones
- Blood pressure/pulse
- Pupils
  - Bilateral fixed dilated – brainstem death, barbiturates, hypothermia
  - Single fixed dilated – coning
  - Pinpoint – pontine lesions, opiates
- Fundi for papilloedema
- Eye movements
  - Doll's head reflex
  - Fixed lateral gaze
- Lateralizing signs
  - Facial drooping
  - Muscle tone
  - Plantar responses
  - Tendon reflexes

Investigations
- Drug screen (urine or blood)
- Serum biochemistry and glucose
- Arterial blood gases
- Thyroid function tests
- Blood cultures
- ECG
- CT scan or MRI of brain
- LP and CSF examination (only after raised intracranial pressure excluded)
- EEG
- Serum cortisol

Immediate management
- Careful observation to detect changes in vital functions or depth of coma
- Protect airway
- Ventilate if necessary

Longer-term management
- Skin care
- Pressure area care
- Oral hygiene
- Nutrition (nasogastric feeding or percutaneous endoscopic gastrostomy tube)
- Eye care
- Urinary catheter only if essential

Table 17.5 Glasgow Coma Scale

Eye opening (E)		Verbal function (V)	
Spontaneous	4	Orientated	5
To speech	3	Confused conversation	4
To pain	2	Inappropriate words	3
None	1	Incomprehensible sounds	2
		None	1
Motor function (M)			
Obeys commands	6		
Localizes to pain	5		
Withdraws	4		
Flexion	3		
Extension	2		
None	1		

Table 17.6 Causes of diffuse brain dysfunction

Drug overdose, alcohol	Adrenal failure
Hypoglycaemia	Hyponatraemia
Hyperglycaemia	Hypernatraemia
Hypoxia	Metabolic acidosis
Hypertensive encephalopathy	Hypothermia, hyperpyrexia
Uraemia	Epilepsy
Hepatic encephalopathy	Encephalitis
CO_2 retention	Head injury
Hypothyroidism	Subarachnoid haemorrhage

BOX 17.2. Status epilepticus

Definition
- Seizures which follow each other without recovery of consciousness

Management
- Nurse the patient in an area with full ventilatory support available if required and with cardiac monitoring facilities
- Give oxygen and monitor pulse, O_2 saturation and BP
- Exclude hypoglycaemia
- Diazepam 10–20 mg i.v. at a rate of 2.5 mg/30 seconds until fitting stops (up to a maximum of 40 mg); beware of respiratory depression
- Loading dose of i.v. phenytoin, 15 mg/kg at a rate 50 mg/minute
- Maintenance phenytoin i.v. or oral depending on patient's ability to take it
- If status continues unresponsive to treatment for more than 90 minutes, the patient needs to be anaesthetized with thiopental or propofol and ventilated

---

Table 17.7 Clinical pattern of epileptic seizures

Generalized tonic-clonic seizures
    Warning – vague
    Tonic phase – body becomes rigid before patient falls (often with a cry), biting the tongue and with urinary incontinence
    Clonic phase – a generalized convulsion with rhythmic jerking of muscles and frothing at the mouth
    Recovery – patient is drowsy or confused, or in a coma for several hours (post-ictal)
Absence seizures
    Patient becomes still and staring and looks pale
    Eyelids may twitch
    Attack lasts a few seconds usually, during which the patient is unresponsive
    No recollection of the event
Partial (focal) seizures
    Aura, e.g. strange smell, tingling in a limb
    Motor (Jacksonian)
    Jerking movements begin at the angle of the mouth or in the hand, spreading to involve the limbs on the side opposite from the epileptic focus
    Patient remains conscious
    Paralysis of the affected limbs may follow for several hours (Todd's paralysis)
    Temporal lobe epilepsy
    May be simple or complex
    Feeling of unreality, often déjà-vu, associated with absence attacks, vertigo or visual hallucinations

Partial
- Simple (e.g. Jacksonian, no impairment of consciousness)
- Complex (impairment of consciousness)

Aetiology
- <30% have a clear underlying cause
- <2% Genetic
- Developmental abnormalities
- 2% Trauma
- Hypoxia
- Surgery (10% of neurosurgical operations)
- Pyrexia (in children, febrile convulsions)
- 3% Intracranial mass
- 15% Infarction (post stroke)
- 6% Alcohol/drug withdrawal
- Encephalitis
- Metabolic abnormalities, e.g. hyponatraemia, hypoglycaemia

Investigations
- EEG (abnormal during seizures, often normal in between)
- CT scan/MRI scan

- Serum biochemistry
- Chest X-ray

Management
During seizure
- Maintain airway and physical safety
- Rectal or i.v. diazepam 5–10 mg if seizure does not stop spontaneously
Prophylactic
- For recurrent seizures
- First-line drugs
  - Sodium valproate
  - Carbamazepine
  - Ethosuximide (petit mal)
- Second-line drugs
  - Phenytoin
  - Clobazam

Toxic drug effects
All drugs
- Ataxia
- Nystagmus
- Dysarthria
Phenytoin
- Gum hypertrophy
- Hypertrichosis
- Osteomalacia
- Folate deficiency
- Polyneuropathy

Driving
- It is illegal to drive if any form of seizure or unexplained loss of consciousness has occurred during the past year
- In the UK, it is essential that a doctor informs patients of the driving regulations; it is then the patient's responsibility to inform the licensing authority

Pseudoseizures
- Often difficult to diagnose
- Prolactin normal (raises following a 'true' seizure)

Other causes of drop attacks, blackouts and episodes of disturbed consciousness

- Diagnosis can usually be determined from the history
- A witness account of an episode is especially valuable

Aetiology
- Syncope, e.g. simple, micturition, hyperventilation
- Transient ischaemic attack
- Panic attack
- Cardiac arrhythmia, e.g. Stokes–Adams attack
- Aortic stenosis
- Hypoglycaemia
- Vertigo

MOVEMENT DISORDERS

Parkinson's disease

- Combination of tremor, rigidity and akinesia
- Gradual development over years

Prevalence
- Increases with age
- 1:200 over 70 years of age
- Less prevalent in smokers

Aetiology
- Idiopathic
- Drug-induced, e.g. phenothiazines
- MPTP (methylphenyltetrapyridine, impurity in illegally synthesized opiates)
- Encephalitis lethargica

Pathology
- Cell degeneration in the substantia nigra
- Loss of dopamine in the extrapyramidal nuclei

Clinical features
- Tremor: 4–7 Hz resting tremor (pill-rolling)
- Micrographia
- Rigidity: increased tone throughout the range of movement
- Cogwheel rigidity (stuttering rigid tone combined with tremor)
- Bradykinesia: poverty of movement
- Falls
- Mask-like facies
- Reduced blinking
- Stooping, shuffling gait (festinant)
- Poor arm swinging
- Monotonous speech, slurring dysarthria
- Normal power
- Brisk reflexes
- Downgoing plantars
- Cognitive function initially preserved; late dementia sometimes occurs

Investigations
- No diagnostic test; diagnosis made on clinical grounds

Management
- Levodopa plus dopa decarboxylase inhibitor, e.g. Sinemet or Madopar; start gradually increasing the dose until adequate response or limiting side-effects (see below)
- Dopaminergic agonists, e.g. bromocriptine/pergolide
- Entacapone – catechol-O-methyl transferase inhibitor
- Selegiline – monoamine oxidase B inhibitor
- Neurosurgery (occasionally for intractable tremor)
- Physiotherapy
- Physical aids

Side-effects of levodopa
Short term
- Nausea and vomiting
- Confusion

- Visual hallucinations
- Chorea

Long term

- End-of-dose dyskinesia – On–off syndrome
- Chorea
- Dystonic movements

Prognosis

- Variable
- Usually worsens over 10–15 years with death from bronchopneumonia

Benign essential tremor

- Common, often autosomal dominant
- Upper limbs, head or trunk
- Alcohol/β-blockers may improve tremor

Huntington's disease

- Autosomal dominant progressive chorea and dementia in middle life
- Mutation of Huntingtin gene (Ch. 4)
- Genetic anticipation: earlier onset with each generation

Prevalence

- 5:100 000

Pathology

- Cerebral atrophy
- Loss of neurones in caudate nucleus and putamen
- Depletion of γ-aminobutyric (GABA), angiotensin-converting enzyme (ACE) and met-enkephalin in substantia nigra
- High somatostatin levels

Clinical features

- Chorea (sudden involuntary jerky semi-purposeful movements, flitting from one part of the body to another)
- Progressive dementia

Investigations

- MRI or CT shows atrophy of caudate nucleus

Management

- Phenothiazines may reduce chorea

Prognosis

- Death 10–20 years after onset

Screening

- Mutation analysis is available for presymptomatic screening in families but no effective treatment is known to alter disease progression

Other causes of chorea

- Sydenham's chorea (rheumatic fever)
- Drugs, e.g. phenytoin
- Thyrotoxicosis
- Stroke
- Systemic lupus erythematosus (SLE)

MULTIPLE SCLEROSIS

- Multiple plaques of demyelination in the brain and spinal cord disseminated in time and place
- Clinical diagnosis: two neurological events separated in time and neurological location

Prevalence
- Increases moving north from the Equator
- 60–100/100 000 in the UK

Aetiology
- 31% concordance among monozygotic twins
- HLA haplotype A3, B7, D2 and DR2 is more common
- Immigrants from law to high risk areas acquire the higher risk

Environmental
- ?Viral infection
- ?Dietary antigens

Pathology
- Plaques of demyelination particularly in
  - Optic nerves
  - Periventricular region
  - Brainstem and cerebellar connections
  - Cervical spinal cord
  - Corticospinal tracts
  - Posterior columns

Clinical patterns
- 80% Acute relapses/remitting
- 20% Chronic progressive

Optic neuropathy/neuritis

Clinical features
- Blurred vision in one eye
- Mild ocular pain
- Recovery within 1–2 months
- Optic disc swelling (optic neuritis)
- Normal disc (retrobulbar neuritis)
- Optic atrophy
- Relative afferent pupillary defect (dilatation of the affected eye when light is transferred from the good eye to the affected eye)

Brainstem demyelination

Clinical features
- Double vision
- Vertigo
- Facial numbness
- Weakness
- Dysphagia
- Pyramidal tract signs
- Nystagmus
- Ataxia
- Cranial nerve defects
- Internuclear ophthalmoplegia

Spinal cord lesion

Clinical features

- Difficulty walking
- Sensory abnormalities
- Electric shock-like pains radiating down trunk and limbs caused by neck flexion (Lhermitte's sign)
- Urinary symptoms (incontinence, retention)
- Spastic paraparesis
- Increased tone
- Weakness
- Brisk reflexes
- Up-going plantars
- Sensory level

Other presentations of MS

- Epilepsy
- Trigeminal neuralgia
- Tonic spasms of a hand
- Organic psychosis
- Dementia

Investigations

Imaging

- MRI brain and spinal cord (visualizes multiple plaques)

CSF

- Oligoclonal bands in 80%
- Raised mononuclear cell count 5–60 cells/mm^3

Visual evoked responses

- Delayed following optic neuropathy

Management

- There is no cure but newer drugs can modify course
- Corticosteroids – i.v. methylprednisolone or ACTH may speed recovery in acute relapses
- β-interferon/glatiramer – reduces relapse rate but not long-term outcome. Oral fingolimod and teriflunomide and mono-clonal antibodies are being used.
- Physiotherapy
- Occupational therapy
  - Walking aids
  - Wheelchairs
  - Car/house conversions
- Speech therapy
- Counselling

Prognosis

- Unpredictable course ranging from grave disability to mild and benign

INFECTIONS AND INFLAMMATORY CONDITIONS OF THE NERVOUS SYSTEM

Meningitis

Aetiology

See Table 17.8.

Table 17.8 Causes of meningitis

Bacteria	Fungi
Neisseria meningitides	*Cryptococcus neoformans*
Streptococcus pneumoniae	*Candida*
Staphylococcus aureus	Chronic inflammatory conditions
Listeria monocytogenes	Sarcoidosis
Haemophilus influenzae	Behçet's disease
Mycobacterium tuberculosis	Syphilis
Treponema pallidum	Malignancy
Viruses	Blood
Enterovirus	Following subarachnoid
Echovirus	haemorrhage
Coxsackie virus	
Herpes simplex	
HIV	
Epstein–Barr virus (EBV)	

Table 17.9 Antibiotics in meningitis

Suspected organism	Antibiotic
Unknown	Cefotaxime
Meningococcus	Benzylpenicillin
	Cefotaxime
Pneumococcus	Cefotaxime
TB	Rifampicin

Clinical features
- Headache
- Neck stiffness
- Fever
- Photophobia
- Vomiting
- Rigors
- Positive Kernig's sign (worsening pain on knee extension when hip extended)
- Petechial/purpuric rash (meningococcal septicaemia)
- Drowsiness/focal signs (suggest complication, e.g. raised intracranial pressure/abscess)

Management
- **Immediate treatment is vital – do not wait for tests**
- Immediate parenteral antibiotics (Table 17.9)
- Further treatment depends on results of blood or CSF culture and sensitivities
- Viral meningitis requires no specific treatment
- i.v. steroids with first dose of antibiotics in adults with pneumococcal meningitis

Investigations
- CT of brain to exclude raised intracranial pressure
- Lumbar puncture (Table 17.10)

Table 17.10 CSF findings in meningitis

	Appearance	Mononuclear cells (per mm³)	Polymorphs (per mm³)	Protein (g/L)	Glucose (% blood glucose)
Normal	Crystal clear	5	Nil	0.2–0.4	>50
Viral	Clear/turbid	10–100	Nil	0.4–0.8	>50
Pyogenic	Turbid/purulent	<50	200–300	0.5–2	<50
TB	Turbid/viscous	100–300	0–200	0.5–3	<30

- Blood cultures
- Blood glucose
- Chest X-ray
- Skull X-ray (if trauma)
- Throat swab for *Neisseria meningitidis*

Prophylaxis
- Meningococcus is notifiable
- Family and very close contacts should be treated with ciprofloxacin or rifampicin to eradicate carriage
- Meningococcal vaccine to close contacts

Tuberculous meningitis

- More chronic course
- Difficult to diagnose
- May demonstrate multiple cranial nerve palsies
- Meningeal enhancement on MRI

Acute viral encephalitis

Aetiology
- Herpes simplex
- Echovirus
- Coxsackie virus
- Mumps
- EBV
- Adenovirus
- Varicella zoster
- Influenza
- Measles
- Rabies

Clinical features
- Often mild and self-limiting
- HSV-1 infection may be more serious
- Headache
- Fever
- Mood change
- Drowsiness
- Seizures

- Focal signs
- Coma

Investigations
- CT scan (may show diffuse oedema)
- EEG (characteristic slow wave changes in HSV)
- CSF (increased mononuclear cells, slightly raised protein)

Management
- i.v. aciclovir for suspected HSV-1

Prognosis
- 20% mortality in serious cases, with many others suffering long-term severe brain damage

Herpes zoster (shingles)

- Recrudescence of varicella zoster virus infection within a dorsal root ganglion

Clinical features
- Typical blistering rash and pain affecting dermatome supplied by the affected nerve root

Trigeminal nerve (ophthalmic division)
- Rash affects the eye and may cause corneal scarring

Facial nerve (Ramsay Hunt syndrome)
- Facial palsy
- Vesicles on ear lobe, external auditory meatus and fauces

Treatment
- Aciclovir

Complications
- Post-herpetic neuralgia

Neurosyphilis

Meningovascular syphilis

Tabes dorsalis
- Subacute meningitis with cranial nerve palsies or paraparesis
- Demyelination of dorsal roots
- Charcot's joints (neuropathic)
- Ataxia
- Stamping gait
- Widespread sensory loss
- Argyll Robertson pupils (small irregular pupil, fixed to light, constricts to accommodation)
- Ptosis
- Optic atrophy

Generalized paralysis of the insane (GPI)
- Dementia
- Weakness
- Tremor
- Brisk reflexes
- Extensor plantars
- Argyll Robertson pupils

Taboparesis
- Congenital neurosyphilis
- Features of tabes dorsalis and GPI in childhood

Management
- Parenteral penicillin for 2–3 weeks

Sporadic Creutzfeldt–Jakob disease (CJD)

Aetiology
- Prion disease (proteinaceous infectious particle)
- Can be passed on from surgical specimens, autopsy material (e.g. corneal grafts) and human pituitary hormones

Pathology
- Spongiform changes in brain

Clinical features
- Slowly progressive dementia develops after age 50

Variant CJD

- First noted in Britain in 1995

Aetiology
- Prion disease
- Linked to ingestion of meat from cattle infected with bovine spongiform encephalopathy (BSE)

Clinical features
- Younger patients
- Early neuropsychiatric symptoms
- Ataxia
- Dementia
- Myoclonus
- Chorea
- Death

Brain abscess

- A focal area of bacterial infection causing an expanding mass lesion in the cerebrum or cerebellum

Aetiology
- *Streptococcus milieri*
- *Bacteroides* spp
- *Staphylococcus* spp
- Fungi
- Parameningeal infection, e.g. ear, nose, paranasal sinuses
- Skull fracture
- Distant infection, e.g. pneumonia, infective endocarditis
- Immunosuppression, e.g. HIV infection

Clinical features
- Headache
- Fever
- Focal signs
- Seizures
- Vomiting
- Drowsiness
- Papilloedema

Investigations
- Imaging (mass lesion on CT or MRI ± hydrocephalus)
- Blood cultures

- Raised ESR
- Raised white cell count
- Look for a local/distant focus of infection
- Lumbar puncture is contraindicated

Management
- Parenteral antibiotics
- Surgical decompression

Prognosis
- Mortality 25%
- Persistent epilepsy common in survivors

INTRACRANIAL TUMOURS (TABLE 17.11)

- Primary intracranial tumours account for about 10% of all neoplasms

Clinical features
- Direct mass effect on function, e.g. hemiparesis
- Raised intracranial pressure (Table 17.12)
- Seizures

Investigations
- CT or MRI scanning
- Brain biopsy

Table 17.11 Intracranial tumours	
Type	**Prevalence (%)**

Metastases
  Bronchus
  Breast
  Stomach
  Prostate
  Thyroid
  Kidney
  Lymphoma (associated with AIDS)
	50

Primary malignant
  Astrocytoma
  Oligodendroglioma
  Lymphoma
  Medulloblastoma
	35

Benign
  Meningioma
  Neurofibroma
	15

Table 17.12 Symptoms and signs of raised intracranial pressure	
Headache	Bradycardia
Vomiting	Decerebrate posturing (coning)
Papilloedema	False localizing signs
Impaired consciousness	VI nerve lesion
Respiratory depression	III nerve lesion

Management
- Reduce cerebral oedema using corticosteroids and/or i.v. mannitol
- Anticonvulsants
- Surgery
- Radiotherapy

Prognosis
- 50% survival at 2 years for high-grade malignant tumours

HYDROCEPHALUS

- Excessive CSF volume
  - Obstruction to CSF outflow
  - Increased CSF production
- Treated by ventriculo-peritoneal shunting or neurosurgical relief of obstruction

HEADACHE AND MIGRAINE

Tension headache

- The vast majority of chronic and recurrent headaches

Clinical features
- Throbbing headache
- Tight band sensation
- Pressure behind eyes

Management
- Avoid precipitating causes
- Simple analgesia (however recurrent analgesic use can induce cyclical headache)

Migraine

- Recurrent headaches associated with visual and gastrointestinal disturbance
- 12% of population report symptoms

Pathology
- Vasodilatation and oedema of blood vessels
- Release of vasoactive substances

Classical migraine

Clinical features
- Prodrome
  - Teichopsia (flashes)
  - Jagged lines
  - Unilateral patchy scotoma
  - Lasts 15 minutes to 1 hour
- Headache hemicranial or generalized
- Nausea and vomiting
- Generally irritable
- Preference for the dark
- Sleeping

Other patterns
- Migraine without aura
- Hemiplegic migraine

Differential diagnosis
- Subarachnoid haemorrhage
- Transient ischaemic attack
- Partial seizures

Management
- Avoid precipitating features

During attack
- Paracetamol
- Antiemetics
- Sumatriptan (5HT$_1$ agonist)
- Ergotamine

Prophylaxis
- Pizotifen, methysergide (5HT antagonists)
- Propranolol
- Amitriptyline (low-dose)

Cluster headaches

- Affect adults in third and fourth decades
- ♂ > ♀

Clinical features
- Recurrent bouts of excruciating pain centred around one eye
- Wakes patient at night
- Vomiting
- Watering and congestion of affected eye
- Transient ipsilateral Horner syndrome

Management
- Usually unhelpful
- Oxygen/sumatriptan during attack
- No analgesia effective for headache
- Verapamil/lithium for prophylaxis

Other causes of headache

- Subarachnoid haemorrhage
- Meningitis
- Sinusitis
- Brain tumours
- Temporal arteritis (see Ch. 7)
- Benign intracranial hypertension
- Head injury

CEREBROVASCULAR DISEASE AND STROKE (TABLE 17.13)

- Stroke is the third commonest cause of death in the UK
- A stroke is a focal neurological deficit due to a vascular lesion lasting >24 hours (if the patient survives)
- A transient ischaemic attack (TIA) is a brief episode of neurological dysfunction due to temporary ischaemia without infarction. NB The arbitrary time of 24hr is not longer used.

Risk factors
- Hypertension
- Smoking
- High alcohol intake
- Lack of regular exercise

Table 17.13 Types of cerebrovascular disease
Thromboembolic infarction
Cerebral and cerebellar haemorrhages
Dissection of carotid or vertebral arteries
Subarachnoid haemorrhage
Subdural and extradural haemorrhage
Cortical venous and dural sinus thrombosis

- Family history
- Hyperlipidaemia
- Afro-Caribbean race
- High-dose oral contraceptive pill

Transient ischaemic attacks

Clinical features
- Focal deficit depends on part of brain affected
- Usually due to microemboli

Carotid system
- Amaurosis fugax
  - Visual loss
- Aphasia (dominant side)
- Hemiparesis
- Hemianopic visual loss

Vertebrobasilar system
- Diplopia
- Vertigo
- Vomiting
- Dysarthria, choking
- Ataxia
- Transient global amnesia

Evidence of source of embolus
- Atrial fibrillation
- Carotid bruit
- Valvular heart disease
- Subclavian artery stenosis

Investigations
- Rapid investigation to identify reversible risks
  - Carotid Dopplers
  - Echocardiogram
  - CT scanning
- Immediate therapy to reduce acute and long-term risk
  - Anti-platelet drugs: aspirin/clopidogrel
  - Statins (irrespective of serum cholesterol)
  - Management of hypertension
- Carotid endarterectomy

Cerebral infarction

Clinical features
- Focal deficit depends on part of brain affected (see below)
- Initially flaccid areflexic weakness followed by spastic tone, brisk reflexes and extensor plantars
- See Figure 17.2 for arterial supply to the cerebral cortex

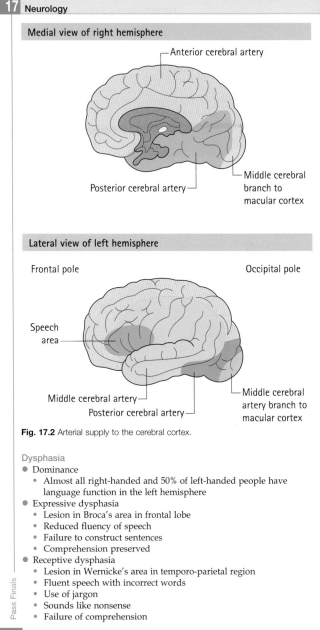

Medial view of right hemisphere

Anterior cerebral artery

Middle cerebral branch to macular cortex

Posterior cerebral artery

Lateral view of left hemisphere

Frontal pole

Occipital pole

Speech area

Middle cerebral artery

Posterior cerebral artery

Middle cerebral artery branch to macular cortex

Fig. 17.2 Arterial supply to the cerebral cortex.

Dysphasia
- Dominance
  - Almost all right-handed and 50% of left-handed people have language function in the left hemisphere
- Expressive dysphasia
  - Lesion in Broca's area in frontal lobe
  - Reduced fluency of speech
  - Failure to construct sentences
  - Comprehension preserved
- Receptive dysphasia
  - Lesion in Wernicke's area in temporo-parietal region
  - Fluent speech with incorrect words
  - Use of jargon
  - Sounds like nonsense
  - Failure of comprehension

Middle cerebral/internal carotid artery (internal capsule stroke);
posterior inferior cerebellar artery (brainstem stroke)

- Hemiparesis (limbs and face)
- Aphasia (dominant side)
- Hemianopic visual loss
- Dysarthria
- Coma, altered consciousness
- Vertigo
- Vomiting
- Dysphagia, choking
- Ataxia
- Contralateral loss of pain on face

Important parts of examination of patients with cerebrovascular disease

- Neurological signs
- Source of embolus (e.g. carotid bruit, atrial fibrillation)
- Blood pressure (in both arms)
- Optic fundi (hypertensive retinopathy, papilloedema)

Investigations
- CT/MRI imaging of brain (see Ch. 5)
  - Demonstrates site
  - Distinguishes between infarct or haemorrhage
- Carotid Doppler scanning
- Magnetic resonance angiography (for possible surgery)
- Blood count
- ESR
- Blood glucose, lipids
- Syphilis serology
- Chest X-ray
- ECG
- Echocardiogram

Management
- Assessment by a regional stroke team
- Thrombolysis in acute stroke (effective if given within 3 hours of onset)
- Aspirin 300 mg initially then 75 mg/day or other antiplatelet therapy
- Identify and treat risk factors where possible
- Antihypertensive therapy
- Anticoagulation (for atrial fibrillation)
- Surgery (internal carotid endarterectomy)

Rehabilitation
- Physiotherapy
- Speech therapy
- Occupational therapy
- Enteral nutrition if unsafe swallow (e.g. percutaneous endoscopic gastrostomy)

Prognosis
- 30–40% survival at 3 years (among initial survivors)
- 10% chance of further stroke within a year

Intracerebral haemorrhage

- Accounts for 10% of strokes

Aetiology
- Rupture of microaneurysms

Risk factors
- Hypertension

Clinical features
- Difficult to distinguish between haemorrhage and infarction
- Haemorrhage may be accompanied by headache and coma

Investigations
- CT head (see Fig. 5.40)

Management
- As for infarction, except avoid antiplatelet and anticoagulant drugs

Prognosis
- 70% death within 2 years

Subarachnoid haemorrhage

- Spontaneous arterial bleeding into subarachnoid space

Prevalence
- 6:100 000/year
- Accounts for 5% of strokes

Aetiology
- Saccular 'berry' aneurysms (70%)
- Arteriovenous malformation (AVM) (10%)
- No lesion (20%)

Clinical features
- Sudden onset of severe occipital headache
- Vomiting
- Loss of consciousness
- Neck stiffness
- Positive Kernig's sign
- Papilloedema and retinal haemorrhages

Investigations
- CT scan
- Lumbar puncture (if CT undiagnostic) – red cells and/or xanthochromia in CSF
- CT/MR angiography

Management
Immediate
- Bed rest
- Treat hypertension
- Dexamethasone
- Nimodipine

Later
- Neurosurgical aneurysm clipping or coil insertion

Prognosis
- 50% mortality at presentation
- 10–20% more die in early weeks

Chronic subdural haematoma

- Accumulation of blood in subdural space following rupture of a vein after head injury (sometimes trivial)

Clinical features
- May be delayed
- Headache
- Drowsiness
- Confusion
- Focal deficits

Management
- Often conservative
- Usually resolve spontaneously without surgical drainage

DEGENERATIVE DISORDERS

Motor neurone disease

- Progressive degeneration of lower motor neurones and upper motor neurones of the cortex, cranial nerve nuclei and spinal cord

Incidence
- 2:100 000 per year
- Slight male predominance

Clinical patterns
- Progressive muscular atrophy – progressive weakness and wasting of arm and hand muscles
- Amyotrophic lateral sclerosis – progressive spastic tetraparesis or paraparesis with wasting and fasciculation
- Progressive bulbar palsy – degeneration of lower cranial nerve nuclei

Clinical features
- Muscle wasting
- Fasciculation
- Reflexes absent or exaggerated
- Dysarthria
- Dysphagia
- Nasal regurgitation of fluids
- Choking
- Bulbar and pseudobulbar palsy (see p. 455)
- Ocular movements are not affected
- Cerebellar or extrapyramidal signs do not occur
- Dementia is unusual
- Sphincter function is usually preserved
- No sensory signs

Investigations
- Diagnosis made on clinical grounds
- EMG – denervation of muscles with preserved motor conduction velocity

Prognosis
Relentlessly progressive course
- Death within 3 years

Management

- Riluzole (sodium channel blocker, inhibits glutamate release) slows progress
- No treatment affects outcome

Friedreich's ataxia

- Progressive degeneration of dorsal root ganglia, spinocerebellar tracts and corticospinal tracts

Aetiology
- Abnormal gene for frataxin (unknown function)
- Autosomal recessive

Clinical features
- Difficulty walking from about 12 years of age
- Ataxia of gait and trunk
- Nystagmus
- Dysarthria
- Absent reflexes in legs
- Optic atrophy
- Pes cavus
- Cardiomyopathy

NEUROPATHY

- A pathological process affecting peripheral nerves

Pathology
- Demyelination
- Axonal degeneration
- Wallerian degeneration (after nerve section)
- Compression
- Infarction
- Infiltration

Mononeuropathies

- Caused by peripheral nerve compression

Carpal tunnel syndrome

- Median nerve compression in carpal tunnel (at wrist)

Aetiology
- Idiopathic
- Hypothyroidism
- Diabetes mellitus
- Pregnancy
- Rheumatoid arthritis
- Obesity
- Acromegaly

Clinical features
- Tingling in fingers (especially at night)
- Weakness of thenar muscles
- Wasting of thenar eminence
- Weakness of abductor pollicis brevis (raising thumb away from palm)
- Weakness of opposition of thumb and little finger

- Tinel's sign (reproduction of tingling by tapping over carpal tunnel)
- Sensory loss of palm and radial three and a half fingers

Management
- Splint wrist
- Surgical decompression

Ulnar nerve compression

- Usually occurs after trauma at elbow

Clinical features
- Wasting and weakness of interossei and hypothenar muscles
- Sensory loss in the ulnar one and a half fingers

Radial nerve compression ('Saturday night palsy')

- Occurs after nerve is compressed against humerus when arm is draped over a hard chair for several hours

Clinical features
- Wrist drop
- Weakness of finger extension

Mononeuritis multiplex

- Multiple mononeuropathies

Aetiology
- Diabetes mellitus
- Leprosy
- Vasculitis
- Sarcoidosis
- Amyloidosis
- Malignancy
- Neurofibromatosis
- HIV infection

Polyneuropathies

Guillain–Barré syndrome
- Acute inflammatory post-infective polyneuropathy
- Follows 1–3 weeks after infection (often trivial, or *Campylobacter* infection)

Incidence
- 3/100 000 per year

Clinical features
- Weakness of distal limb muscles ± numbness
- Weakness ascends over days for up to 3 weeks
- Can affect respiratory and facial muscles in 30%
  Variants
- Autonomic neuropathy
- Miller–Fisher syndrome (affecting ocular muscles with ataxia)

Investigations
- Diagnosis is made on clinical grounds
- Nerve conduction studies (demyelinating neuropathy)
- CSF (cell count normal, protein raised 1–3 g/L)

Management
- Measurement of respiratory function (arterial blood gases, vital capacity, FEV_1)

Table 17.14 Other polyneuropathies	
Metabolic	Thalidomide
Diabetes mellitus	Vincristine
Uraemia	Cisplatin
Porphyria	Vitamin deficiencies
Amyloidosis	Thiamin (B₁)
Toxic	Pyridoxine (B₆)
Alcohol	Vitamin B₁₂
Drugs	Nicotinic acid
Phenytoin	Non-metastatic manifestation of
Isoniazid	malignancy
Metronidazole	

- Assisted ventilation if necessary
- High-dose i.v. γ-globulin
- Plasmapheresis
- Subcutaneous heparin for prevention of thromboembolism

Prognosis
- Spontaneous gradual recovery
- 15% disability or death

Other polyneuropathies

See Table 17.14

Thiamin deficiency (Wernicke–Korsakoff syndrome)
Clinical features
- Ocular signs
  - Nystagmus
  - Bilateral rectal palsies
  - Fixed pupils
- Ataxia
- Confusion (amnestic syndrome, with loss of short-term memory)

Investigations Reduced red cell transketolase
Management
- Parenteral thiamine

Vitamin B₁₂ deficiency (subacute combined degeneration of the cord)

Aetiology
See p. 371, Table 15.3.
Clinical features
- Distal sensory loss
  - Light touch
  - Vibration sense
  - Joint position sense
- Absent ankle jerks
- Extensor plantars
- Optic atrophy
- Dementia

Investigations
- Reduced serum B$_{12}$
- Macrocytosis
- Megaloblastic bone marrow

Management
- Parenteral B$_{12}$

Peroneal muscular atrophy (Charcot–Marie–Tooth disease)

- Inherited sensorimotor neuropathy
- Several types: autosomal dominant and recessive

Clinical features
- Distal limb wasting and weakness
- Inverted 'champagne bottle' legs
- Pes cavus
- Clawing of toes
- Loss of sensation
- Loss of reflexes

Autonomic neuropathy

Aetiology
- Diabetes mellitus
- Guillain–Barré syndrome
- Amyloidosis

Clinical features
- Postural hypotension
- Retention of urine
- Erectile dysfunction
- Diarrhoea
- Diminished sweating
- Cardiac arrhythmias

MUSCLE DISEASE

Aetiology
See Table 17.15.

Myasthenia gravis

- Disorder of the neuromuscular junction

Table 17.15 Causes of myopathies	
Type	**Example**
Inflammatory	Polymyositis
Metabolic	Cushing syndrome
Myasthenic	Myasthenia gravis
Hereditary	Duchenne muscular dystrophy
Myotonias	Myotonic dystrophy
Channelopathies	Periodic paralysis

Prevalence

- 4:100 000
- ♀ > ♂ (2:1)
- Age of onset about 30 years

Aetiopathogenesis

- Unknown aetiology
- IgG antibodies to acetylcholine receptor
- Immune complex deposits on postsynaptic membrane
- Destruction of acetylcholine receptor
- Thymic hyperplasia in 70%
- Associated with
  - Thyroid disease
  - Rheumatoid arthritis
  - Pernicious anaemia
  - SLE

Clinical features

- Weakness and fatigability of muscles
  - Proximal limb
  - Extraocular
  - Speech
  - Facial expression
  - Mastication
- Ptosis
- Reflexes preserved but fatigable

Investigations

- Serum acetylcholine receptor antibodies (positive in 90%)
- Mediastinal imaging for thymoma (chest X-ray, CT, MRI)

Management

- Oral anticholinesterases, e.g. pyridostigmine
- Thymectomy (improves prognosis)
- Corticosteroids
- Azathioprine
- Plasmapheresis

Lambert–Eaton myasthenic-myopathic syndrome

- Non-metastatic manifestation of small cell carcinoma of the bronchus due to defective acetylcholine release at the neuromuscular junction

Clinical features

- Muscle weakness and absent reflexes which improve with contraction

Myotonic dystrophia

- Autosomal dominant inheritance

Clinical features

- Cataracts
- Frontal baldness
- Ptosis
- Facial weakness
- Progressive distal muscle weakness
- Mild intellectual impairment

- Cardiomyopathy
- Hypogonadism
- Glucose intolerance

CRANIAL NERVE DEFECTS

See Table 17.16.

Specific cranial nerve and brainstem defects

Optic pathway
See Figure 17.3.

Bell's palsy
- Common acute, isolated facial nerve palsy
Aetiology
- Viral infection (often herpes simplex) causes swelling of nerve within petrous temporal bone
Clinical features
- Unilateral lower motor neurone facial weakness and droop
- Loss of taste on anterior two-thirds of tongue
Investigations
- Diagnosis made on clinical grounds
Management
- Prednisolone 60 mg reducing to zero over 10 days plus aciclovir
- Closure of eyelid to protect cornea
Prognosis
- Spontaneous improvement begins during second week
- Recovery takes up to 12 months
- Less than 10% have residual severe weakness

Bulbar palsy
- LMN weakness of cranial nerve nuclei within medulla (IX, X, XI, XII)
Aetiology
- Motor neurone disease
- Syringobulbia
- Poliomyelitis
- Myasthenia gravis
Clinical features
- Weakness of elevation of palate
- Loss of gag reflex
- Paralysed vocal cords
- Dysphagia
- Nasal regurgitation of fluids
- Choking

Pseudobulbar palsy
- Bilateral upper motor neurone lesion of lower cranial nerve nuclei
Aetiology
- Motor neurone disease
- Multiple sclerosis
- Multi-infarct dementia
- Severe head injury
Clinical features
- Stiff, slow, spastic tongue (not wasted)
- Dysarthria

Table 17.16	Cranial nerve defects	
Nerve	**Causes**	**Features**
I	Head injury	Loss of smell (anosmia)
II	Optic neuritis Optic nerve compression Visual pathway lesion	See MS Tunnel vision (if at chiasma) See Figure 17.3
III	Coning Aneurysm of posterior inferior carotid artery Diabetes	Ptosis Eye points down and out Fixed dilated pupil
IV	Rare	Diplopia looking away and down
V	Brainstem lesion Acoustic neuroma Cavernous sinus thrombosis	Sensory loss (face and tongue) Loss of corneal reflex Deviation of jaw towards lesion
VI	MS Glioma Raised intracranial pressure	Convergent squint Diplopia looking towards lesion

VII	Upper motor neurone lesion
	  (infarction)
	Lower motor neurone lesion
	  (Bell's palsy, Ramsay
	  Hunt syndrome, parotid
	  gland disease)
		Lower facial muscle weakness
		
		Upper and lower facial
		  weakness + Loss of taste
		  on anterior two-thirds of
		  tongue

VIII	Acoustic neuroma Meningitis Head injury Drugs – gentamicin	Sensorineural deafness Vertigo Nystagmus
IX and X	Brainstem infarct Motor neurone disease Carcinoma of nasopharynx	Weakness of elevation of pharynx Loss of gag reflex Hoarseness Dysphagia Bulbar or pseudobulbar palsy
XI	Syringobulbia Motor neurone disease Carcinoma of nasopharynx	Weakness of sternomastoid and trapezius

XII	Brainstem infarct
	
	Motor neurone disease
	
	Carcinoma of nasopharynx
		LMN lesion; unilateral wasting,
		  weakness and fasciculation
		  of tongue
		UMN lesion; stiff, spastic
		  tongue

(A)

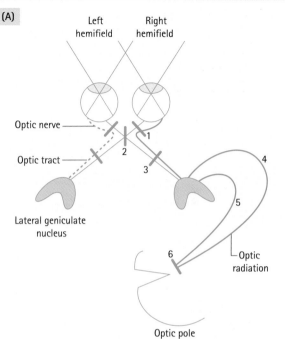

Fig. 17.3 Lesions of the visual pathway. (a) Optic nerve tracts and lesions.

Continued

- Dry gravelly voice
- Preserved gag reflex
- Exaggerated jaw jerk
- Emotional lability

Horner syndrome
- Lesion of the cervical sympathetic pathway

Aetiology
- Brainstem stroke
- Coning
- Syringomyelia
- Apical lung cancer (Pancoast's tumour)
- Cervical rib
- Brachial plexus trauma

Clinical features
- Ptosis
- Myosis (constricted pupil)
- Enophthalmos
- Loss of sweating on side of face

(B)

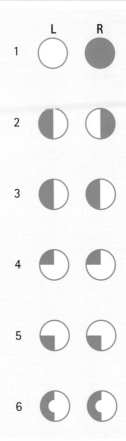

Fig. 17.3—cont'd (b) Visual field defects caused by lesions in the optic pathway. Lesion 1: This is analogous to losing an eye. One eye is completely blacked out. Lesion 2: Here only inputs from the nasal retinas are cut, so peripheral vision is lost on both sides. This can be caused by a pituitary tumour. (The pituitary lies just under the optic chiasm.) Lesion 3: Homonymous hemianopia: loss of the left hemifield. Both eyes are blind to anything on the left side of the world (assuming the eyes are pointed straight ahead). Lesion 4: The lower optic radiations are carrying information from the upper visual world so vision is lost in the upper quadrants of the left hemifield. Lesion 5: Here the parietal portion of the optic radiations are cut, so the lower visual world is affected on one side. Lesion 6: When the cortex itself is lesioned, vision at the fovea is spared, perhaps because there is such a large representation of the fovea in the cortex, or perhaps due to overlapping blood supply. The loss of vision is not a complete hemifield, then, but a notched hemifield. This is called macular sparing.

Table 17.17 Causes of spinal cord compression	
Within the cord	Outside the cord
Spinal cord neoplasms	Vertebral neoplasms
Transverse myelitis	(metastases, myeloma)
In the meninges	Disc lesions
Epidural abscess	Vertebral collapse
Epidural haemorrhage	
Ependymoma	
Meningioma	

SPINAL CORD DISEASE

Spinal cord compression

Aetiology
See Table 17.17.

Clinical features
- Radicular pain
- Spastic paraparesis or tetraparesis
- Sensory loss to level of compression
- Sphincter disturbance (retention of urine and incontinence)

Investigations
- Plain spinal X-rays
- Chest X-ray
- MRI
- Myelography

Management
- Surgical decompression if possible

Syringomyelia and syringobulbia

- A fluid-filled cavity (syrinx) within the cervical spinal cord (syringomyelia) or extending up into the brainstem (syringobulbia)

Aetiology
- Arnold–Chiari malformation
- Spina bifida
- Hydrocephalus
- Intrinsic cord tumours

Pathology
- The expanding cavity within the cord destroys spinothalamic neurones, anterior horn cells, lateral corticospinal tracts, sympathetic trunk, trigeminal, IX, X XI and XII nuclei

Clinical features
- Loss of pain and temperature sensation in upper limbs
- Painless burns
- Trophic changes
- Normal light touch sensation
- Loss of upper limb reflexes
- Wasting of small muscles of hands
- Spastic paraparesis

- Neuropathic joints
- Brainstem signs, e.g. bulbar palsy, Horner syndrome

Investigations
- MRI

Management
- No effective treatment or surgery

SELF-ASSESSMENT QUESTIONS

Multiple choice questions (single best answer)

1. In epilepsy:
   A. Generalized convulsions are characterized by maintenance of consciousness
   B. Absence seizures are generalized
   C. Absence seizures are commonest in adults
   D. Temporal lobe seizures may affect the myocardium
   E. Todd's paralysis follows temporal lobe seizure
2. In epilepsy:
   A. The EEG is usually diagnostic between fits
   B. All generalized seizures should be treated immediately with intravenous diazepam
   C. It is the doctor's responsibility to inform the driving authorities when a patient is diagnosed with epilepsy
   D. Ataxia usually signifies drug toxicity
   E. Phenytoin causes alopecia
3. Which of the following statements is true in Parkinson's disease?
   A. Smoking predisposes to Parkinson's disease
   B. Males are more commonly affected
   C. There is dopamine loss in the pyramidal nuclei
   D. Incidence is 1:200 over 70 years of age
   E. It may be caused by alcohol abuse
4. Common features of Parkinson's disease:
   A. Intention tremor
   B. Cogwheel rigidity
   C. Dementia
   D. Characteristic findings on CT brain scan
   E. Extensor plantar reflexes
5. Which of the following is true about Huntington's disease?
   A. It is inherited in an X-linked recessive manner
   B. It is caused by a mutation on chromosome 5
   C. It is associated with rheumatic fever
   D. It is characterized by involuntary movements
   E. It is associated with a higher than average IQ
6. The following are features of multiple sclerosis:
   A. It may cause afferent pupillary defect
   B. There is no concordance between monozygotic twins
   C. The pathology is characterized by neurofibrillary tangles
   D. Invariably leads to severe disability
   E. Is associated with recent *Campylobacter* infection
7. The following are features of motor neurone disease:
   A. Muscle hypertrophy
   B. Ophthalmoplegia

C. Frontal balding
D. Cerebellar ataxia
E. Bulbar palsy

8. Causes of mononeuritis multiplex include:
   A. Diabetes mellitus
   B. Sarcoidosis
   C. Vitamin B_{12} deficiency
   D. HIV infection
   E. All of the above

9. A 45-year-old man was seen with pain and numbness in his hands and feet. On examination there was sensory loss to touch in a glove and stocking distribution and wasting of the thigh muscles with reduced power. What is the most likely diagnosis?
   A. Acute intermittent porphyria
   B. Thalidomide therapy
   C. Thyrotoxicosis
   D. Chronic alcohol misuse
   E. Motor neurone disease

10. Which of the following is a characteristic of autonomic neuropathy?
    A. Hypertension
    B. Erectile dysfunction
    C. Polydipsia
    D. Diarrhoea
    E. Infertility

11. The following statements about cerebrospinal fluid (CSF) are correct:
    A. It normally contains 5–10 red cells
    B. In bacterial meningitis the lymphocyte count is raised
    C. In viral meningitis glucose is lower than one-third of blood glucose
    D. In subarachnoid haemorrhage, xanthochromia occurs after 18 hours
    E. In Guillain–Barré syndrome protein is normal with a raised cell count

12. Which of the following statements about CNS infections is true:
    A. Herpes zoster causes a symmetrical rash
    B. Prion diseases are transferred by droplet spread
    C. Acute viral encephalitis is commonly caused by rotavirus
    D. Meningococcal septicaemia causes a vesicular rash
    E. Tuberculous meningitis is associated with high CSF protein

13. The following statements about Creutzfeldt–Jakob disease (CJD) are true:
    A. It is caused by a herpes virus infection
    B. It can be acquired during prosthetic heart valve replacement
    C. New variant CJD is more common in vegetarians
    D. It causes spongiform changes in the brain
    E. It is treatable with antiretroviral drugs

14. The following are aetiologically linked with brain abscess:
    A. Glue ear
    B. Lumbar puncture
    C. Nasal bone fracture
    D. Bacterial meningitis
    E. Diabetes insipidus

15. The following are symptoms and signs of raised intracranial pressure:
    A. Headache
    B. Tachycardia
    C. Papilloedema
    D. Non-dominant hemiplegia
    E. Pronator drift

16. Which is the most important risk factor for cerebrovascular disease:
    A. Diabetes mellitus
    B. Hypertension
    C. Asian race
    D. Family history
    E. Hypothyroidism

17. Aetiological factors in transient ischaemic attacks include:
    A. Atrial fibrillation
    B. Deep venous thrombosis
    C. Aortic sclerosis
    D. Warfarin therapy
    E. Polycystic kidney disease

18. Chronic subdural haematoma:
    A. Is due to arteriovenous malformation in 10% of cases
    B. Is usually precipitated by severe head injury
    C. Is characterized by a classical 'lucid period'
    D. Most often requires surgical drainage
    E. None of the above

19. A 69-year-old man was referred with a 2 hour history of left arm weakness. A CT scan of the head was normal. What is the most appropriate initial therapy?
    A. Oral streptokinase
    B. Intravenous clopidogrel
    C. Oral aspirin
    D. Oral simvastatin
    E. Subcutaneous fondaparinux

20. An 18-year-old woman was seen in the Emergency Department. She was reported to be drowsy. On examination she was not opening her eyes to verbal command or stimuli. She localized to painful. What is the best estimate of her Glasgow Coma Score?
    A. 3
    B. 5
    C. 7
    D. 12
    E. 15

21. A 26-year-old man was brought in by ambulance after having been found on the street unconscious. What is the most important first step in his management?
    A. Assess his airway, breathing and circulation
    B. BM Stix assessment of blood glucose
    C. Intravenous naloxone
    D. CT scan of the head
    E. Assessment of papillary reflexes

Extended matching questions

Question 1 Theme: Difficulty walking/limb weakness

A. Embolic stroke
B. Spinal cord compression
C. Guillain–Barré syndrome
D. Foot drop
E. Phenytoin toxicity
F. Motor neurone disease
G. Multiple sclerosis
H. Parkinson's disease
I. Huntington's disease
J. Friedreich's ataxia
K. Hysteria

For each of the following questions, select the best answer from the list above:

I. A 34-year-old housewife presents with difficulty walking due to weakness in her legs, 2 weeks after recovering from a bout of food poisoning. Examination shows absent tendon reflexes and ⅘ power in both legs. What is the most likely diagnosis?

II. A 70-year-old right-handed hypertensive smoker presents with sudden onset of weakness in the left leg and difficulty speaking. What is the most likely diagnosis?

III. A 61-year-old solicitor presents with a 1-year history of increasing difficulty walking. His wife has noticed his hands shaking and his secretary finds his handwriting has become too small to read. What is the most likely diagnosis?

Question 2 Theme: Headache

A. Migraine
B. Temporal arteritis
C. Primary brain tumour
D. Hypertension
E. Subarachnoid haemorrhage
F. Meningitis
G. Encephalitis
H. Tension headache
I. Trigeminal neuralgia

For each of the following questions select the best answer from the list above:

I. A 24-year-old student presents with recent onset of flu-like symptoms, headache, vomiting, photophobia and neck stiffness. He is pyrexial (38.7°C), with a purpuric rash on the trunk. What is the most likely diagnosis?

II. A 32-year-old female legal secretary has a 6-month history of episodic throbbing right-sided headaches associated with nausea, often on Saturday mornings. What is the most likely diagnosis?

III. A 51-year-old Afro-Caribbean female with chronic kidney disease and diabetes presents with a 3-week history of headache and blurred vision. Fundoscopy reveals retinal haemorrhages and papilloedema. What is the most likely diagnosis?

Question 3 Theme: Loss of consciousness/coma

A. Grand mal epilepsy
B. Vasovagal faint
C. Hyperglycaemia

D. Hysteria

E. Hypothermia

F. Head injury

G. Drug overdose

H. Meningoencephalitis

I. Septicaemia

J. Stroke

K. Alcohol excess

L. Hypoglycaemia

For each of the following questions select the best answer from the list above:

I.   A 48-year-old female diabetic is found unconscious in bed. Her husband died recently and she was last seen arguing with her son the previous day. She visited her GP complaining of insomnia a week ago. What is the most likely diagnosis?

II. A 75-year-old female is found unconscious in bed and smells of urine. She is pyrexial (38.5°C) and a urine dipstick shows positive nitrites. What is the most likely diagnosis?

III. An 88-year-old female not seen for several days is found unrousable in her front room on New Year's Day. On examination her pulse is 58 and regular, her BP is 90/60, there are no focal neurological signs but tendon reflexes are depressed. The ECG shows J waves. What is the most likely diagnosis?

Psychiatry is the study and management of disorders of mental function. Psychological medicine or liaison psychiatry is concerned with psychiatric and psychological disorders in patients who have physical conditions or complaints (Box 18.1).

THE PSYCHIATRIC HISTORY

The psychiatric history is different in some ways from standard history-taking. Corroboration and additional details should be sought from a relative or friend. The history should include the following:

Reason for referral

- Why and how the patient came to the attention of the doctor

Complaints

- As reported by the patient

Present illness

- Detailed account of the illness from its beginning to the present
- Include the degree of insight on the patient's part

Family history

- Family atmosphere in childhood
- Early stresses (death or separation)
- Mental illness in family members

Personal history

- Short biography of childhood, school, jobs, marriage/divorce and children
- Present housing, social and financial situation

Personality

- Attitudes, beliefs, moral values and standards
- Leisure activities and interests
- Usual reaction to stress and setback

Medical history

- Health in childhood
- Menstrual and sexual history
- Previous mental health and past medical history
- Drug history, including use of alcohol, drugs and tobacco as well as over the counter and prescribed therapies

Box 18.1. The approximate prevalence of psychiatric disorders in different populations

	% (approx.)
Community	20
Neuroses	16
Psychoses	0.5
Alcohol misuse	5
Drug misuse (total in community 20% due to co-morbidity)	2 (an underestimate)
Primary care	25
General hospital outpatients	30
General hospital inpatients	40

(Reproduced from Kumar P, Clark M. Kumar and Clark's Clinical Medicine, 8th edn. Edinburgh: Elsevier; 2012, with permission from Elsevier.)

Forensic history

- Legal problems or contact with the police or courts
- Note any violent or sexual offences (risk assessment)

EXAMINING THE MENTAL STATE

Appearance/general behaviour

- Can give information about mood
- Facial appearance, eye contact, colour of clothes
- Posture
- Movement

Speech

- Disorders of thinking are recognized from speech

Pressure of speech
- Varied ideas arise in abundance
- Characteristic of mania
- Occurs in schizophrenia

Poverty of speech
- Patient reports lack/absence of thoughts
- Characteristic of depression
- Occurs in schizophrenia

Thought blocking
- Abrupt and complete interruption of stream
- Strongly suggests schizophrenia

Disorders of form of thought

Flight of ideas
- Quickly moving from topic to topic
- Distracted by clues in the immediate environment
- Clang associations (using words with similar sounds)

- Punning
- Rhyming

Perseveration
- Persistent and inappropriate repetition
- Occurs in dementia and other conditions

Loosening of associations
- Lack of clarity
- 'Knight's move' thinking
- 'Word salad'

Mood

- Affect/feeling/emotion

Changes in nature of mood

- Depression
- Anxiety
- Elation

Changes in fluctuation of mood

- Loss of emotion (apathy)
- Reduced variation in mood (blunted)
- Rapidly and excessively changeable mood (labile)

Inappropriate mood

- Incongruous mood such as laughing when describing death of close relative

Thought content (worries and preoccupations)

Obsession
- Recurrent persistent thoughts

Compulsion
- Repetitive, seemingly purposeful action
- Must be carried out
- Urge to resist

Insight
- Degree to which patient recognizes own illness

Abnormal beliefs and interpretation of events (delusions)

- Delusions are abnormal beliefs arising from distorted judgements
- They are:
  - False
  - Held with absolute conviction
  - Not modifiable by reason/experience
- Persecutory delusions – paranoid thoughts
- Delusions of worthlessness/grandeur
- Nihilism
- Thought insertion – the belief that thoughts are implanted from outside
- Thought withdrawal
- Thought broadcasting – the belief that unspoken thoughts are known to others

Abnormal experience referred to the environment, body or self

- Illusions
- Hallucinations
- Depersonalization – the patient feels 'unreal'/detached/remote
- Derealization – the external environment feels unreal/remote

Cognitive state/memory

- Assessed using cognitive function testing ('Folstein score') (see Chapter 3)

ORGANIC MENTAL DISORDERS

Delirium/toxic confusional state

- Impairment of consciousness associated with abnormalities of perception and mood

Aetiology

See Table 18.1.

Clinical features

- Acute – clears within days
- Fluctuant with lucid periods
- Worse at night
- Visual hallucinations may occur
- Patient is frightened, suspicious, restless and uncooperative
- More common in elderly patients

Investigations

- To determine underlying cause
- Bloods
  - Full blood count (FBC)
  - Urea and electrolytes (U&E), glucose, liver function tests (LFTs), calcium
  - Vitamin B_{12}
  - Thyroid function tests

Table 18.1 Causes of delirium

Infection
  Any infection, particularly
    if high fever
Metabolic disturbance
  Electrolyte upset
  Hepatic/renal failure
  Hypoxia
Endocrine
  Hypoglycaemia
  Cushing syndrome
Intracranial
  Trauma
  Tumour
  Abscess
  Subarachnoid haemorrhage
  Epilepsy
	Drug intoxication
	  Anticonvulsants
	  Anxiolytics/hypnotics/
	    antidepressants
	  Opiates/dopamine agonists
	  Digoxin
	Drug/alcohol withdrawal
	Postoperative states
	Vitamin deficiency
	  Thiamine (Wernicke–Korsakoff
	    syndrome)
	  Nicotinic acid (pellagra)
	  Vitamin B_{12}

- Blood and urine cultures
- ECG
- Chest X-ray
- CT of brain

Management

- Treat underlying cause
- Nurse carefully in a well-lit area
- Communicate clearly and concisely
- Give repeated information to orientate (family/carers can be useful for this)
- Ensure adequate hydration
- Sedate only if necessary, e.g. haloperidol i.m.
- Paracetamol if febrile
- Review all drugs and stop all but essential ones

Management of the agitated patient

- Agitated patient who is likely to harm him/herself or others

Emergency treatment

- Talk calmly to patient: if this fails, get help to restrain him/her
- Check blood sugar, oximetry, coma scale and for focal neurological deficit
- If not hypoglycaemic or hypoxic and has good coma scale with no focal neurology, then consider sedation with 5 mg i.m. haloperidol (repeat up to 20 mg if needed)
- If alcohol or benzodiazepine withdrawal likely, then use lorazepam 2 mg

Initial investigations

- Bloods – FBC, U&E, glucose, calcium, LFTs
- Blood and urine cultures if sepsis suggested
- Measure arterial blood gases
- ECG
- Chest X-ray

Dementia

- Progressive decline of cognitive function in the absence of clouded consciousness

Aetiology
See Table 18.2.

Differential diagnosis
- Depression

Investigations

- Blood
  - FBC
  - U&E, glucose, LFTs, calcium
  - ESR, C-reactive protein
  - Red cell folate, vitamin B_{12}
  - Thyroid function tests
  - Syphilis serology
  - HIV antibodies if indicated and patient counselled
- Chest X-ray
- CT/MRI

Table 18.2 Causes of dementia

Degenerative	Intracranial
Alzheimer's disease (65%)	Subdural haematoma
Dementia with Lewy bodies	Tumour
(25%)	Toxic
Frontotemporal dementia	Alcohol
Huntington's disease	Occupational
Parkinson's disease	Lead or mercury poisoning
Normal pressure hydrocephalus	Traumatic
Primary progressive aphasia	Boxing (punch drunk
Vascular	syndrome)
Cerebrovascular disease	Vitamin deficiency
Cerebral vasculitis/cranial	Thiamine
arteritis	Vitamin B_{12}
Metabolic	Infections
Uraemia	Creutzfeldt–Jakob disease
Hepatic failure	HIV
Paraneoplastic syndromes	Syphilis
Endocrine	Whipple's disease
Hypothyroidism	Psychiatric
Hypocalcaemia	Pseudodementia

Alzheimer's disease

Neuropathology
- Neuronal loss
- Neurofibrillary tangles
- Senile plaques
- Amyloid deposition

Aetiology
- Early onset – may be familial linkage to chromosomes 1, 14 and 21
- Late onset – apolipoprotein E gene

Clinical features
- Inability to learn new information or recall previously learnt information
- Decline in language, particularly names
- Apraxia – unable to carry out motor functions
- Agnosia – unable to identify/recognize objects
- Impairment of organizing/sequencing
- Behavioural change – wandering, agitation, aggression
- Paranoia and loss of insight

Management
- Cholinesterase inhibitors and drugs blocking glutamate transmission slow the rate of decline slightly but their use is clouded by complex cost–benefit arguments

Dementia with Lewy bodies

Clinical features
- Second commonest cause of dementia
- Fluctuating cognition with pronounced variation in attention/alertness

- Memory loss uncommon in early stages
- Sleep disorders, visual hallucinations, delusions and transient loss of consciousness

Management
- Avoid neuroleptic drugs

Vascular dementia/multi-infarct dementia

Clinical features
- History of transient ischaemic attacks or stroke
- Features depend on the site of ischaemic damage

Management
- Stroke prevention measures including antiplatelet drugs

SCHIZOPHRENIA

- Abnormal integration of emotional and cognitive functions

Epidemiology
- 2–4/1000 annual incidence
- 1% lifetime risk

Aetiology
- Genetic – lifetime risk in patients with a parent affected is 12%
- Altered neurotransmitters
  - ↑ Dopamine activity
  - Altered serotonin metabolism
- Environmental triggers
  - Cannabis use is a possible risk factor

Clinical features
- Peak onset early 20s
- ♀ = ♂

Diagnosis
- Based on presence of first-rank symptoms:
- Auditory hallucinations
- Thought withdrawal
- Thought insertion
- Thought broadcasting
- Delusions
- External controlled emotions
- Somatic passivity and feelings (feeling that thoughts and acts are due to the influence of others)

Subtypes
Positive schizophrenia
- Acute onset
- Prominent delusions and hallucinations
- Good response to neuroleptics
- Better prognosis

Negative schizophrenia
- Insidious deterioration in personality
- Relative absence of acute symptoms
- Delusions and hallucinations absent
- Increasing apathy and eccentricity

- Slow withdrawal from society
- Poor response to neuroleptics

Management
- Combination of drug and social treatment delivered by multidisciplinary team

Drugs
- Antipsychotics/neuroleptics
  - Dopamine antagonists (chlorpromazine, haloperidol); unwanted side-effects are shown in Table 18.3
  - Atypical anti-psychotics (clozapine, risperidone, olanzapine) have less extrapyramidal side-effects

Psychological treatment
- Reassurance and support

Social treatment
- Structured work and social programme

MOOD (AFFECTIVE) DISORDERS

- Spectrum of disorders ranging from depression through to mania
- Patients who suffer attacks of both have bipolar disorder (Fig. 18.1)

Aetiology

Physical
- Genetic – monozygotic twin concordance 30–60%, higher in bipolar disorders

---

Table 18.3 Unwanted effects of neuroleptic drugs

Common effects	Rare effects
Motor	Hypersensitivity
Acute dystonia	Cholestatic jaundice
Parkinsonism	Leucopenia
Akathisia (restless, repetitive	Skin reactions
and irresistible need to	Others
move)	Precipitation of glaucoma
Tardive dyskinesia	Galactorrhoea
(mouthing and smacking	Amenorrhoea
of the lips, grimaces and	Cardiac arrhythmias
contortions of the face/	Seizures
neck)	Neuroleptic malignant syndrome
Autonomic	Hyperthermia
Hypotension	Muscle rigidity
Failure of ejaculation	Tachycardia
Anticholinergic	Labile BP
Dry mouth	Pallor
Urinary retention	Elevated white cell count,
Constipation	creatine kinase, liver function
Blurred vision	tests
Metabolic	Treatment: lower temperature,
Weight gain	bromocriptine, dantrolene

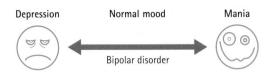

Fig. 18.1 Bipolar disorder.

- Neurotransmitter imbalance – downregulation of 5 HT receptors in depression
- Hormonal
  - Cortisol (Cushing syndrome induces depression and corticosteroids alter mood, moreover hypercortisolaemia occurs in patients with depression
  - Oral contraceptives/pregnancy/premenstrual
- CNS abnormalities – brain MRI/PET studies show:
  - Increased ventricular volume, frontal lobe atrophy and altered blood flow
  - Volume reduction in the hippocampus

Psychological
- Maternal deprivation
- Learned helplessness

Social
- Stressful life events, e.g. divorce, unemployment
- Sexual abuse in childhood

Clinical features

- See Table 18.4
- Range of severity (Fig. 18.2)
  - Severe life-threatening disease
  - Minor forms

Differential diagnosis

Mania
- Drug-induced psychosis
  - Amphetamines/ecstasy/cocaine
  - Long-term cannabis use
  - Steroids
- Acute schizophrenia
- Hyperthyroidism/Cushing syndrome

Depression
- Malignancy
- Hypothyroidism/hyperparathyroidism
- Cushing syndrome
- Neurological diseases (multiple sclerosis, Parkinson's)
- Cerebral ischaemia or tumour
- Heart failure
- Porphyria

Table 18.4 Clinical features of depression and mania

Characteristic	Depression	Mania
Mood	Depressed	Elevated
	Miserable	Labile
	Unhappy	Irritable
Talk	Slow	Fast
	Impoverished	Pressurized
	Monotonous	Flight of ideas
Energy	Reduced apathetic/lethargic	Excessive
Ideation	Feelings of:	Grandiose
	Futility	Self-confident
	Guilt	Delusions of:
	Self-reproach	Wealth
	Unworthiness	Power
	Hypochondriasis	Influence
	Worrying	Religious significance
	Suicidal thoughts	Persecutory delusions
	Delusions of guilt	
	Nihilism	
	Persecution	
Cognition	Impaired learning	Disturbance of registration of memories
	Pseudodementia if elderly	
Physical	Early waking	Insomnia
	Poor appetite	Weight loss
	Weight loss	
	Constipation	
	Loss of libido	
	Erectile dysfunction	
	Fatigue	
	Bodily aches and pains	
Behaviour	Poverty of movement/expression	Disinhibition
	Retardation/agitation	Increased sexual interest
Hallucinations	Auditory	Excessive drinking/spending
	Hostile	Fleeting auditory
	Critical	Occasionally visual

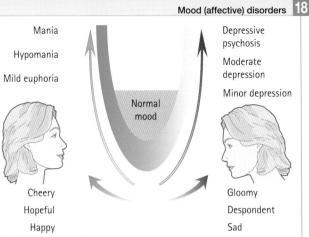

Mania

Hypomania

Mild euphoria

Depressive psychosis

Moderate depression

Minor depression

Normal mood

Cheery

Hopeful

Happy

Gloomy

Despondent

Sad

Fig. 18.2 Continuum of normal and abnormal mood.

Table 18.5 Clinical features of normal grief reaction and depressive illness after bereavement (morbid grief reaction)

Characteristic	Normal bereavement	Morbid grief reaction
Onset	Immediately after loss	Delayed for weeks/months
Duration	Weeks	Months/years
Pattern	Slow acceptance and adjustment	Denial of loss and refusal to accept implications
Grief	Expressed openly	Expressed with difficulty
Guilt	Mild regret in early stage	Marked guilt often present

- Drugs
  - Steroids
- Psychiatric disorders
  - Schizophrenia
  - Alcohol/drug (e.g. amphetamines) misuse or withdrawal
  - Borderline personality disorder
  - Dementia
- Normal bereavement reaction (Table 18.5)

Management

Physical

- Stop depressing drugs including alcohol
- Regular exercise (good for mild/moderate depression)

Depression (Fig. 18.3)

- Drugs – choice depends on side-effects and safety
  - Serotonin reuptake inhibitors, e.g. fluoxetine
  - Tricyclic antidepressants (TCAs), e.g. amitriptyline; see Table 18.6 for unwanted effects
  - New generation antidepressants, e.g. venlafaxine – serotonin and noradrenaline receptor blocker, mirtazapine increases both noradrenaline and selective serotonin transmission noradrenaline reuptake inhibitors, e.g. reboxetine
  - Monoamine oxidase inhibitors, e.g. phenelzine – used 2nd line
- Electroconvulsive therapy (ECT)
  - Used in life-threatening depression

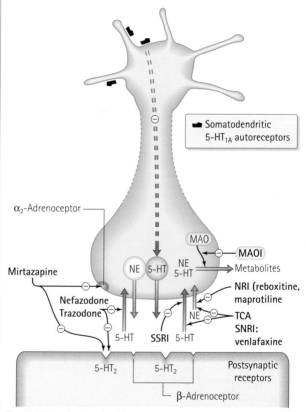

Fig. 18.3 Sites of action of antidepressants with examples. *(From Waller DG, Renwick A, Hiller K, (eds). Medical Pharmacology and Therapeutics. Edinburgh: Saunders; 2010, with permission)*

Table 18.6 Unwanted effects of drugs used in affective disorders

Tricyclic antidepressants	Lithium

Anticholinergic effects
  Dry mouth
  Constipation
  Tremor
  Blurred vision
  Urinary retention
  Postural hypotension
	GI symptoms
	Hypothyroidism
	Fine tremor
	Weight gain (increased appetite)
	Polyuria/polydipsia
	Toxic symptoms
	Drowsiness

Cardiac effects
  ECG changes
  Arrhythmias
	Blurred vision
	Tremor
	Ataxia

Lowered seizure threshold	Dysarthria
Weight gain	Convulsions
Sedation	Coma and death
Mania	

Mania

Acute attacks
- Atypical antipsychotics
- Lithium – Table 18.6 lists unwanted effects
- Neuroleptic drugs for severe hyperactivity, e.g. haloperidol

Prophylaxis
- Lithium
  - Regular check on drug levels (narrow therapeutic window)
  - Regular check on renal function (renal excretion)
  - Regular check on thyroid function
- Carbamazepine
- Valproate

Psychological
- Psychotherapy
- Cognitive/behavioural therapy

Social
- Assistance with social problems
- Group support
- Stress management
- Family/carer support

PUERPERAL AFFECTIVE DISORDERS

- Childbirth has a higher relative risk of depression than life events or physical illness
- Treatment of these disorders is as for any other affective disorder

Maternity blues

Clinical features
- Brief episodes of emotional lability, irritability and tearfulness
- Occurs in 50% of women 2–3 days postpartum
- Resolves spontaneously

Postpartum psychosis

Clinical features

- 1 in 500–1000 births
- Onset usually within 2 weeks of birth
- Classical features of affective psychosis plus confusion and disorientation
- If severe, patient may have delusions that the child is deformed, evil or affected in another way which can lead to suicide or infanticide
- Responds well to treatment
- 20–30% recur in next puerperium

Postnatal depression

Clinical features

- Depression occurs in 10% of mothers in first postpartum year
- Clinically similar to other depressive illness
- Recovery after a few months

SUICIDE AND DELIBERATE SELF-HARM

Suicide

Risk factors

- Living alone
- Immigrant status
- Recent bereavement/separation/divorce
- Unemployment/retirement
- Male sex
- Older age
- Family or previous history of
  - Affective disorder
  - Suicide
  - Alcohol abuse

Table 18.7 For deliberate self-harm patients – indications for referral to psychiatrist

Absolute indications
  Clinical depression
  Psychosis
  Clearly pre-planned suicide attempts
  Persistent suicidal intent
  Violent method used
Relative indications
  Alcohol/drug abuse
  Patients with risk factors for suicide (see above)
  Patients with family history of suicide
  Patients with serious (particularly incurable) physical illnesses
  Those in whom there is a major unresolved crisis
  Persistent suicide attempts
  Any patient giving concern

- Previous suicide attempt
- Drug/alcohol addiction
- Severe depression/early dementia
- Incapacitating, painful physical illness

Deliberate self-harm (DSH)

- ♀ > ♂
- Most patients <35 years
- 90% involve self-poisoning
- Formal psychiatric disorder is unusual
- 1–2% kill themselves in the following year
- Assessment procedure (see Ch. 3)
- Indications for referral to psychiatric team (Table 18.7)

NEUROSES AND STRESS-RELATED/SOMATOFORM DISORDERS

Anxiety disorder

Clinical features
See Table 18.8.

Differential diagnosis
Psychiatric disorders

- Depression
- Obsessive compulsive disorder
- Schizophrenia
- Dementia
- Drug/alcohol dependence
- Benzodiazepine withdrawal

Table 18.8 Clinical features of anxiety	
Physical	**Nervous system**
Gastrointestinal	Fatigue
Dry mouth	Blurred vision
Dysphagia	Dizziness
Epigastric pain	Headache
Flatulence/aerophagy	Sleep disturbance
Diarrhoea	Tremor
Respiratory	**Psychological**
Sensation of chest	Apprehension and fear
constriction	Irritability
Difficulty inhaling	Difficulty concentrating
Over-breathing	Distractibility
Cardiovascular	Restlessness
Palpitations, awareness of	Sensitivity to noise
missed beat	Depression
Chest pain	Depersonalization
Genitourinary	Derealization
Frequency	
Failure of erection	
Lack of libido	

Physical disorders
- Hyperthyroidism
- Hypoglycaemia
- Phaeochromocytoma

Management

Psychological
- Reassurance about physical symptoms
- Relaxation techniques
- Anxiety management training
- Biofeedback
- Behaviour therapies
- Cognitive behavioural therapy

Drugs
- Selective serotonin reuptake inhibitors (SSRIs)
- β-blockers for physical symptoms
- Short courses of benzodiazepines

Obsessive compulsive disorder

- Characterized by obsessional thinking and compulsive behaviour with varying degrees of anxiety/depression and depersonalization

Clinical features
- Persistent and intrusive obsessions/compulsions
- Functioning impeded
- Constant need to check
- Repetitive/superstitious actions

Management
- Behaviour therapy
  - Response prevention
  - Modelling
- Serotonin reuptake inhibitors (may need higher doses than those used in depression)

Dissociative (conversion) disorder (previously known as hysteria)

- Characterized by
  - Absence of physical pathology
  - Unconscious production
  - Triggered by an unresolved conflict or life event
  - Absence of sympathetic overactivity

Clinical features
- ♀ > ♂
- Rarely occurs in those >40 years
- See Table 18.9
- May confer advantage (secondary gain)
- Patients' emotional distress is less than expected

Management
- Psychotherapy

Somatoform disorders

- Patients
  - Repeatedly present with physical problems

Table 18.9 Common dissociative/conversion symptoms	
Dissociative (mental)	**Conversion (physical)**
Amnesia	Paralysis
Fugue	Gait disorder
Pseudodementia	Tremor
Dissociative identity disorder	Aphonia
Psychosis	Mutism
	Sensory symptoms
	Globus hystericus
	Hysterical fits
	Blindness

- Have repeatedly negative findings on clinical investigation
- Have no demonstrable physical cause

Clinical features
Hypochondriasis
- Preoccupation with ill health
- Disproportionate and unjustified concern

Somatization disorder
- Repeatedly present with a variety of medical symptoms
- Undergo repeated investigations/operations
- May have medical connections

Management
- Explain and reassure
- Explore psychological/social problems
- Avoid repeated investigations
- Graded exercise programmes
- Trial of an antidepressant

Acute stress reaction and post-traumatic stress disorder

- Occur in individuals in response to exceptional physical or psychological stress

Acute stress reaction
- Lasts a few hours/days
- Initial state of 'daze'
- Then a phase of either
  - Withdrawal/stupor *or*
  - Agitation/over-activity
- Commonly associated with autonomic signs of anxiety

Post-traumatic stress disorder
- Delayed/protracted response to a stressful event
- 'Flashbacks'
- Intense distress in/avoidance of situations resembling the event (including anniversaries)
- Emotional blunting/numbness
- Detachment from others
- Hypervigilance
- Insomnia

- Anxiety and depression
- Occasionally suicide

Management
- Counselling

DRUG AND ALCOHOL MISUSE AND DEPENDENCE

- Current figures in the UK show 10% of women and 20% of men drink in excess of the recommended safety limits for long-term health risk

Alcohol dependence syndrome

Clinical features
- Compulsive need to drink
- Altered alcohol tolerance
- Stereotyped pattern of drinking
- Drinking takes primacy over other activities
- Repeated withdrawal symptoms
- Relief drinking to avoid withdrawal, e.g. early morning drinking
- Rapid relapse if patient drinks again following a period of abstinence

Management
Psychosocial support and group therapy
- Example: Alcoholics Anonymous

Drugs (effects are enhanced by combining them with counselling)
- Naltrexone reduces the risk of relapse into heavy drinking and the frequency of drinking
- Acamprosate alters neurotransmitters and reduces drinking frequency
- Disulfiram reacts with alcohol to form acetaldehyde which produces unpleasant symptoms to discourage drinking

Drug misuse

- For commonly used illicit drugs the desired and adverse effects are shown in Table 18.10

Management
- Withdrawal programmes, e.g. using methadone
- Psychosocial support to help the addict live without drugs

EATING DISORDERS

Anorexia nervosa

Aetiology
- Genetic
- Childhood sexual abuse
- Dietary problems in early life
- Social factors
  - Higher social class
  - Occupation – ballet dancers/nurses

Clinical features
- BMI (body mass index) <17.5
- Intense wish to be thin
- Morbid fear of fatness
- Amenorrhoea in women
- ♀ >> ♂

Table 18.10 Desired and adverse effects of commonly used 'illicit' drugs

Drug	Desired effects	Adverse effects
Solvents ('glue sniffing')	Euphoria Floating sensation	Amnesia Visual hallucinations Inhalation of vomit Bone marrow/brain/liver/kidney toxicity Tolerance
Amphetamines	Stimulant Euphoria	Psychological dependence Restlessness Over-activity Paranoid psychosis
Cocaine	Stimulant Hyperarousal	Dependence Paranoid ideation Fits Coronary artery spasm/disease Perforation of nasal septum if inhaled
Cannabis	Exaggeration of pre-existing mood	No definite withdrawal syndrome or tolerance Psychosis
MDMA ('Ecstasy')	Psychedelic effects	Hyperpyrexia Acute hepatic/renal failure Possible chronic brain damage
Hypnotics (e.g. benzodiazepines)	Relaxation Sleep induction	Dependence Withdrawal syndrome Respiratory depression
Narcotics (morphine, heroin, codeine, methadone, pethidine)	Calm Slight euphoria Analgesia Flattening of emotions	Marked and rapid tolerance Withdrawal syndrome Respiratory depression Complications of injecting: Infection (e.g. HIV/hepatitis B and C/endocarditis) Vein thrombosis

- Onset in adolescence, rare >30 years
- Previous history of chubbiness/fatness
- Relentless pursuit of low body weight
- Distorted image of own body
- Eats little
- Avoids carbohydrates
- Vomiting/excess exercise/purging
- Loss of sexual interest
- Lanugo hair

Management

- Behaviour therapy – goal setting/reward for weight/dietary intake
- Psychotherapy
- Family therapy

Bulimia nervosa

Clinical features

- Binge eating
- Self-induced vomiting
- Laxative abuse
- Misuse of drugs, e.g. diuretics, thyroxine, anorectics
- ♀ >> ♂
- Often associated with anorexia nervosa
- Premorbid personality – neurotic traits
- May be associated with
  - Depression
  - Alcohol dependence
- Fluctuation in body weight
- Periods irregular

Consequences of vomiting

- Cardiac arrhythmias
- Renal impairment secondary to low K^+
- Muscular paralysis
- Tetany – hypokalaemic alkalosis
- Swollen salivary glands
- Eroded dental enamel

Management

- Cognitive behaviour therapy
- SSRIs

Box 18.2. The basis of mental health laws for detention or commitment

1. The individual to be detained must be suffering from a defined mental illness.
2. Detention is for the purposes of observation and refinement of the diagnosis and/or to actively treat the disorder (i.e. detention is a means to an end).
3. Attempts to treat the individual on an outpatient basis have failed.
4. The offer of a voluntary admission to hospital has been refused or is impractical.
5. Treatment in hospital is necessary:
   - because it will benefit the outcome of the illness
   - to protect the patient from harm (in terms of physical health, mental health and abuse or manipulation at the hands of others)
   - to protect others from harm that the patient might cause them passively (neglect) or actively.

PSYCHIATRY AND THE LAW

Compulsory section under the Mental Health Act

Conditions

- For a patient to be held against his/her will under the Mental Health Act, he/she must be:
  - Suffering from a defined mental disorder
  - A risk to his/her and/or other people's health or safety
  - Unwilling to accept hospitalization voluntarily

Sections

See Box 18.2 for details.

SELF-ASSESSMENT QUESTIONS

Multiple choice questions (single best answer)

1. Of these first-rank symptoms of schizophrenia which also occurs in mania?
   A. Thought broadcasting
   B. Thought withdrawal
   C. Thought insertion
   D. Auditory hallucinations
   E. Persecutory delusions

2. In dementia the following is correct:
   A. Consciousness is clouded
   B. Multi-infarct dementia is the commonest cause
   C. Depression is a differential diagnosis
   D. Dementia with Lewy bodies accounts for 40%
   E. A CT scan is not indicated

3. The following management strategy in toxic confusional state may exacerbate the problem:
   A. Establish a corroborative history from a witness
   B. Nurse the patient in a darkened room
   C. Prescription of appropriate intravenous fluids if not drinking
   D. Minimize polypharmacy
   E. Prescription of antibiotics

4. In depression:
   A. Patients sleep well
   B. Patients usually have increased sexual interest
   C. Patients may have auditory hallucinations if disease is severe
   D. Monozygotic twin concordance is only 10% for unipolar depression
   E. Most patients are treated with psychotherapy alone

5. The following feature of mania may also be seen in thyrotoxicosis:
   A. Delusions of wealth
   B. Weight loss
   C. Excessive drinking
   D. Flight of ideas
   E. Critical hallucinations

6. Lithium:
   A. Is used to prevent depression
   B. 50% undergoes renal excretion
   C. Causes hyperthyroidism

    D. Needs therapeutic drug level monitoring

    E. Is used to treat acute attacks of depression

7. The following are factors that increase the risk of suicide:
   A. Female sex
   B. Young age
   C. No previous history of depression
   D. Living with a large extended family
   E. A family history of suicide

8. In deliberate self-harm:
   A. 75% is by self-poisoning
   B. There is often an associated psychiatric disorder
   C. Patients with depression should be referred to a psychiatrist
   D. A violent method makes suicide less likely
   E. Patients who planned to be discovered are at higher risk of suicide

9. The following are physical symptoms of anxiety disorder except:
   A. Chest pain
   B. Diarrhoea
   C. Erectile dysfunction
   D. Urinary frequency
   E. Jaundice

10. Anorexia nervosa:
    A. Patients often have a BMI of over 30
    B. Patients have usually been thin since childhood
    C. Is more common in higher social classes
    D. Amenorrhoea occurs late in the disease
    E. Patients think they are thin

11. Regarding the Sections of the Mental Health Act:
    A. Section 2 allows patients to be held for 6 months
    B. Section 3 is for psychiatric assessment only
    C. Section 5(2) relates to patients already in hospital
    D. Section 5(2) allows the patient to be detained for 6 hours
    E. Section 2 requires the signatures of one doctor and a social worker/relative

12. The following statements are correct:
    A. Obsessive compulsive disorder responds to low-dose serotonin reuptake inhibitors
    B. Paralysis is a common symptom of a conversion disorder
    C. Conversion disorder is produced consciously
    D. Post-traumatic stress disorder occurs immediately after a stressful event
    E. In acute stress reaction bradycardia is usual

13. The following are effects of illicit drugs:
    A. Cocaine causes hyperarousal
    B. Amphetamines induce sleep
    C. Cannabis use is associated with a withdrawal syndrome
    D. The development of tolerance to heroin is slow
    E. MDMA has no long-term side-effects

14. The following statements are correct about alcohol withdrawal:
    A. Delirium tremens occurs within hours of alcohol cessation
    B. Seizures can be treated as an outpatient
    C. Acamprosate will help tremor

    D. Prevention with Disulfiram is usually effective

    E. Drugs to prevent alcohol dependence are enhanced by combining them with counselling

15. Antidepressant drugs:

    A. Are safe in overdose

    B. SSRIs are used in all patients

    C. Choice of drug depends on the side-effect profile

    D. Tricyclic antidepressants are effective within a few days of starting treatment

    E. Venlafaxine has no effect on serotonin

Extended matching questions

Question 1 Theme: Agitation

A. Acute confusional state

B. Acute mania

C. Puerperal psychosis

D. Schizophrenia

E. Obsessive compulsive disorder

F. Alzheimer's disease

G. Anxiety disorder

H. Alcohol withdrawal syndrome

I. Cocaine abuse

J. Somatization disorder

For each of the following questions, select the best answer from the list above:

I. A 59-year-old female smoker who lives with her husband presents with agitation. On direct questioning she can remember details of the distant past but her short-term memory is poor. She has lost weight but there are no other physical signs or symptoms. What is the most likely diagnosis?

II. A 23-year-old female who was born in Jamaica but has lived in the UK since the age of 8 attends the A&E department alone; she is agitated. She appears to have threatening auditory hallucinations. She also says that she is having difficulty sleeping. The casualty records show a previous attendance at a psychiatric outpatient clinic 2 years ago. The limited physical examination she allows is normal. What is the most likely diagnosis?

III. A 48-year-old male presents with agitation. On direct questioning he admits to visual hallucinations. He has a previous history of gastrointestinal bleeding. On examination he is sweaty and the pulse rate is 110/min. Blood tests reveal the following: Hb 14.4, MCV 101. What is the most likely diagnosis?

Question 2 Theme: Hallucinations

A. Acute confusional state

B. Acute mania

C. Puerperal psychosis

D. Schizophrenia

E. Obsessive compulsive disorder

F. Alzheimer's disease

G. Anxiety disorder

H. Alcohol withdrawal syndrome

I. Amphetamine abuse

J. Somatization disorder

For each of the following questions, select the best answer from the list above:

I. A 26-year-old man who lives with his mother presents with auditory hallucinations. He has recently been made redundant after he was said to be acting strangely at work. There are no physical signs or symptoms. He reports that he thinks people can hear his thoughts. On direct questioning his hallucinations are persecutory in nature. What is the most likely diagnosis?

II. A 33-year-old male attends the A&E department alone and agitated. He appears to have paranoid auditory hallucinations. He also says that he is having difficulty sleeping. The A&E records show a previous attendance 2 years ago with an overdose of benzodiazepines. He denies problems with alcohol use now or in the past. The physical examination shows a tachycardia and raised blood pressure. What is the most likely diagnosis?

III. A 45-year-old male presents with agitation and complaining that he cannot sleep. He has recently been dismissed from his job. His wife is very upset and is accusing him of spending huge amounts of money and of having an affair. On direct questioning he admits to fleeting auditory hallucinations. He has lost weight and reports increased libido. What is the most likely diagnosis?

Question 3 Theme: Psychiatric treatments

A. A tricyclic antidepressant
B. A selective serotonin reuptake inhibitor
C. ECT
D. Lithium
E. A monoamine oxidase inhibitor
F. Venlafaxine
G. Cognitive behavioural therapy
H. Carbamazepine
I. Chlorpromazine
J. Clozapine

For each of the following questions, select the best answer from the list above:

I. A 59-year-old female who lives with her husband presents with symptoms of depression. Her husband has just been diagnosed with lung cancer. She is overweight but there are no other physical signs or symptoms. What would be the most appropriate choice of treatment?

II. A 22-year-old female presents with an episode of hyperventilation. She describes panic attacks when trying to leave the house. The limited physical examination she allows is normal. You diagnose an anxiety disorder. She is not keen to take any drug treatment. What would be the most appropriate choice of treatment?

III. A 48-year-old man is known to have bipolar disorder. He had been on lithium but was recently found to be hypothyroid so the lithium had been stopped. He requires another drug for his returning symptoms of mania. What would be the most appropriate choice of treatment?

The epidemiology of a disease is a description of the demographics of the affected population and the environment from which they originate. Statistical analysis is the manipulation of data about a population sample designed to reveal similarities or differences between groups of differing patients or between treatment types. Statistical analysis is also used to describe details about a population.

TYPES OF DATA

Nominal

- Mutually exclusive groups
  - Male (♂) or female (♀)

Ordinal

- Ranked exclusive groups
  - Mild/moderate/severe

Continuous

- Numerical values that may be anywhere along a continuum
  - Age

Descriptional statistics

- A method of describing a population or a sample from that population

Mean

- The mathematical average of a set of numerical data

Mode

- The most commonly occurring value

Median

- The middle number when the dataset is arranged in numerical order
- If there is an even number of values it is the mean of the middle two

Sample mean

- The mathematical average of a variable measured in a sample

Population mean

- The mean calculated if the entire population under study were measured
- *Note*: this is rarely achievable

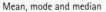

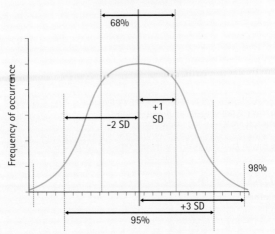

Fig. 19.1 Gaussian or normal distribution. This is symmetrical about the mean. A total of 68% of all values in the dataset fall within ±1 standard deviation (SD), 95% between ±2 SD and 99% between ±3 SD. This is often described as the bell-shaped curve.

Distribution

- The pattern of spread of values
- Many biological values fit a 'normal' or Gaussian distribution, a bell-shaped curve

Normal distribution

- A symmetrical 'bell-shaped' curve distribution where the mean, mode and median are the same (Fig. 19.1)

Skewed distribution

- Very high or low values may result in an asymmetrical distribution leading to a positive (high value) or negative (low value) skew (Fig. 19.2)

Variance

- Describes the spread of values either side of a mean

Standard deviation

- Gives the range of values within which a certain proportion of the sample will lie
- 68% will lie ±1 SD from the mean
- 95% will lie ±2 SD from the mean
- 99% will lie ±3 SD from the mean

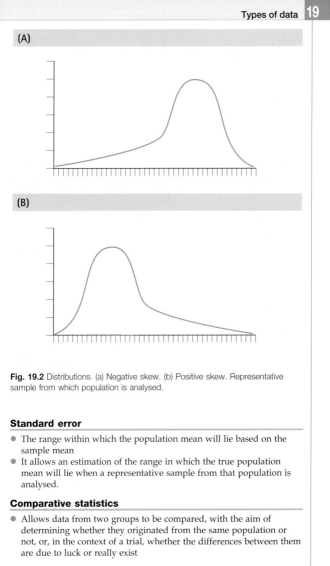

(A)

(B)

Fig. 19.2 Distributions. (a) Negative skew. (b) Positive skew. Representative sample from which population is analysed.

Standard error

- The range within which the population mean will lie based on the sample mean
- It allows an estimation of the range in which the true population mean will lie when a representative sample from that population is analysed.

Comparative statistics

- Allows data from two groups to be compared, with the aim of determining whether they originated from the same population or not, or, in the context of a trial, whether the differences between them are due to luck or really exist

Hypothesis

- The concept being tested

Null hypothesis

- That no difference exists between the two samples being analysed

Bias

- Inequalities between the groups being compared that lead to incorrect conclusions being reached

Errors in experimental design that cause incorrect results

Type 1 error
- A false positive result
- A difference is found between two groups where one does not exist

Type 2 error
- A false negative result
- No difference is detected although one does exist

Parametric data

- Data values fit a 'normal distribution'

Statistical tests

- Tests that provide a probability value
- The 'p' value is the probability that the two sets of data being compared are from the same population, i.e. that no difference exists between them
- Statistical significance is stated to be a probability of less than 1 in 20 that the two groups are the same ($p < 0.05$)

Parametric tests

- Used on data following a normal distribution, e.g.
  - Student t-test
  - Paired t-test

Non-parametric tests

- Used on non-normally distributed data
  - Unpaired: Mann–Whitney
  - Paired: Wilcoxon

Nominal tests

- If data can be placed in a 2×2 square, e.g. the response to a treatment or placebo (Fig. 19.3) – then a Chi-squared test (χ^2-test) can be used

	Disease present	Disease absent	Totals
Treatment given	9	41	50
Placebo given	39	11	50
Totals	48	52	100

Fig. 19.3 The 2×2 table. If you consider a disease for which a treatment is given, 100 patients enter a study and are randomized to receive the treatment or a placebo. The groups are mutually exclusive. An individual cannot be in more than one group. A 2×2 table can then be drawn up of the outcomes. In this example, 50 patients received the treatment and 41 were cured, as were 11 of those who received the placebo. Analysis of this data can be carried out using a Chi-squared test in order to determine whether the treatment is statistically better than the placebo.

95% confidence intervals

- The 95% confidence interval (CI) is the range of values around the mean within which the true population mean will lie in 95% of cases
- It is calculated from the standard error. We can state that in 95% of cases, the population mean will lie ±2 standard errors from our sample mean
- Data can therefore be expressed as a mean and 95% confidence interval, the values being the range provided by the mean ±2 standard errors

Correlation and regression (Fig. 19.4)

Correlation coefficient

- Reports on the relationship between two variables
- A value of 1 suggests a completely linear relationship
- 0 suggests that no relationship exists between them

Regression

- Allows calculation of the equation of a line drawn when two variables are plotted against each other
- Once this equation is defined, the value of one variable can be calculated when the other is known

Accuracy of test values

Normal range

- For any variable there is usually a range of normal values, usually defined as the mean value ±2 or 3 standard deviations

Sensitivity

- The ability of a test to report an abnormal result when the disease is present
- It reports on what proportion of patients with a disease will have a positive test

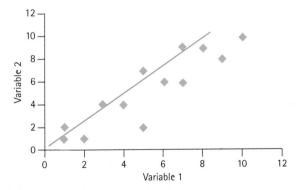

Fig. 19.4 Correlation and regression. When two variables are plotted against each other, a scatter plot results. A line of best fit can then be drawn through these points and the accuracy of the relationship between the two variables can be calculated based on the variance between each data point and the best fit line. This is the correlation coefficient.

Specificity

- The ability of a test to return a normal result when the disease is absent
- It reports on what proportion of patients without the disease will have a negative test

Positive predictive value (PPV)

- The proportion of positive tests where the disease is actually present
- A high PPV suggests that if the test is positive, then the disease is present, i.e. there are few false positives

CLINICAL TRIALS

- Designed to compare the effect of a therapy with either a placebo (i.e. an inactive substance) or another therapy

Power (calculation)

- A calculation of the numbers needed in a trial to confidently measure a stated difference between the two groups to '$p < 0.05$'

Randomization

- Each patient entered into the trial has an equal chance of being in each of the therapy groups in the trial

Controlled trial

- Comparison of one therapy against another or a placebo

Blinded

- Patients do not know which therapy they are receiving

Double blind

- Neither the doctor nor the patient knows which therapy is being received

Bias

- Inequalities between the two groups other than the difference in therapy that they are receiving

Publication bias

- Failure of negative trials to be published, so only positive data about a therapy reaches the public domain

Intention to treat

- The analysis of the trial data includes all patients entered, irrespective of whether they completed the treatment course

Cross-over trials

- Each subject undergoes both types of therapy, one after the other
- A comparison can then be made for each individual patient

Endpoints

- Primary endpoint: the main measurement aim of the trial – this is used in the power calculation to determine the number of subjects
- Secondary endpoints: other measurements reported in the trial. The trial may not be sufficiently powered to test these without a type II error

EVIDENCE-BASED MEDICINE

Definition

- The conscientious, explicit and judicious use of current best evidence in making decisions about the care of individual patients

Role

- EBM leads to patient care guided by the best available data on therapies available, but it is specific to the patient; in other words it aims to take into account differences between individual patients
  - If a trial on hypertension were carried out in male Caucasians, its results may not be true of African women.

Resources

Cochrane Collaboration
- A collection of critical appraisals of trials on specific therapies

Medline/Pubmed/Index Medicus
- Databases of biomedical studies published worldwide

Critical appraisal

- The analysis of all the trials that have studied the same therapy in the same disease with a conclusion about the overall role of that therapy
- In general, only randomized controlled, preferably blinded trials are included and an intention to treat analysis is carried out

Relative risk (RR)

- The percentage change in the probability of an event occurring due to the therapy given
- If the chance of a stroke *on* aspirin is 2% and the chance *off* aspirin is 4%, the relative risk of a stroke *on* aspirin is 50% (the proportion of strokes that would have been avoided)
- A relative risk of 100% ($\equiv 1$) suggests that the risk in each group is identical

Absolute risk

- The proportion of all patients who would benefit from the therapy
- In the above example, the chance of a stroke *off* aspirin is 4% while *on* aspirin it is 2%; therefore the absolute reduction in risk from taking aspirin is: $4\% - 2\% = 2\%$

Number needed to treat

- An estimation of the number of patients who would need to receive a therapy in order for a defined event to be avoided
- In the example, 2 in every 100 patients taking aspirin will be prevented from having a stroke; to avoid 1 stroke, therefore, 50 patients have to be given aspirin

SCREENING AND SURVEILLANCE

Screening

- The investigation of a population in order to identify those who have a specific disease

Surveillance

- The investigation of an individual in order to detect recurrence of a disease

Ransom's criteria

- Criteria for an appropriate screening test
- That there is a safe and sensitive test for the disease with a high positive predictive value; the test should not have a high complication rate
- The yield of the test needs to be high enough to merit the cost of the test and the inconvenience and discomfort for both those in whom the disease is detected and those in whom it is not
- Earlier treatment of the disease has to have a benefit to the patient compared with late treatment; in other words, an effective therapy has to be available

Number needed to screen

- The number of individuals who have to be screened in order to prevent one death due to the disease

Lead time

- The time difference between detection of a disease by screening and the point at which it would have presented by causing symptoms

EPIDEMIOLOGY

- The study of disease and the way it is distributed within the population
- The risk of developing a specific disease can depend on a wide variety of factors

Genetic predisposition

- Genetic variation between individuals alters their susceptibility to a disease
  - HLA-B8 DR3 increases the risk of autoimmune disease

Exposure to causative agent

- Increased exposure to an infectious agent, carcinogen or other agent may be a function of geographical location, immediate personal contacts, work environment or personal habits such as diet, alcohol or smoking

Availability of healthcare

- Availability and utilization of healthcare resources impacts upon prevention of disease (e.g. vaccination) and the stage at which a disease presents; this may have a large impact on outcome

Social and cultural beliefs

- The response to disease is modified by an individual's perceptions of illness and his or her society's approach to disease management

Definitions in epidemiology

Incidence
- Number of new cases arising during a defined period of time
  - 300 per year

Prevalence
- Total number of cases in a population per unit time

Prevalence rate
- Prevalence per unit population

Mortality
- Death rate per unit time

Mortality rate
- Death rate per unit population per unit time

Age-standardized mortality
- Correction of the mortality rate for a disease for age

Standardized mortality ratio
- Ratio of deaths observed in a cohort to the number expected across the whole population
- For example the mortality in any specific age range in smokers is higher than that for the population as a whole

AUDIT AND GOVERNANCE

- Audit is a method of monitoring performance and standards in healthcare
- Governance is the mechanism by which standards are maintained

Stages of audit

- Describe the variable to be audited
- Choose an appropriate standard to be used as a benchmark for performance
- Collect the data on local performance
- Compare local results with the standard
- Identify ways of improving local performance
- Repeat audit after implementation of the new protocols in order to assess their effect

Rules

- Audit should be non-confrontational and non-judgemental
- Individuals should not be openly targeted
- However, an individual doctor who is under-performing should be encouraged to improve practice and supported in doing so

Governance

- The means by which organizations ensure the provision of quality clinical care by making individuals accountable for setting, maintaining and monitoring performance standards
- Involves individuals and groups of healthcare workers in identifying best practice and how it may be achieved

SELF-ASSESSMENT QUESTIONS

Multiple choice questions (single best answer)

1. A study of a pulse rate in an adult population of 500 people is carried out. Which one of the following would be the most appropriate method of describing the dataset that results?
   A. Mean and standard deviation
   B. Mode and range
   C. Median and interquartile range
   D. Mean and standard error
   E. Median and 95% confidence intervals

2. A clinical trial of a new drug is carried out and an 'intention to treat' analysis performed. What is the best description of this form of analysis?
   A. All patients who completed the trial are included
   B. All patients who were considered for the trial were included
   C. All patients who were randomized in the trial were included
   D. All patients who took the drug rather than placebo were included
   E. All patients who dropped out of the study were excluded from the analysis

3. A study looking at 1-year survival in patients randomized to one of two forms of drug treatment was carried out. What would be the most appropriate analysis tool to compare the treatments?
   A. Student *t*-test
   B. Mann–Whitney test
   C. Paired *t*-test
   D. Chi-squared test
   E. Regression analysis

4. Which one of the following is the best definition of 'population screening'?
   A. Investigation of symptomatic patients for the underlying cause
   B. Assessment of a patient with a previous diagnosis for recurrence of the disease
   C. Assessment of patients with a disease for evidence of an associated condition
   D. Assessment of asymptomatic patients for a disease
   E. Random selection of a sample from a population for inclusion in a trial

5. Which one of the following defines prevalence?
   A. Number of patients with a disease seen in the hospital setting
   B. Number of patients with a disease expressed as a proportion of the total population
   C. Number of new patients presenting each year with a disease
   D. Number of new cases of the disease per 100 000 people per year
   E. Total number of cases within the total population per year

Appendix A

Answers to MULTIPLE CHOICE QUESTIONS

4. Pharmacology and therapeutics
1. FTFTF
2. TFFFF
3. TFFFF
4. FFFFT
5. TTFTT
6. TTFFF
7. A
8. A
9. C
10. A
11. D
12. D

5. Radiology
1. TTFTF
2. TFFTT
3. C
4. B
5. C
6. D
7. C
8. B

6. Clinical chemistry
1. D
2. C
3. C
4. E
5. A
6. E
7. A
8. C
9. A

7. Infectious diseases
1. TFTTT
2. TFTFF
3. FFTFF
4. TTFTF
5. TTTTF
6. TFTTT
7. TFTTT
8. TFTFF
9. TTFTF
10. TFTFF
11. FTTFT
12. TTTTT
13. TFTTT
14. TTFFT
15. TTTFT
16. FFTTF
17. TTTTT
18. FTTFF
19. TFFTF
20. TTTFF
21. D
22. A
23. E
24. A
25. B
26. C
27. C
28. D
29. E

8. Respiratory medicine
1. A
2. B
3. A
4. D
5. E
6. E
7. A
8. E
9. B
10. A
11. B
12. B
13. A
14. B
15. B

9. Cardiology
1. C
2. A
3. B
4. B
5. E
6. A
7. B
8. C
9. A
10. D
11. B
12. B
13. E
14. A
15. A
16. D
17. E
18. A
19. B
20. B

10. Gastroenterology and hepatology
1. E
2. A
3. D
4. E
5. A
6. C
7. A
8. C
9. C
10. D
11. D
12. B
13. A
14. A
15. D
16. C
17. B
18. B
19. E
20. D
21. B
22. B
23. A
24. C
25. A
26. D
27. A

28. FTTFF
29. FFTTT
30. TTFTT
31. FTTFT
32. TTTFT
33. TTTFF
34. FTTFF
35. TTFFT
36. TTTFT
37. TTFTT
38. TFTFF
39. TTFTT
40. TFFTT

11. Rheumatology
1. B
2. D
3. B
4. D
5. E
6. C
7. C
8. B
9. D
10. E
11. A
12. D

12. Dermatology
1. E
2. C
3. C
4. C
5. B
6. D
7. C
8. E
9. C
10. C

13. Endocrinology
1. C
2. A
3. C
4. C
5. E
6. C
7. B
8. E
9. E
10. B
11. E
12. E

13. C
14. B
15. A
16. C
17. D
18. E
19. C

14. Renal medicine
1. B
2. A
3. D
4. A
5. E
6. E
7. B
8. D
9. B
10. D
11. B
12. B
13. E
14. A
15. E
16. B
17. B
18. A
19. D
20. E

15. Haematology
1. FTTTT
2. TFFTF
3. TFTTT
4. TFTTF
5. TFFFT
6. TTTTT
7. B
8. C
9. B
10. C

16. Oncology and genetic disease
1. TTTTT
2. FTFFT
3. TFTTF
4. FTFFF
5. FTTFF
6. FFTTF
7. C
8. D
9. D

10. B
11. C
12. D

17. Neurology
1. B
2. D
3. D
4. B
5. D
6. A
7. E
8. E
9. E
10. B
11. D
12. E
13. D
14. E
15. D
16. B
17. A
18. E
19. C
20. C
21. A

18. Psychological medicine
1. E
2. C
3. B
4. C
5. B
6. D
7. E
8. C
9. E
10. C
11. C
12. B
13. A
14. E
15. C

19. Statistics and evidence-based medicine
1. A
2. C
3. D
4. D
5. D

Appendix B

Answers to EXTENDED MATCHING QUESTIONS

4. Pharmacology and therapeutics
   1. K
   2. I
   3. A
   4. H
   5. D
   6. J
   7. I

5. Radiology
   1. I. F. PA chest is the classical test but CT is more accurate.
       II. I.
       III. K. Much more sensitive than CT for liver lesions.
       IV. D. 'Pepperpot' skull lytic lesions are seen.

6. Clinical chemistry
   1. I. C. Confusion is nonspecific. Oedema suggests right heart failure.
       Hypokalaemia is an unwanted effect of loop diuretics. Renal
       failure could be secondary to heart failure or unwanted effect
       of diuretics.
       II. I. Hypokalaemia, hypomagnesaemia, dehydration and normal
       anion gap metabolic acidosis all result from electrolyte and
       water losses from high ileostomy outputs.
       III. D. Hypoxia and low PCO_2 suggests respiratory problem, fever
       suggests infection. Low sodium is a result of syndrome of
       inappropriate ADH (SIADH) and is associated with
       pneumonia.
   2. I. H. Hypercapnia and hypoxia suggest type II respiratory failure.
       II. F. Metabolic acidosis with respiratory compensation (low PCO_2)
       in a patient with diabetes who is unwell and vomiting is very
       suggestive of diabetic ketoacidosis.
       III. C. Metabolic acidosis with high anion gap is compatible with
       aspirin overdose.
   3. I. A. All three are markers of acute cardiac muscle damage.
       II. D. Lymphadenopathy and an elevated LDH give the diagnosis.
       III. E. Normal LFTs with a low Hb and elevated bilirubin point to
       this answer.

7. Infectious diseases
   1. I. E. There is evidence of immunocompromise and/or reactivated
       TB (chest X-ray, lymphadenopathy, fever).
       II. J. Rust-coloured sputum and peri-oral HSV are associated with
       Strep. pneumoniae.
       III. F. Hepatosplenomegaly, jaundice, a fever and low platelets are
       all characteristic of malaria.

2. I. L. Liver ultrasound would demonstrate cholecystitis (thickened inflamed gallbladder) and cholangitis (gas in biliary tree, stones or an obstructed biliary tree). CT would be the second choice.

   II. B. The clinical picture is that of malaria.

   III. G. The data suggest infective endocarditis. Multiple sets of blood cultures are needed to detect the organism and derive the antibiotic sensitivities.

8. Respiratory medicine

1. I. B. Eczema suggests atopy in a young woman. Spirometry results suggest an obstructive defect. These, together with history, make asthma very likely.

   II. A. Breathlessness with clubbing and weight loss strongly suggest lung cancer, especially with progressive symptoms.

   III. H. Normal chest X-ray and pulmonary function tests exclude many of the answers. NSAIDs (e.g. ibuprofen) cause GI ulceration and iron deficiency particularly in elderly patients.

2. I. A. *Strep. pneumoniae* is the commonest cause of pneumonia and is associated with rusty coloured sputum.

   II. E. The marked hypoxia with normal chest X-ray suggests *Pneumocystis pneumonia* in this immunocompromised patient.

   III. F. *Staph. aureus* pneumonia cavitates and is associated with flu outbreaks.

3. I. F. The clue is the fact that she gets better when she is away from the farm; extrinsic allergic alveolitis symptoms are worst at the time of antigen exposure.

   II. A. Cough and bilateral lymphadenopathy is a common presentation of sarcoid.

   III. H. His exposure to asbestos, the presence of chest pain and the chest X-ray findings make mesothelioma likely.

9. Cardiology

1. I. D. The presence of different blood pressures in each arm, interscapular pain and Marfan's point to a dissected thoracic aorta.

   II. B. This is exercise-induced angina in a patient with risk factors (diabetes mellitus and smoking).

   III. A. The age and the relationship to food are suggestive of a gastrointestinal rather than cardiac cause.

2. I. B. The right heart failure and cardiomegaly in a drinker suggest alcoholic cardiomyopathy.

   II. C. Deep vein thrombosis with a pulmonary embolus – recent travel with a swollen leg and breathlessness.

   III. C. The history of diabetes and the presence of an ulcerated area could be cellulites or vascular insufficiency. The history favours the former.

3. I. B. The rate of 160 b.p.m. and no 'P' waves in a smoker suggest AF.

   II. I. The tachycardia is due to the β-agonist (it also causes tremor). If the patient was not on inhalers consider thyrotoxicosis.

   III. D. The symptoms are all due to anxiety-related hyperventilation – shortness of breath and tingling of the fingers and mouth.

10. Gastroenterology and hepatology
  1. I. D. Autonomic neuropathy due to diabetes mellitus links the symptoms.
      II. H. The mucus and low potassium suggest a tubulovillous adenoma. The mucus is very potassium rich and can be profuse.
      III. G. Ulcerative colitis (anaemia, fever and diarrhoea) all point to severe disease.
  2. I. E. The risk factors of diabetes and heart disease, combined with pain and diarrhoea after food, suggest mesenteric ischaemia.
      II. G. Ulcers, weight loss and anaemia, plus erythema nodosum, all point to inflammatory bowel disease and therefore Crohn's in this question.
      III. H. Irritable bowel – the alternating bowel habit, bloating and left iliac fossa pain are suggestive and the weight gain discounts other pathologies.
  3. I. B. Growth failure with GI symptoms points towards coeliac disease, Crohn's or cystic fibrosis. The latter is unlikely to present as late as this.
      II. A. Pernicious anaemia – the low vitamin B_{12} and the history of autoimmune thyroid disease point to this.
      III. E. The history suggests chronic pancreatitis – steatorrhoea and chronic alcoholism.
  4. I. B. NSAIDs markedly increase the risk of gastric ulceration.
      II. H. The change in bowel habit and weight loss suggest that a carcinoma is the most important diagnosis to rule out.
      III. J. Bright red rectal bleeding suggests a rectal or anal cause, and in this age group haemorrhoids are the most likely.

11. Rheumatology
  1. I. D. Syndesmophytes are suggestive of ankylosing spondylitis and the ESR and HLA status support this.
      II. B. Osteoarthritis is a common cause of back pain. Normal bloods and no erosions on X-ray make the other diagnoses unlikely.
      III. A. Recent wrist fracture in a post-menopausal woman with normal bloods is highly suggestive of osteoporosis. She may have had steroids for her asthma, making osteoporosis more likely.
  2. I. D. Elevated urate suggests gout. The distribution of the joint symptoms is compatible with gout.
      II. F. Rash, joint pains and raised inflammatory markers with a positive ANA is strongly suggestive of SLE.
      III. B. Heberden's nodes with normal ESR suggests osteoarthritis.
  3. I. H. Recurrent miscarriages are the key here.
      II. C. The MCP joint erosions and a systemic illness point to rheumatoid.
      III. A. Anticentromere antibodies are associated with systemic sclerosis.

12. Dermatology
1. I. I. Raised, purple, painful red areas on the legs suggest erythema nodosum, which is associated with Crohn's disease.
    II. A. History of atopy. Distribution suggests eczema (flexural).
    III. F. Yellow crusts strongly suggests *Staph. aureus* infection.
2. I. F. An ulcer which is rapidly increasing in size in a patient with Crohn's disease is highly suggestive of pyoderma gangrenosum.
    II. A. The pigmentation and brown colour suggest venous ulceration.
    III. B. Being a gardener suggests UV exposure. The appearance and hard node suggests SCC rather than malignant melanoma.
3. I. G. Infection with *Corynebacterium minutissimum*.
    II. F. Jaundice and itching = biliary obstruction.
    III. A. Iron deficiency is associated with itching.

13. Endocrinology
1. I. D. She has multiple endocrine neoplasia type I (a parathyroid adenoma causing hyperparathyroidism, associated with a pancreatic tumour). The high calcium resulting from this is causing the constipation and polyuria.
    II. B. She has Sheehan syndrome – a pituitary infarction following a postpartum haemorrhage – leading to diabetes insipidus. This is rare.
    III. A. There is a metabolic acidosis (low bicarbonate), thirst, polyuria and weight loss – classical early onset diabetes mellitus.
2. I. A. She has autoimmune disease already, so her risk of a further autoimmune disease is increased. Anxiety, palpitations, diarrhoea and weight loss are all pointing towards thyrotoxicosis.
    II. E. The palmar pigmentation, abdominal pain and postural hypotension suggest Addison's disease (in this case due to adrenal tuberculosis suggested by sweats, weight loss and foreign travel).
    III. B. 50% of coeliac disease presents with iron deficiency. Weight loss and abdominal pain support this. The southern Irish origins increase the risk of coeliac.

14. Renal medicine
1. I. C. The history of gout increases the risk of renal stones. The colicky pain and sudden onset in the absence of indicators of infection support this.
    II. H. The chest signs point to a pneumonia. The urinary abnormalities may be due to an atypical pneumonia (e.g. mycoplasma or legionella).
    III. E. There is an association between polycystic kidney disease and berry aneurysms that result in subarachnoid haemorrhage. The pain is probably due to bleeding into one of the renal cysts.

2. I. A. The presence of liver cirrhosis with new acute renal failure favours hepatorenal syndrome as the cause.
   II. F. Haemolytic-uraemic syndrome results from *E. coli* O157 and occurs after food poisoning with this organism. The anaemia and thrombocytopenia are as a result of the haemolysis.
   III. I. The mass in his pelvis is his bladder. This is a classical presentation of acute retention due to prostatic enlargement.

15. Haematology
    1. I. A.
       II. D. Sickle results in sickled red cells and regional hypoxia causing severe pain.
       III. B. Although both B_{12} and folic acid deficiency cause macrocytosis, only B_{12} requires the stomach to be present to be absorbed.
    2. I. I.
       II. J.
       III. H. Both reticulocytes and platelets increase after blood loss but platelets do not have nuclei.
    3. I. C. O = 44%, A = 45%, B = 8%, AB = 3%.
       II. A.
       III. F. The mother must be RhD negative. A first RhD positive fetus induces anti-D antibodies. The second suffers the syndrome.

17. Neurology
    1. I. C. The distal progressive weakness and areflexia are typical of Guillain–Barré. The history of a recent GI infection supports this.
       II. A. The smoking and hypertension are key risk factors for ischaemic stroke. This is a non-dominant side event with dysphasia.
       III. H. The shuffling gait, micrographia and resting tremor all point to Parkinson's.
    2. I. F. The rash, photophobia and fever all suggest meningitis (probably meningococcal).
       II. A. The combination of abdominal symptoms and unilateral headache, probably initiated by alcohol, points to migraine.
       III. D. The retinal changes suggest malignant hypertension, and are not features of diabetic retinopathy.
    3. I. G. All the elements are here for a benzodiazepine overdose, using drugs prescribed by the GP. She could be either ketoacidotic or hypoglycaemic but the history points to deliberate self-harm due to reactive depression.
       II. I. Septicaemia due to urinary sepsis.
       III. E. Hypotension, bradycardia and, in particular, J waves on the ECG all point to hypothermia.

18. Psychological medicine
    1. I. F. The pattern of memory loss is compatible with early dementia.
       II. D. She has first rank symptoms of schizophrenia. Her ethnicity increases the risk of this disease.
       III. H. High MCV suggests alcohol excess. Visual hallucinations, sweating and tachycardia occur in alcohol withdrawal syndrome.

2.   I. D.   Persecutory ideation and thought broadcasting suggest schizophrenia.

    II. I.   Paranoia and agitation with a history of drug addiction points to amphetamines.

    III. B.   Sleep loss, increased libido and spending beyond one's means are suggestive of mania.

3.   I. B.   Tricyclics cause weight gain and so would be relatively contraindicated. SSRIs are useful in reactive depression.

    II. G.   Anxiety disorders are usually effectively treated with CBT.

    III. H.   Carbamazepine is a useful second-line drug in bipolar disorders.

Appendix C
Normal reference ranges:
Normal values for laboratory tests

These may vary from hospital to hospital.

Test	Abbreviation	Normal range	Units
Full blood count			
Haemoglobin	Hb	Males 13.5–17.7 Females 11.5–16.5	g/dL g/dL
Mean corpuscular volume	MCV	80–96	fL
Mean corpuscular haemoglobin	MCH	27–33	pg
Mean corpuscular haemoglobin concentration	MCHC	32–36	g/dL
Reticulocyte count	Retics	0.5–2.5%	
Red cell count	RCC	Males: 4.5–6 Females: 3.9–5.0	$\times 10^{12}$/L $\times 10^{12}$/L
White cell count	WCC	4–11	$\times 10^{9}$/L
Basophils		0.01–0.1	$\times 10^{9}$/L
Eosinophils		0.04–0.4	$\times 10^{9}$/L
Lymphocytes		1.5–4.0	$\times 10^{9}$/L
Monocytes		0.2–0.8	$\times 10^{9}$/L
Neutrophils		2.0–7.5	$\times 10^{9}$/L
Platelets		150–400	$\times 10^{9}$/L
Haematinics			
Serum B_{12}	B_{12}	160–925	ng/L
Serum folate		2.9–18	µg/L
Ferritin	Fe	Male: 20–260 Female: 6–110	µg/L µg/L
Iron		13–32	mmol/L
Total iron binding capacity	TIBC	42–80	mmol/L
Other haematology			
Erythrocyte sedimentation rate	ESR	<20	mm/hour
Coagulation			
Bleeding time		3–9	minutes
Active partial thromboplastin time	APTT	23–31	seconds

Continued

Test	Abbreviation	Normal range	Units
Prothrombin time	PTPT	12–16	seconds
International normalized ratio	INR	1.0–1.3	
Urea and electrolytes			
Sodium	Na^+	135–146	mmol/L
Potassium	K^+	3.5–5.0	mmol/L
Chloride	Cl^-	95–106	mmol/L
Urea		2.5–6.7	mmol/L
Creatinine		79–118	µmol/L
Liver function tests			
Alanine aminotransferase	ALT	5–40	IU/L
Aspartate aminotransferase	AST	12–40	IU/L
Gamma glutaryl transpeptidase	gT	10–40	IU/L
Alkaline phosphatase	ALP	39–117	IU/L
Bilirubin	Bili	<17	µmol/L
Other biochemistry			
Glucose (fasting)		4.5–5.5	mmol/L
Glycosylated haemoglobin	HbA_{1c}	3.7–5.1	
Calcium	Ca^{2+}	2.20–2.67	mmol/L
Phosphate	$PO4^{3-}$	0.8–1.5	mmol/L
C reactive protein	CRP	<10	mg/L
Urate		0.18–0.42	mmol/L
Lipids			
Cholesterol	Chol	3.5–6.5	mmol/L
HDL cholesterol	HDL	Male: 0.8–1.8 Female: 1.0–2.3	mmol/L mmol/L
Triglycerides	Trig	Male: 0.7–2.1 Female: 0.5–1.7	mmol/L mmol/L
Arterial blood gases			
Arterial partial oxygen pressure	P_aO_2	10–13.3	kPa
Arterial partial carbon dioxide pressure	P_aCO_2	4.8–6.1	kPa
pH	pH	7.35–7.45	
Bicarbonate	HCO_3	24–28	mmol

Index

Illustrations are comprehensively referred to from the text; therefore, significant material in illustrations and tables have usually only been given a page reference in the absence of their concomitant mention in the text referring to that figure.